PLANET MEDICINE

FROM STONE AGE SHAMANISM
TO POST-INDUSTRIAL HEALING

RICHARD GROSSINGER

North Atlantic Books,
Berkeley, California

Planet Medicine: From Stone Age Shamanism to Post-Industrial
Healing

Copyright © 1980 1982, 1985, 1987, 1990 by Richard Grossinger

ISBN 1-55643-093-0
Published by North Atlantic Books
    2800 Woolsey Street
    Berkeley, California 94705

Cover Art: Section of a painting by Pablo Amaringo, from *The Ayahuasca Visions
    of a Peruvian Shaman* by Pablo Amaringo and Luis Eduardo Luna,
    North Atlantic Books, 1991.

Cover Design: Paula Morrison

Planet Medicine was originally published by Doubleday/Anchor Books and later
republished by Shambhala/Random House in a revised edition. This is the second
revised edition to be published by North Atlantic Books.

Planet Medicine is sponsored by the Society for the Study of Native Arts and
Sciences, a nonprofit educational corporation whose goals are to develop an ecological and crosscultural perspective linking various scientific, social, and artistic
fields; to nurture a holistic view of arts, sciences, humanities, and healing; and to
publish and distribute literature on the relationship of mind, body, and nature.

Library of Congress Cataloging in Publication Data
Grossinger, Richard, 1944–
  Planet medicine.
  Bibliography: p.
  Includes index.
  1. Therapeutic systems—History. 2. Healing—
History.   3. Medical anthropology—History.
4. Medicine—Philosophy. I. Title.
R733.G76   362.1   82–50278
ISBN 1-55643-093-0 (pbk.)

PLANET
MEDICINE

Contents

I dedicate the revised edition of this book to those healers who taught me the principles on which it is based: Paul Pitchford, Polly Gamble, Ian Grand, Randy Cherner, Richard Strozzi Heckler, Ben Hole, Marcus Laux, Carol Lee, George Quasha, Michelle Haviar, Bruce Burger, Peter Ralston, and Ron Sieh.

Preface

This is a book about healing: its origin in primary and ancient systems of human knowledge, its basis as a social category, and its diverse meanings and values, from culture to culture and through human history. Our starting point is the oldest medical images and activities. Though we cannot know these exactly, we imagine them by comparison with our own modes of perception and idea formation, we reconstruct them from Ice Age remnants, and we find their equivalents practiced by tribal peoples in Africa, Australia, Asia, and the Americas. Literacy and civilization bring with them complex medical philosophies and new models for the behavior of the doctor. This book examines hermetic and elemental medicine, medicine of the vital force, and medicine reconciling mind and body. Contemporary thought holds two different images of the evolution of medicine. From the perspective of progressive technology and global culture, we have arrived at a universal industrial medicine. But, from the perspective of the unknown quanta of disease and cure, we must return to primary processes and reinvent a working medicine we no longer have.

Disease perception and healing both touch the core of our human meaning. How we locate disorder, and remedy it, is an aspect of how we imagine our existence as body and mind. Each person's "struggle" with his biological being is recorded in his health. This state of relative health or disease has a priority that ideas and attitudes, which merely emerge from it, cannot. That is, there are deep and urgent collective images, both personal and cultural, which cannot be expressed except as variations and difficulties of health. Their "philosophical" meaning is akin to that of the genes themselves, which also carry a biological message into the human world.

People rarely notice the real profundity and intricate variability of health and disease that they nonetheless experience. They may sense, at times, that all is not well, that they have a sickness, that they are confused, that there must be a way out; at other times, that a sickness has gone away, that something else is wrong, that they do not know whether anything is wrong. This is the intrinsic dilemma of flesh and mind, heaped upon its own cellular and psychic formation. The isolated treatment of certain diseases is an outcome of sociological categories, and it does not alter the more pagan domain of the ailment or the cure. This book is a statement of the cultural and metaphysical status of all medicine and is an attempt to revise assumptions, both academic and popular, about what the process of disease and cure is.

Although this is not a book specifically about alternative medicine, it falls into the context created by the new American holistic philosophy, a context of revision and revolution. But I have not accepted the rhetoric or internal terminology of these systems. I have arrived at them anew by an analysis of their origins, their philosophical and cultural premises, and their political and economic ramifications. The danger of accepting the alternative medicine movement in the innovative and modern terms in which it tends to view itself is that we get a false and shallow sense of newness and breakthrough. There *is* a present momentum and invention that are different from anything else we have seen and represent a break with certain aspects of tradition, but the methodological roots lie deep in Western thought and even deeper in the pre-Western arcanum. How we inherit certain methods and choose them from among the vastness of possibilities is a fundamental issue of this book. What is new becomes more significant when we see how it was shaped in what is ancient. In order to understand the radical in contemporary terms, we must perceive it as seeds, as primal imagination of body and mind.

While they go about attempting to cure people and challenging the medical establishment, the new medicines also raise basic questions of the laws of nature and the meanings and goals of human life. When they are explained in terms of simple rationales and methodologies, as they are in a great many books on holistic health, their exact activities may be clear, but their consequences and relationships to any concrete event are totally open to interpretation. When unique and bizarre elements are resolved only in terms of internal mythology, belief or disbelief becomes a matter of faith.

Just about any current book on the new medicine plunges the reader into the dilemma. A style of language replaces explanation. "We are not only bodies," we are invariably told. "We are fields of energy, processes, radiant matter. Nothing has a reality separate from mind. Our minds influence the production of cells in our bodies and pass on the messages which become diseases. The universe itself resembles a giant mind. All medicine must speak to our inner wisdom."

The objection to this is certainly not that it is "wrong," or even unappealing. But certain instances of holistic jargon are too sweet and holier-than-thou, and there is a tendency among advocates to fall back on derivative concepts from theosophy, quantum physics, and parapsychology in place of a precise and hard-won logic or even vision. The real objection is that if it is the answer, what is the question? What does knowing all this about ourselves, or pretending to have images for our innermost life, tell us about how to live, who we are, why we get sick, and how we get better?

In our optimism, we are often inclined to accept the holistic cure (because it is, by name, entire) without knowing what it is we want to have cured and whether it is holistic by the same definition. It solves nothing to say that everything is holistic, or that we have radiant psychic bodies, for it is the definition of these things that makes them real.

The cynicism and pessimism of the other side—in this case, of the materialistic doctors of the establishment—go no further toward answering those questions. It is the other side of the same tyranny. And the tyranny itself removes us from our individual difficulties and the complexities of our real perceptions. Too many books on new medicine and holistic health give "answers," so this book will primarily be an asking of the question.

In its collectivity, the new medicine is one of the major political and philosophical statements of our time. The modern thinkers Alfred North Whitehead, Maurice Merleau-Ponty, and Jacques Derrida, among others, have touched on the major paradoxes of mind, matter, and language that underlie healing systems. The incredibly complex and interrelated dynamics of disease and cure are parallel to the equally complex dynamics of linguistic analysis and the philosophical inquiry into nature. At the same time that medicine treats specific complaints—actual disease—it examines the over-all epistemological and social framework in which human beings exist. It has a simultaneous pragmatic and philosophical reality, but its meaning emerges from its act of curing. If it is existential, semantic, nihilistic, or phenomenological, it states its case as technique alone. When survival or well-being are at stake, the mind generally has little room for ideas. The mind must, in a sense, give up. The response of the disease itself to the application of a remedy is a system's harshest and only critic.

The philosophical and linguistic complications are also extraordinarily important. An appreciation of them can have a curative effect in itself, as the psychoanalytic philosophers now tell us. Unfortunately, most people are not well enough to enter into the dialogue nor educated enough to entertain it in its traditional complexity. Wilhelm Reich, for all his raw methodology, may get at a more central meaning than the infinitesimally more delicate and comprehensive meanderings of Derrida and Jacques Lacan, and their "French Freud." After all, it is not that we don't understand. We have virtually exhausted ourselves watching every action twice and three times over. It is that we understand and cannot change things. That is when action speaks louder than words—unintellectual, lower-class action. It does not matter that action limits complexity, for it generates another kind of complexity. Somatic therapy, for instance, misses many philosophical subtleties, but it does face the animal basis of our humanity. The alternative medicines do not generate specific philosophies, except in the style of biological mysticism I noted above; however, they do a far more radical thing: they change people. And this in itself transforms our knowledge.

When we talk about the "new medicine," there is a possible problem of terminology. I use the terms "alternative medicine," "new medicine," "holistic medicine," and "holistic health" almost interchangeably. There are, however, some differences of connotation. "Alternative medicine" describes the general and continuous emergence of systems of treatment in opposition to a universal technological medicine. It includes various ancient and folk medicines, that reassert themselves from era to era, as well as new medicines that may well come, at least in part, out of aspects of the scientific model. When I speak of the "new medicine," I mean particularly the present collection of alternative practices that emerged during the 1960s and 1970s in the United States. Although many of these practices are quite old, they share a new political and ideological thrust as well as an often unstated social and economic alliance. I use "holistic medicine" to suggest the significant similarity between the "new medicine" and traditional medicine as it was practiced in prehistoric and ancient times. In both stone-age tribes and countercultural clinics, medicine is simultaneously an art, a philosophy, a science, and a craft; it deals with the human being as a single entity of mind and body in a biological and cultural circumstance from which he cannot be extricated. "Planet medicine" is the name I have given this phenomenon because it is the medicine of most of the people on the Earth through most of human history. "Planet medicine" comprises systems that ask basic and original questions about the human condition while treating disease as a fundamental disorder of meaning and spirit. This would include not only shamanism, voodoo, and faith healing, but also homoeopathy, acupuncture, and herbalism. "Planet medicine" is both prehistoric and contemporary; it has been with man during the whole of his time on the Earth and has evolved beside him. I do not deny that scientific medicine is a branch of "planet medicine"—it is, but only in its exact techniques for curing the sick, not in its establishment of a universal system of health in the image of progressive science.

"Holistic health" is the term I have, more or less, replaced because it has been used as a trade name for various coalitions using new medicines or groups of conventional practitioners wanting to be identified as sympathetic to a revolution in the treatment of disease. It has a slightly ironical connotation, since it can designate the fad and its various excesses and abuses, as well as the provinciality of the movement. Insofar as I use all these terms interchangeably, I am documenting a series of events which reflect and resemble each other across cultures and through all of human history.

My discussions of the past and of other cultures also require a clarification. I seem to be talking about facts of ancient and tribal medicine, but a closer reading will show that I am exploring modern issues. Even our own sense of who we are, historically, genetically, ecologically, is a contemporary image of events that have taken place over millions of years. Our perception of other cultures and their medicines is born of present reality and bias. There is no actual account of the peoples of this planet. We have only a series of current images, for anything—the origins of healing as much as the origins of life or the first languages.

In fact, the images of non-Western medicine have arisen in the same context as the alternative medicines themselves. Although the events are separated by millennia, as are shamanism from Rolfing, the forms of knowing them are contemporaneous. Our futurism is inextricably linked to our classicism. In some cases, new medicines are launched, unconsciously, from actual documents or oral accounts of ancient or remote practices. The new thing is the old thing reborn, a thing uniquely suited to our own situation and needs. The reconstructions of African medicine, to take one example, are "fictions" of exactly the same order. They retain some element of the truth, but their real use is in our own transformations of them into new forms.

So, when this book does not deal explicitly with the new medicine, it deals with the quest for the primary structures and the roots of healing itself. By analyzing the very nature of ethnomedical thought, it provides a context for understanding not only present medical systems but also the possible structures of forms which have yet to be invented. It is anthropological and historical, but, more than that, it is meta-anthropological and transhistorical. It does not rest on concrete facts or their documentation, but takes into account *this* society and all its modes of inquiry (medical, anthropological, historical, political). They all happen at the same time and in consequence of the same meanings and gaps of meaning.

In a book on fundamental structures of healing, we cannot take anthropological accounts of American Indian or African healing as gospel. We must discuss them also in a medical context—as if each were a symptom of an unknown condition. This would be to take our information about medical practices on the same level of seriousness as we take the medical practices. As there is a politics of medicine, there also may be a medicine of politics. Many systems which purport to show the origin and meaning of practices are themselves variations in the natural world which those practices treat. Why should political systems have the last word? They can also be symptoms and aspects of diseases. The political power of the shaman may be identical to his methodology of cure.

The integrity of the book rests on this continuous search for contexts and origins. Even what we take for granted at the beginning, in order to begin at all, must be called into question by the end.

As must be clear from this description, this book does not fit into any one academic field, though it certainly uses elements of anthropology and psychology, as well as traces of literary, mythological, religious, and philosophical analysis. In this way, I have taken such various folk as Claude Lévi-Strauss, Marshall Sahlins, Jacques Derrida, Frances Yates, Charles Olson, Michel Foucault, Alfred North Whitehead, Owen Barfield, Carl Sauer, and Rudolf Steiner into the changing texture of my definitions and explorations. Others are so directly involved in the main plot that they have become my characters: Samuel Hahnemann, Sigmund Freud, Wilhelm Reich, Carl Jung, Carlos Castaneda.

I consider medicine a great unexplored territory. Historians and physicians give us one side of the picture. Religion, metaphysics, and hermeticism give us a different side. Yet it is almost impossible to match or merge the two. Anthropology and psychology are our best bridges, for they literally have stanchions on both sides of the stream. But each of them has settled on something less than the full problem. Anthropology at least establishes the basis for cultural relativism as an antidote to absolutist models of cure. But the sorry fact is that most anthropologists still prefer Western definitions of healing, and medical anthropology has not shown one tenth the courage of the early ethnographers and explorers, preferring instead to stay close to the sources of research money in the public health bureaucracy. The academically archaic field of ethnomedicine has more to offer us about the real issues of native medicines and cures.

Twentieth-century psychology has unveiled some of the mechanisms not only of human systems of healing but also of unconscious healing structures within organisms. It has lacked the cross-cultural perspectives of anthropology, so its images of externalizations and healing technologies are ethnocentric. It also lacks a concrete subject matter, like the atoms of physics or the cells of biology. Anthropology lacks a clearcut object too, for that matter, but its territory is so exteriorly vast as not to require it. Psychology suffers the vagueness of "mind" in a way that anthropology does not suffer the abstractions that arise from "culture."

One of the more obvious things I have done in this book is to bring anthropology and psychology together around matters of healing, giving simultaneous sympathy to theoreticians who are implicitly protagonists, such as Lévi-Strauss and Reich. It is anthropology that allows us to talk about early man and the disease spirits of Bali, but it is psychoanalysis that takes us inside the methodology of the shaman. The relationship between ethnomedicine and psychoanalysis is potentially a fertile one, and I have tried to make it explicit. It is something that almost everyone who has written on this subject has suggested, but it is also something that has almost never been worked through.

Our hermetic and artistic legacies are also keys to this book. I trust their ancient wisdom, and I do not believe that modern scientific thought has advanced so far that it can do without them. If contemporary science were as lucid as it seems to claim, and as beyond paradox, I would be forced to go along with it all the way. It is not. Science is like a reforming politician with plenty of dirty linen of his own. I hope that this orientation of mine, set long before the writing of this book, will not keep anthropologists and scientists from reading this book or taking it seriously. However, my experience has taught me that one gives up part of one's audience and some of one's credibility by entertaining ostracized modes of thought. I believe I have been true to the best of anthropology and science in this century, but that belief, so stated, will hardly convince, or even charm, most of my critics.

Specifically, I believe that such poets as William Blake and Charles Olson, such spiritualists as G. I. Gurdjieff and Rudolf Steiner, and various parapsychologists and others of similar background have an invaluable contribution to make to such a difficult subject matter. They present the type of alinear, synchronous, and metaphorical thinking that sheds new light on famous riddles. But even if they did not, they bring a cosmic and a human dimension without which the world would be a sterile place. It is virtually a fanaticism of this century and its professional life to leave out the inside of things. I take this as an economic event. People have staked their reputations and occupational integrity on the fields of inquiry as they are presently constellated. To bring in materials that cannot be categorically assigned by the academic mind is to threaten the corporate security of the individual disciplines. But I do not take that security to be any more deep, in most circles, than the fact of and the continuity of employment. Few academics and scientists fully live out the vision they present professionally (if it is vision at all), and it is exactly that difference between the vision, the actual lives, and the argument presented in academic terms that concerns

me. For it is in the lives of people that issues of life and death, disease and health, are established. Just because academicians and
bureaucrats were unaware of the ecological viewpoint for so long does
not mean that ecological issues were not being decided by them in
the absence of a conscious imperative.

Some of the material in this book evolved from my own graduate
work in anthropology, which included brief studies of Indian and
European culture in Arizona in 1967 and an extended study of
Maine coast fishermen conducted on and off between 1969 and 1972.
An even larger part of this book was gathered during fifteen years of
independent research into the various phenomena described. The actual text was written between 1977 and 1979, except for some of the
sections in the chapters on homoeopathy, which were written during
1976.

The number of people to whom I am indebted in the preparation
of this material is too great for a list. Many of them are mentioned
in the chapter notes, but I would like to thank some of them specially here: Angela Iadavaia-Cox, my editor at Doubleday, who read
and criticized this text in its original outlines and drafts, all with
good sense and sympathy; Bob Bagwell, my colleague for several
years at Goddard College, now working for the Mental Health Division of the government of the state of Oregon, who read drafts of
the early chapters and wrote extensive notes on them; Randy Neustaedter and Dana Ullman, who made it possible for me to work in
California's Bay Area homoeopathic community and who were generous in their time and insights; Margaret MacKenzie, who was my
liaison with the world of medical anthropology and the University
of California at Berkeley; Roy Rappaport, who taught me my anthropology, and how to think and write it; Bob Callahan, who gave
me insights into the context of the whole book and who was un-
erring in his political characterizations and geographical references;
Sheppard Powell and Diane di Prima, for primary wisdom; and my
students at Goddard from 1972 to 1977, who changed and shaped my
own subject matter and found for me the threads I had lost. I would
also like to thank the National Endowment for the Arts, for giving
me a Writer's Fellowship to work in the Bay Area in 1976.

RICHARD GROSSINGER

The Epistemology and Ethics of the Cure

I

More than ten years have passed since I began writing *Planet Medicine* in 1976, and by now I realize the degree to which the book is a reflection of paradoxes and riddles rather than a proof or a critique — its validation lies only in our ongoing experience. We unconsciously suffer such a profound ambivalence vis a vis disease categories and their treatment it is as though we had experienced a kind of cultural amnesia in which antitheses are now able to replace one another seemingly at will. In effect, we are in collective psychoanalysis, and the terminology of medicine serves as both the static crust of our resistance and the active medium of our transference. Our language of illness and remedy is itself a transparent symptomology.

Planet Medicine is a guide not to systems of holistic medicine as such but to the ethical and epistemological issues that are externalized as we encounter the inner turmoil of disease and apply contemporary logic and technology to their resolution. Specifically, the book represents my own odyssey from 1976 to 1982 when I was able to combine a personal quest into homoeopathy, bioenergetic therapy, and internal martial arts with a book contract from Doubleday and some abandoned graduate work on ethnomedicine and ethnopsychiatry.

Planet Medicine then began a nine-year project of research and writing that led to two subsequent works as well: *The Night Sky: The Science and Anthropology of the Stars and Planets* and *Embryogenesis: From Cosmos to Creature — The Origins of Human Biology*. This trilogy explores the reciprocal syntaxes of atoms, stars, cells, tissues, animals, and symbols, and the moral and epistemological dilemmas of science — which is, after all, the language by which the twentieth century addresses itself.

I had one prior opportunity to rethink the presentation of this material — in early 1982 during the change in publishers from Doubleday to Shambhala. At that point I restored some sections of the text to their original form (prior to imposed Doubleday editorial changes), and I wrote the Epilogue, "How to Choose a Healer." In the Doubleday edition, by not making pragmatic distinctions between medicines and by keying my value system to millennial time, I left practically-oriented readers in a quandary. Individuals do not seek doctors in millennial time; they must choose from among available alternatives, even if these systems arise from transitory categories and offer only ambiguous solutions. The Epilogue transposes this relativism into a hierarchy of therapeutic strategies.

The crisis of medicine and health care that underlies this book is primarily a crisis of definition. First of all, we have the most basic difficulty understanding and articulating the nature of the disease process, and finding—or even imagining—acceptable cures. Then, we encounter complex systems of medicine and healing operating at different levels of concreteness and contradicting one another's definitions of the same processes and terms—while at the same time each proposing universal holism. *Planet Medicine* begins by reexamining our quiescent categories in such a way that their contradictions become energetic, at least on the level of language.

Reexamination *must* be participatory and phenomenological. I do not believe that a sociological or philosophical overview does anything more than repackage traditional categories in the illusion of new paradigms. For instance, a decision to review medicine anthropologically does not eliminate cultural bias or guarantee universal ethics. Likewise, the deconstruction of therapy by conceptual and psycholinguistic models undermines its basis in raw experience; the result is an intellectualized argument rife with its own rigid symptomology (despite the fact that the model may also critique its self-evoked disease). I finally prefer the exercises of Wilhelm Reich to the much more exquisitely reasoned diagnoses of Jacques Lacan et al. if only because the former submerge the body in the somatic criteria of its survival whereas the latter are always subject to the clever manipulations and evasions of the professional persona.

Yet, to by-pass both the medical and academic authorities and to pretend to resolve the crisis by making it spiritual, "holistic"—or both—is a naive overvaluation of our ability to redefine and thereby alter our condition. This overvaluation is the credo of the "holistic health" movement and the reason why *Planet Medicine* is not a "holistic health" book. I am in sympathy with even many of the jazzier alternative systems, but I have trouble with their tendency to present themselves as if coming from authority and as adjudicating all intermediate issues of level and meaning. It is as though, by definition, a vitalistic medicine, like homoeopathy or shamanic chanting, encounters and activates the life force of the organism, which then distributes its "elixir" to every region of body, mind, and spirit. I do not think this is generally true (if true at all). I also do not think its "lie" negates the value of certain so-defined treatments; it does, however, entail simplification of their exaggerated mythologies.

I consider all the present talk (vintage, 1987) about channels, mediums, extraterrestrials, shamanic trances, healing crystals, and chreodes to be relevant and exciting, but I resist being told exactly what any of these things mean, and particularly how they relate on a one-to-one literal basis to our evolution, personal or planetary. Such spiritual authoritarianism is *always* someone else's interpretation of their own experience for their own reasons.

Perhaps these visitations or visions are archetypes of modern chaos perceived in crisis. Perhaps the so-called entities from the Pleiades and elsewhere represent realms of our own being whose manifestations we cannot accept, so project outward into the bigness of outer space. But even if there are real "intruders," I doubt that our situation will be clarified or resolved by science-fiction escapades or harmonic convergences. If aliens cloned our species from their own "protoplasm," as some claim, we have since become so interwoven in the molecular and viral fabric of the Earth we are now inextricable.

In matters of healing, absolutes are inevitably simplistic and counterproductive. People are self-maintaining organisms in continuous interaction with their environment, so, clearly, no illness will ever be one-hundred-per-cent cured, i.e., excised from their living system. We are charged quanta of tissue, energy, trauma, scars, immunity, aura; every trace of *everything* radiates through the zones of our wholeness, forever.

From the standpoint of modern medicine we are catastrophic diseases in temporary remission, so allopathy is usually a matter of how long to attempt to sustain life; it is almost never a question of meaning. Yet, even as we can never be cured, we are continuously in the process of self-healing. The most fundamental medicine is our own metabolism. Day by day, through our movements, our thoughts, our food—and by night, through the autonomous by-products of our sleep and dreams—we are healing, and that is *always* a question of meaning; i.e., it is a process intrinsic to the individuation of our organism. Even the most heroic medicine merely stimulates and supports that.

For instance, surgery and drugs represent explicit attempts to remove pathologizing agents; their prescribers don't even pretend to affect the heart of the defense mechanism. It is no accident that the largest expanding category of lethal diseases includes those that directly attack our immune response, that dampen or eliminate the power of self-cure in our bodies. AIDS, lupus, arthritis, diabetes, asthma, allergies—even cancer—alert us to turn away from the traditional tools of allopathy, which are mere postponements—treatments often more toxic than their diseases—and toward the vital and immune-oriented systems of homoeopathy, anthroposophy, acupuncture, bioenergetics, and the like.

But whatever we tell ourselves about psyche and spirit, the biophysical aspect of our existence will terminate. We are involved in an esoteric process that transcends ideology and purity of intent. Disease is our metabolic interface with the universe, so indelibly it is the signature of our responsiveness and individuality. It maintains our necessary separateness from the unity of substance at the same time that it is the revolt of nature *against* our exclusivity—an unrelenting attempt to return our body-minds to the anonymous flow. It is our education, unto death.

Anything, after all, is potentially lethal, anything potentially curative, even AIDS and nuclear weapons. As deep as we sink into pathology, that deeply (by definition) are we mobilizing a defense response. Medicine is a cultural and symbolic aspect of that response. But ultimately the treatment transcends its symbols in order to enter unconscious and biological realms.

For us in the twentieth century, technology is the most deadly mirage distracting us from our crisis and its seriousness. It is not only the direct effects (radiation leaks, toxic industrial wastes, antibiotics breeding exotic new germs, etc.) that make us sick, and then keep us from getting well; it is the degree of our mesmerization with the *concept* of technology that prevents us from approaching the problem in an intrinsic way. This is hardly an idiosyncratic failing of medicine. We need look only at the effects of automobiles on habitation and land-use and of nuclear weapons on general political life to see that we invariably prefer a powerful, energy-consuming device to bind the status quo. The collective residue of all our displacements and postponements of responsibility show up in our health — automobiles and nuclear weapons internalized along with everything else — so of course (paradoxically) we want to enact their same machine "magic" on our bodies. This vast, undifferentiated addiction replaces the sanctity and individuation of our own experience.

We declare, "Get rid of this disease!" as though the locus of its interaction with us could be concretized, isolated, and severed. Then (we tell ourselves) we will feel better. Often we simply feel less, thus feel less disease. Often, too, the disease is an externalized aspect of the healing process, and without it we are sicker.

Because disease is always our intrinsic response to an invasion rather than the invasion itself, it delineates our degree of susceptibility and distortion. Because medicine treats personal experience directly and because it embodies the most powerful metaphor for transformation we have, healing becomes a paradigm for both social revolution and self-development, and cannot be simplified or packaged and programmed into shortcuts.

However, when the day-to-day functioning and economic health of society are viewed in terms of static machines, we picture ourselves as unchanging algorithms too — our organs as separately functioning sites in an assembly-line. A check-up becomes a tune-up. It is hard to envision where the epiphenomenon of "mind" is located in such a schema. To the doctor it is probably a troublesome by-product, the alias of systemic activity in the patient; in himself, it is mostly an unexamined version of his professional ego. To the patient the self is usually an innocent observer trapped in a sophisticated vehicle of meat.

The cumulative effect of such latent beliefs in a profit-oriented society is disastrous. Hospitals have come to view patients primarily as investments. A sick individual is not only a mechanism like a clock; he or she is a commodity, a product on an assembly-line. If too much "care" and time are put into the product, the hospital's profit-margin is reduced. The fewer resources that are put into a product, the better the bottom line. So, the goal of treating patients humanely is not only *one step* removed by the mechanization of biology, it is removed *a second step* by the commodization of the machine. If a sick person's insurance profile does not match the disease prognosis, i.e., does not indicate that there will be money available to pay for the full treatment, doctors are advised not to admit the patient if at all possible. A good doctor, by some present definitions, is one who knows how to churn out as many patients in as short a time as possible, and also how to spot unprofitable patients for rejection. Only those patients whose disease conditions fit the model of expensive high-technology diagnosis and remediation are desirable, and then only if either they or their insurance can afford them.

The cures that take place under such a regime are not only symptomatic and mechanical, they are the *cheapest* symptomatic and mechanical solutions that can be legally perpetrated. (It is a supreme irony that Andy Warhol, who turned the assembly-line image into art, was killed by assembly-line health care.) It is not impossible to get adequate and compassionate treatment in this situation, but such treatment would be entirely incidental to the institutional goals — and a certain indigent percentage of the population would be denied even this skimpy and shoddy mode of care.

Near our home is an oral surgeon who recently performed exquisitely as the malefic physician. I met him several years ago when he was recommended by our dentist as the most convenient person to remove the wisdom teeth of our son Robin. We were uncertain that the operation was necessary, but could get no clear opinion either way from a "holistic" dentist. My wife, Lindy, went for the first consultation and must have communicated that I was the more difficult one, for, through her, the surgeon extended an invitation to me to visit him for a quiet chat. In the waiting room he entertained me with a philosophical discussion about medicine, including a virtual litany of holistic catch-words. "I'm your neighbor," he added. "You can call on me night or day."

I was swayed by his humane persona and agreed to the procedure. Then, for the relatively simple operation, Robin was overdosed with sedatives (while the needle-bearing nurse teased him with comments so spooky he had nightmares for months afterwards: "Where's your big vein hiding, Robin?"). He was returned to us unconscious, and remained half-asleep for days, during which time our "friend" either refused to return our calls or berated me for the "primitive belief-system" I had shown in his office. The sale had been made, so the mask was off. Beneath his relentless suaveness dwelled only the rigid allopathic quack, the type of person who never would have become a physician before the era of automation.

I was not overly shocked when, a few weeks ago, a writer who has cancer of the mouth told me of a recent visit to my "neighbor" to have part of his jaw removed. Despite the fact that he was in great pain, the surgery was postponed until October 31st in order to accommodate the doctor's vacation schedule. My friend arrived for the operation to find the surgical assistant dressed in a Halloween costume, sequins on her face. He was not fully sedated because of the danger he might choke on the bone being removed, and during the operation he heard the doctor say: "This job pays for my trip to Tahiti," and "Be sure to get this guy's money before he leaves."

As my friend described it, the surgeon was breaking off chunks of his jaw with a tool about as sophisticated as a pair of pliers and at the same time talking about him as though he couldn't hear.

"Maybe he didn't think I was too bright," he told me. "I guess that's because of the way I was dressed and the state of my finances. If he were a little smarter he would have known that fools don't dress this way either. I felt like the computer HAL, you know in *2001.* They might just as well turn me off. At one point when they were cracking through the jaw, the assistant tells him, 'Now you're cookin.' I looked at her fingernails and saw little skulls painted on them. I felt as though I were suddenly part of some occult ritual. I was of course; it's this bizarre ritual called American culture."

Dehumanization, however, is a superficial — and even indulgent — response to the complexity of machines and their origin in the collective psyche; it is one more symptom of our general materialism. Modern technology is ultimately a great riddle, and a dismissal of its modes would be an evasion of many of our most profound and disturbing discoveries about the universe and ourselves. These revelations, ranging from the explosive conditions of galaxy formation to chromosomes determining heredity, may prove, one day, to be no more than skewed and partial truths, but they will never be proved "wrong." Furthermore, there is an enlightened and healing aspect to technology (why else have we promoted progress so devotedly these last few centuries?). Unless our destiny as a species (and a planet) points to an ecological "stone age" following a cataclysm instead of journeys to the stars, we should not reject progressive science in its birth throes. In fact, as noted throughout this book, we are inseparable from its crisis and have long ago passed the failsafe point, when renunciation was possible—so we are far better off including a version of technology in our quest for new medicines and meanings.

Holistic medicine is modern medicine too, and it often partakes of the false authority and materialism of technology. I was reminded of this recently when visited by a German practitioner of a form of energetics. He had a machine that combined the diagnostic aspects of Chinese acupuncture, the circumstantial "proof" of Kirlian photography, and the curative mode of Reich's orgone therapy. It was a very provocative and optimistic machine, and probably a useful one. What was intolerable, though, was its bearer's claim that it healed absolutely everything and that other methods of bodywork, polarity, acupuncture, and herbs were now obsolete. When I tried to offer a more subdued assessment, he told me, kindly and patronizingly, that I was simply not informed and thus ignorant of the implications of the breakthrough.

Such claims leave no room for individuality and doubt; they are orthodoxies equal to allopathy. Human beings are not machines or templates that can be spontaneously vitalized, medicinalized, chi-ed, or shamanized into their own higher beings. They are extremely conservative organisms, and their mere contact with a medium, or their reading a book about reincarnation or chanting, or doing a weekend's shamanic or EST exercises, is not going to transform their lives, or even affect each person in the same way. Very concrete, almost miraculous things are possible, but only in subtle ways and with great attention to details and idiosyncrasies. There is not yet a universal medicine or a catchall metaphor for change.

Despite the literal implication of the word "holistic," the human organism is a fragmented entity and must be treated level by level, persona by persona (some levels and personae will not even appear in a lifetime, and cannot be treated). Surgery and drugs effectively treat one level; gestalt therapy, another; Bach flower remedies, another; chiropractic, another; and so on. But because these levels are actually interpenetrating fields—oscillating flows of biomorphic and psychic "energy"—medicines and meanings introduced into one will be transmitted to all. That is the optimism and legitimate promise of holism. However, a medicine will be directly curative only in the level at which it is introduced. What it translates to other levels may be curative insofar as those levels shift within mind-body awareness and call out for their own treatments. One hopes that a homoeopathic or chiropractic treatment will also clear the mind and lead the individual to seek a psychoanalytic or spiritual treatment to continue the healing process, and vice versa. It is possible, though, that a very effective treatment, even a vitalistic one, may have pathological consequences if it introduces too much energy into a persona that cannot contain and integrate it. Perhaps this is why Edward Whitmont, who is both a homoeopath and a Jungian psychologist, prefers not to use homoeopathy separate of psychoanalysis: He is concerned about setting in motion forces that the personality will then either cathect neurotically or suppress.

In direct answer to the question, can a homoeopathic remedy remove layers of Reichian armor from the forehead and belly?, I would say, no. I think that somaticized trauma is structured deeply and rigidly in the mind/body and can be removed only by a process of breathing, exercise, and imaging akin to the pathways by which it was incorporated. However, a homoeopathic remedy could alleviate a digestive ailment associated with belly armor and thereby participate in the bioenergetic process of its removal. A potency might also release the miasmatic and dermatological aspect of a "mask" and so energize the dissolution of facial armor.

Cases of such mutually interactive healing, even including coarse allopathic treatments, are probably more prevalent than people realize, because our most fundamental holistic responses are profoundly unconscious, creating their own presemantic symbols and constructs. All treatments are equalized, their effects optimized homeostatically. Somewhere within, surgery, flower potency, breath, and dream meet, and converge. Despite the medium, all healing is finally spiritual in consequence. That's *how* it works and *why* it works. Many so-called holistic and spiritual treatments merely enact a metaphor of this fact in their attempts to maintain ideological exclusivity. Sometimes everything else about a treatment fails, except an inner transformation.

The so-called mind-body split that we work holistically to unify is probably better described as a split between the mind of the body and the mind of the mind. It is not mind-body as such because we are *always* separated from the vast unconscious archetypal body. The problem is that we are often pathologically separated from the mind of the body as well. Meditation, various forms of bodywork (like that of Feldenkrais, Alexander, Lomi School, etc.), some forms of psychoanalysis, and, even occasionally, more "physical" therapies like chiropractic and herbs address the mind as body (or the body as mind), that is, open a channel through our moment-to-moment proprioception into the patterns of energy and substance in our organs. If the process is successful, physical and mental change are simultaneous.

This dynamic might be made clearer by our distinguishing between the intellectual mind, which objectifies itself from the phenomena it experiences (in one of its most sophisticated forms, it is the scientific mind), and the mind of the body, which uses its subjective experiences to develop an internal language of feelings and functional connections. When we speak abstractly of the heart and love for instance, we are not attributing characteristics to the physical aorta; we are identifying the charge we feel from the pumping of blood and the deep oxygenation of the organs *and* our capacity to contain and integrate that charge, to translate it into feelings about another person and acts of emotional exchange. The aikido master identifies the same "love" with the harmony of spirals between *uke* and *nage*. When one puts his or her heart into an act, the projection is far more complex than either the semantic metaphor or the life-giving actions of the circulatory system.

Certainly a major failing of Western culture, and industrial civilization in general, is that it cuts off everyone—capitalists as well as workers—from the mind of the heart, i.e., cuts them off not only from the healing but the acts of compassion that arise from there.

II

Not long after I wrote the Epilogue to this book, my wife and I went through a baffling two-year-long ailment with our daughter Miranda, then nine years old. Throughout it I found myself almost back at the beginning, without resources or any conviction of how to proceed. It doesn't finally matter what one either believes or resists believing. Events create their own ideology:

Miranda's ailment surfaced in September of 1983 with a boil (sty) on her left eye after a cold. It took two weeks of soaking to break it open; a fairly typical "pink eye" infection followed, spreading to both eyes. When the infection persisted for another week, we took her to our GP, a doctor sympathetic to homoeopathy and other alternative treatments and, in fact, an editor of holistic health books. He prescribed an antibiotic (Erythromyocin), after which the visible "pink eye" improved. However, her eyes never really felt right; they itched and were red in the mornings. She had times, especially at school, when she wanted to close them, so that we periodically had to come and take her home. Since it was a new and difficult school for which she wasn't fully prepared, we and the GP gave some consideration to a psychological aspect of the condition. (She has large, light blue eyes that have always attracted attention; because of them, people have tended to regard her as a spacy Aquarian child when she is actually more of a wry extrovert. Certainly her eyes have been the place at which the world chooses to meet and define her.)

One Sunday morning in February Miranda got shooting pains in both eyes. They were so uncomfortable that she rolled on the floor. Instead of taking her to the emergency room, we met a substitute for our GP at his office. He could find no visible sign of infection but, in testing her vision, found that it had deteriorated significantly since September. He sent us to the only opthamologist who would see her at once—in other words, someone not necessarily selected for quality. We ended up at a crowded clinic filled with mostly young children and elderly people. After a several hour wait, the doctor examined her with slit lamps and eye charts. Based on her poor vision at the time, he was mainly interested in prescribing glasses. He did see signs of an infection, but he downplayed it as secondary to her vision and prescribed a stronger antibiotic with a steroid. He assured us the infection would go away in two weeks.

Although Miranda had no further acute attacks in those two weeks, her eyes still bothered her. She described it mainly as a sensation of something being stuck in them, a dryness. She did not want to open them in bright light, and often when we were outdoors, she would pretend to be blind and ask to be led—a game that amused her and frightened us.

We kept our two-week appointment, and the opthamologist declared the infection cured and wanted to proceed with glasses. We decided to wait. Meanwhile, Miranda's problems continued. The physician mother of one of her friends told us that we should be concerned about serious systemic diseases, and we were spooked enough to call a relative who is a gynecologist in San Francisco. He recommended an opthamologist from New York who, he said, was the best children's eye-doctor in the Bay Area, and he even set up the first appointment for us within a week.

This prominent opthamologist seemed both compassionate and knowledgeable. He said almost immediately, "This is a very uncom-

fortable little girl and for good reason." After a thorough and painful examination, he told us that the original opthamologist didn't
know what he was talking about: Miranda had an extensive infection that had left disease products in her eyes and mottled the cor-
neas. He prescribed regular cleansing of the vicinity around the eyes
with a Q-tip and shampoo (the brand name No Tears, which Miranda
came to call More Tears), and a stronger antibiotic with cortisone.

To this point we had made no attempt to find an alternative physician. The disease was in a risky area, had begun as a "simple" infection, and had created its own trail of doctors. We were not naive
about the real causes, but much of life is spent not dealing with the
real cause of things. Miranda was in a situation of having to catch
up in school, and there seemed little room in which to experiment,
especially with her eyes. This is typical of the situation in which most
health care is sought and dispensed; it is like walking into the nearest
fast-food outlet when you're hungry because there is only an hour
before you're due back at work. It's why most people postpone self-
inquiry and personal change, often forever. One is inattentive until
they are in such a serious dilemma they are jolted to responsiveness.

When systemic illness became a possibility, my first panicked
thought was homoeopathy. However, when the new opthamologist
dismissed the possibility of any more serious disease, and later
confirmed his dismissal by lab tests, I returned to my distracted state.
The continuation of an antibiotic, now amplified by cortisone, was
certainly disturbing by any holistic or homoeopathic standards, but
we resolved to use it for as brief a time as possible. The credentials
of our doctor led us to believe that the disease would soon be resolved.

Miranda began the daily regimen of cleaning and applying the
antibiotic. The improvement was minor, but at least she did not have
any recurrences of acute painful attack. In the summer she complained about her eyes sweating and traffic fumes and even perfume
which, she said, caused them to "go crazy," and drove her either in-
doors or into outraged jigs. She was still painfully hypersensitive to
light. We finally made another appointment in August, and the opthamologist examined her thoroughly and said, despite her complaints,
that he saw no further sign of infection. It was only a matter of time,
he felt, before all effects of the disease disappeared. He told us to
continue the cleaning scrupulously

During the first weeks of school Miranda's problems got much worse. She ended up sitting by the side with her eyes closed on several occasions, and either Lindy or I had to rescue her. We insisted on another appointment, which we took her to directly from school one day. The charming old physician was definitely frayed; he accused us of not following through on his treatments because we believed in alternative medicines and insisted that her relapse was our fault (he did finally agree that the infection was still virulent). He referred us immediately to a San Francisco clinic specializing in infectious diseases of the eye.

Miranda's examination and culture there cost $200, and we were told that she had an allergological reaction to an underlying infection. There was no cure for the complex, but it could be treated hygenically. This meant continuing the shampoo treatments, but extending them to the nostrils and the sides of the nose. The doctor at the clinic emphasized that all of our previous treatments had been either wrong or incomplete. The original Erythromyocin was the only antibiotic to which the bacteria were susceptible, and the antibiotics prescribed by both opthamologists were incorrect and, in the case of the cortisone, contraindicated and potentially blindness-causing! The cleaning would work only if she got all the infected zones, which meant her entire face and scalp. Otherwise bacteria would simply spread again from the ignored pockets.

Still stung by the earlier doctor's accusations, we implemented that treatment rigorously for three and a half months into December. The condition improved enough that Miranda was able to stay at school and keep her eyes open, but she was unable to participate in outdoor sports in direct light (thus sat on the side), and still had very red eyes in the morning and a great deal of difficulty getting them open. At this point we assumed that allopathy could make no further headway, and we allowed a lay homoeopath to take her case. He prescribed *Pulsatilla* on a constitutional basis. He asked us to discontinue the topical antibiotic for at least ten days to see the results, warning us that she might experience an immediate aggravation. She developed a heavy cold, but her eyes neither improved nor got worse.

Later in the month we were in northern rural California and visited a macrobiotic naturopath we already knew. He typically enough suggested eliminating all dairy products and carrying out a mild saltwater bathing of the eyes twice daily, including snorting of saltwater through her nostrils. He felt her sodium balance was off, and he specifically prescribed a complete mineral salt to improve that balance as well as to make up for what-he-called other trace element deficiencies. He said that homoeopathy, for using just one substance at a time, could never fulfill the range of needs in her system. It was a misunderstanding of homoeopathy, but even mutually vitalistic systems tend to be incompatible.

After two weeks her eyes were itchy and red and it was time for her to return to school; we were at a definite impasse. We did not want to antidote the homoeopathic treatment, but we needed something to control the discomfort, so we returned to the Erythromyocin while continuing the bathing and restrictive diet. A few days later the right eye was clear and the left eye was swollen almost shut. We called the clinic and they said there was nothing we could do but persist in the treatment. We called the prominent opthamologist, and he said that the swelling was an infection in the gland and to continue soaking it. At this point we were back where we had begun and with a much worse situation.

I phoned an out-of-town homoeopath and described Miranda's history and condition in detail. With much reservation about remote prescribing he mailed us *Tuberculinum 30* and included a letter in which he described her condition as a deep-seated inherited psoric miasm and warned that use of the remedy with the antibiotic would eventually cause mutual aggravation. Within days after we gave the remedy, the sty went down, but a second sty formed on the upper eyelid and swelled to the size of a marble. We continued to soak it for several days, but there was no improvement and she could not go to school.

We returned to our GP in desperation. He felt that whatever else was true that he had to prescribe an oral antibiotic to deal with the immediate infection. She took Tetracycline, and the sty eventually broke, although two months later it was still present in reduced form. During those months she continued the hygenic treatment and occasionally used topical Erythromyocin. (The out-of-town homoeopath later attributed the failure of the remedy to the fact that we gave it twice — in his mind a very dangerous action. "It's lucky," he said, "it was her eye and not her heart.")

In early March the situation escalated to another crisis. Miranda bumped into her brother Robin in the hall and hit her eye. The pain was so bad that she screamed for ten minutes and said she wanted to die. Under the pressure of this new and frightening deterioration,

I called my gynecologist cousin and reviewed the alternatives. He agreed that we could go no further down any of the past roads. We had to find some way to act more decisively. The next morning he called me back, having gotten us an appointment with a research opthamologist who did not ordinarily see patients but nonetheless would meet us in his laboratory that afternoon.

He was a distinguished-looking older man, more gentle with Miranda than any of the practicing physicians had been. He ran her through the battery of slit lamps, dyes, and cultures with a graduate student, and then heard out our whole history, which included naturopathy and homoeopathy. (For instance, he read our letters from the out-of-town homoeopath.) He said he knew the condition well and could understand our series of blind circles. The disease was essentially—as the clinic had explained—a special reaction to ordinary bacteria. But he was more precise: It wasn't an infection of the eye in the usual sense and certainly should not have been treated as conjunctivitis; it was the result of a preadolescent acne so slight as to be almost imperceptible except for an oiliness and slight scaling around the nose. The bacterial by-products of the skin got into the eyelids, lashes, and onto the cornea itself, causing the scarring. Through his magnifying lenses I could see the stained surface of Miranda's cornea with pits and streamers of irritation. "Deep-seated psoric miasm indeed," he mused. "The language is not contemporary, but the diagnosis is essentially correct. I wouldn't say anything when my student was here because he'd have my head. Graduate students are so narrow these days. But she has inherited a complex to which she is unable to generate a normal immune response." Later, I surmised that it was perhaps my mother's skin, my wife's father's eyes— incompatible in one person—but that was spontaneous myth as much as genetics.

We went back to the regimen of washing and using a topical ointment, with the difference that Miranda visited the laboratory every other week; her vision was tested, the surface of her eyes mapped, her face photographed, and a culture taken. "I'm the star," she said during one session with typical acerbic wit. But another time she added, "I heard what he said. There's no cure. I'm going to be like this forever. He'll have a photo album of my whole life."

Soon there was gradual but not overwhelming improvement in the surface of the cornea and discomfort. The photophobia and pinkness remained. Her vision stabilized at the level to which it had initially declined, serious enough for glasses if it remained but not debilitating in most circumstances.

After three months she suddenly developed acne rosaceae, which quickly became a fullblown facial eruption. We were now truly trapped between systems of medicine. A visiting homoeopath said that we had to let the acne run its course because it was the external-ization of the disease into less vital organs. The research opthamolo-gist said, "Hogwash! The acne is the source of the infection, and it is now rampant. Unless we treat this immediately with an internal antibiotic her sight will be threatened."

The idea of an internal antibiotic concerned me because of its possible longterm consequences — the homoeopathic warning was direct. However, if we did not pursue that treatment, the optha-mologist would not see her anymore. We were at a true crossroads.

We agreed to let her take Tetracycline. For his part the opthamolo-gist promised the smallest possible amount, "an almost homoeopathic dose," he joked. At the same time we went to see the one homoeo-path in our area who would work with patients using allopathic drugs. On the day Miranda started the Tetracylcine, he took her entire case carefully and prescribed an individualized homoeopathic remedy — *Mercurius*. It was a very low potency — 6C — but he had her take it three times daily. He also prescribed homoeopathically prepared microdoses of Tetracycline, to diminish negative side effects from the drug. I asked him the obvious questions: wasn't the skin ailment a movement outward of the disease?, won't the antibiotic and po-tency aggravate each other?, isn't giving repeated doses dangerous? He had the same answer to all of them: "I'm not an ideologue."

He said he was interested only in treating Miranda as she was. Her sight was threatened, so she should be taking an antibiotic. A good homoeopathic treatment wasn't interested in rules; it was involved only in restoring her actual vital force. He had never had any prob-lem with antibiotics or multiple doses, and he considered such ortho-dox homoeopathy superstitious.

During a month of travel on the East Coast, Miranda took all three remedies — a foul tasting fungus and two sugar pills containing only spiritual essence — and continued to scrub. She experienced the most dramatic improvement yet. Her skin cleared completely, she was able to be outside in bright sunlight for the first time in months, and, when we returned, her bacteria level was way down and her cornea less aggravated. The opthamologist thought the Tetracycline did it, but admitted he didn't know how. "I gave it to her in subtherapeutic doses, and she missed a number of days at that. It's really a black box. Maybe homoeopathic mercury is the answer, but I won't write that down anywhere. Who cares, as long as she's better?"

I remarked that it was too bad we couldn't tell what had cured her. "Oh Son of Man, thou canst not know," he said with a smile.

That spring he expressed some disappointment that, despite other improvement, the cornea was still pitted and Miranda's vision hadn't improved. Meanwhile, she had developed plantar's warts, and they had spread and become quite painful. With reduction of sensitivity in her eyes, she had begun ballet, and the warts made it difficult. Lindy and I locked horns here. Lindy wanted to have a dermatologist treat them, as was done in her childhood; I felt that they were somehow connected to the antibiotic and the eyes and I wanted the homoeopath to see her.

We compromised. Miranda went first to a dermatologist, who said that the warts were deep-seated and would be difficult to remove without surgery. The next day she went to the homoeopath. In taking her case anew he repetorized a remedy that covered both scarring of the cornea and plantar's warts (*Silica*), and he prescribed it with the observation that *Mercurius* had been selected primarily for photophobia, which it seemed to have already handled.

Within twenty-four hours the plantar's warts had turned black and begun to fall off; a week later the opthamologist found her cornea remarkably cleared, and on the eye chart she shot right through the 20–20 line and kept on going until he said, with a smile, it was good enough.

The actual course of this disease and its treatments is a map of something unknown. Since we have no information about how either subtherapeutic Tetracycline or microdoses of *Mercurius* and *Silica* work in tissue, or how Miranda's own metabolism and individuating psyche affected all this, we can resolve nothing vis a vis competing systems, nor do we have any guarantee the cure will be sustained, that the medicines won't have side-effects, or that we will know how to proceed the next time.

But this is the state of our civilization anyway.

PLANET
MEDICINE

Origins and Definitions

I

Disease and Cure: Image and Process in Medicine

We live on a planet of seas and vapors, mud, fire, and dust. We are suspended in a field of attractions cast by heavy objects which go on eternally, nesting in each other so that the smallest things we know are in continual touch and influence from the largest and from things beyond visibility. We have no simple beginning, no precedent, no explanation.

We live too in a sea of light pouring from a sun-star many thousands of times the size of our world. This light is so full and rich that we are bathed in it at all times. It has penetrated the planet so long that our bodies are made of its deposits. It is the yellow oils of buttercup and the volcanic embers; it is the rain, and it is also the snow. The heat of the ground, of every breath and organism comes from it. Our very thought and civilization is a by-product of sun.

In the clear daytime sky we see the absolute condition of atmosphere like a painting—temperatures and relations of winds strung out in clouds. Each clump of trees breathing carbon dioxide, each lake evaporating, every perspiring city, mountain deflecting currents of air, every yarn of density in the cloud matter itself, registers again in the sky as mottles, streaks, and whips within the prism blue.

At night, when sunlight is bent out of the prism, we see a universe. There is no sense of *where* it is, only that it is held together by instantaneous lines and attractions. There are stars where matter and gravity build them; blackness elsewhere. Each object is a world of some sort, composed as this one is. If creatures inhabit any of them, they live outside our entire reality and history, outside even our biology; yet we silently share the creation. From any one world, the other worlds appear as points of light, each the size and brilliance of its makeup and remoteness from the viewer. There is no self-apparent reason for distance and space, but things are distributed in this way, and we come into being as spatial creatures, from the minute geometries of the genes to the raw bloody topology of our flesh and the birth canal to the geography of the senses and the brain. All is arranged, as it were, in a river of time which enfolds the creation.

We are inside this condition. We *are*, in fact, the inside of this condition—the only inside we know. As big and dense and distributed as the universe is, our senses give it to us as normal and inhabitable, even cozy. We do not question our presence here. We assume we are natives. The amount of everything does not overwhelm and destroy us because we know it as ourselves. We contact it within us and not out there where it is.

We swim in the cool mountain pool; sun-warmed currents blend with underground rivulets of ice; waves pass through our nervous system, changing our feelings, reviving memories. Our nerves and tissues see the light sparkling on the surface; they create relations of currents and rivulets.

We live in such a pool, a pool so sensitive that these words and images, as they pass through consciousness, change my present chemistry as I write them, yours as you read them.

When the surf echoes and crashes out to the horizon, its whorls repeat in similar ratios inside our flesh. The ocean and sky are vast; we know this because our awareness of them is vast in a whole other way. Their raw infinity cannot touch us without destroying us, so we will never know *it*.

Yet, all the time, that thing we are, which does this feeling, seeing, knowing, imagining what it is, is that same water, mud, dust, and fire. Even if we were predestined to arise from matter—a common religious interpretation of science—we have done so only by the chemical properties of that matter, without shortcuts, without discontinuity, and in full accord with the absolute laws of nature. We are extremely complicated, but our bloods and hormones are fundamentally seawater and volcanic ash, congealed and refined. Our skin shares its chemistry with the maple leaf and moth wing. The currents our bodies regulate share a molecular flow with raw sun. Nerves and flashes of lightning are related events woven into nature at different levels.

We are a particular form in a larger pattern, shaped within it, hewed to it, held there by the invisible contour of being. Our consciousness is a natural feature of creation. We cannot extract it, exceed it, or evade it; we cannot duck it or be driven outside it. Our evaluations of it fail, for they must always be a part of the thing they are about.

Everything we see, is. We see fiery and watery and empty conditions only where they are: the Milky Way where primal hydrogen is thickest and hottest, twenty miles of dandelions in a field in Maine, a clump of phlox in the backyard, giant rocks the glaciers have rolled into Quebec, and stones the ages have formed from protean lava. Billions of ant eggs spawn and bird nests appear in the trees. Villages emerge along Indian trails that were once buffalo migration routes. The furnaces smoke. No invention can eliminate that smoke; it may be changed only into some other thing.

There is only this one world, this one creation. Even so-called supernatural events must occur within it, for there is no other place in which they could happen.

In certain periods of history and in certain regions, things may be consigned to another world because they do not seem right where they occur. The "other world" is a way of expressing the complexity and paradox of their relation to us and the more familiar world. They do not require another universe. The universe we are in is vast enough to contain them too.

Matter itself does not challenge us or intend our defeat. It is the cutting edge of our being, and it keeps processing us, as perception and mass, through the thing of which we are made.

We have solid-seeming bodies and live in a world of definitive events. Yet our actual being is a shimmering, multidimensional thing, embodying, in its ongoing cellular life and continuum of perception, the first cell and the beginning of thought. Our contemporary life repeats and re-experiences ancient moments while giving birth to them anew. This is our profundity and our sense of our own meaning. The process that brings creatures into the world, in body and in senses, sustains and reproduces those creatures in exactly the same way that it invented them.

Categories of medicine are inseparable from definitions of life and consciousness. Disease occurs as organisms do: in the living chemistry of tissue and the cognizance of mind. It has no intrinsic meaning and no guarantee of remedy. Individual systems of medicine explain this in their individual ways, usually giving the appearance of order, understanding, and correctly selected cures. But disease is no more explicable than life itself. Any one system, like any one metaphysical inquiry, solves some problems but fails to arrange a perfect match between its explanations and remedies and the diseases themselves. Any one system is limited by its tools and its cultural context. By choosing a path of explanation and defense, it must neglect others, so it must always be regional or provincial.

This is a basic point to all discussion of medicine. For medicine is both a craft and a philosophy. It provides meanings and explanations for illnesses, and it also proposes to cure them. Unlike most philosophies, it cannot dawdle in the paradoxes; it must choose a path, even if that path is inadequate and partial. Many practices resolve crises but with profound secondary consequences. Other methods explore the profundities of cure and cosmos at the expense of decisive and explicit action. These poles mark medicine's ever-present struggle with both action and meaning.

There is no universal methodology. How one treats disease depends on what one considers the nature of man and the universe to be. Different cultures express unique aspects of the human condition, and, although skills can often be transmitted, definitions cannot. On the level of craft, doctors can reduce specific dangers and ease life-threatening situations. Even so, the patient is never completely cured, for he is changed by the disease, and he must proceed on a new course. How that change is integrated into future life, whether it prevents or spawns new illnesses, is a function of how the particular culture or style of treatment prepares the patient. And this has much more to do with the ethics and cosmology of the group than with the absolute nature of either the disease or the cure. It is as true in our own civilization as it is in the most primitive hunting band: a doctor alleviates the immediate distress as best as he can; then both he and the society prescribe the appropriate course for the patient's life. There is no final court of right or wrong, except the populace which allows itself to be treated in this manner. In a certain sense, medical treatment expresses how a society distinguishes itself from raw, pagan nature (or, in many cases, how it identifies itself with such nature).

The basic categories in this book are disease, remedy (or cure), and medicine as a profession.

We can define disease in a number of ways. First, and most obviously, it is a disruption of the biological well-being of the organism.

But disease can also be anything which a group considers deviant, including ways of behaving, menstruation, or aging itself. When societies do not distinguish between biological disruption and social taboo, their systems of medicine do not either, with the result that every society, including our own, has a difficult time defining what disease is and in assigning legal or supernatural responsibility, as the case may be.

Modern holistic health disciplines attempt to engage and integrate that difficulty, so they tend, unofficially, to consider as disease anything which limits the freedom and/or potential of the organism. Some biological disturbances are then considered creative changes, while many behavioral problems are treated as equivalent if not identical to organic malfunctions.

The remedy (or cure) is caught on the horns of the same dilemma. It can be the substance, activity, or event which helps restore biological functioning and harmony (or intends to), but it can equally be the substance or process which leads to culturally desired behavior. In some cases, it is the agent which helps promote the change of which the disease is an aspect. Throughout this book, we will consider two degrees of cure: one which has a limited and predetermined goal in relation to a particular ailment and one which ignores or minimizes the ailment in an attempt to bring an over-all state of well-being and freedom to the organism. The two degrees are really incompatible, since the practitioners of either one consider the other to be a promotion of pathology rather than health.

Medicine is the general inquiry into disease. It can involve the explanation of disease, the curing of disease, or both. Many systems throughout history have passed as medicines, and the basic issue of what is fake and nonfunctional (i.e., quackery) and what is sincere, educated medicine continues to be debated in contemporary American society. This debate may well be one of the things which shapes our era, for it underlies many political, economic, and ecological issues.

From the origin of man as a species, there have been two separate traditions of the practice of medicine. One is the art of healing, which may be exactly that: an art, practiced through sympathy and intuition; it more usually involves its own difficult training and techniques and parallels the other tradition in requirements of skill and education. The latter tradition we can call technological-scientific medicine, meaning by that the first primitive skills of surgery and pharmacy as well as the sophisticated forms they have taken in current global culture.

Throughout history, the two traditions have interacted; each has supplied the other with elements that it lacked. In some situations their identities merge in one system or individual; at other times they are in active opposition. Sometimes their identities are so confused that one actually passes for the other (we may find homoeopathy to be a dramatic case of this instance). At all times, though, information from the systems passes back and forth between them, and they necessarily develop in relation to one another. If they were totally separate, the confusion would be less, but each one claims to be the universal medicine. The art of healing often views technology as a shallow imposter, and the mainstream of technology views the art of healing as an archaic uninformed troublemaker. Even some of the severest critics of technological medicine argue that only better technology is needed and that to adopt the various forms of healing offered as alternative would be like going back to the bow and arrow and stone tools.

The relationship between these traditions is one of the major topics of this book. However, before we get any further into systems of medicine and healing, let us go back to the matter of disease and re-examine it from an individual and phenomenological perspective.

There is no clear moment in the organism's life at which sickness begins. Even the result of disease is recognized only some time after it has occurred. A sick person remembers the moment at which the discrepancy demanded his attention, but not the moment it crystallized in his system, though that moment also may have sensory correlates.

The fact is that at each moment, health and illness are in balance with each other and inseparable. The doctor who works to change the illness simultaneously works to change the health. That is, he changes the body and all things that are in it, even if he has no effect on his specific target. Many of these changes may be random and trivial; they may also not be trivial—they may be more important than the intended "cure."

At the same time the doctor is working on them, both health and illness are being influenced by events inside and outside the body, events which do all the things that medicines do, though maybe not with the same intensity and singular locus. Personal chemistry, dreams, feelings, daily relationships with other people, weather, food, and air all permeate the plane on which the doctor is working. These are not specific drugs prescribed by a physician in the context of a goal, but there is nothing such prescribed medicines can do that natural "medicines" cannot. This does not endanger the status of pharmacy, for rarely does the flux of daily events produce a concrete and lasting cure; however, it does suggest the busy context in which drugs must operate. Everything else does not stop in order to listen to the medicine. Medicines must speak to the body the same way that everything does. There is no medicine that obviates all other conditions, and there is no medical treatment that breaks the continuity of organism and environment without creating worse disease or destroying life itself. Healing has always worked in a din of overwhelming static, but with powerful fundamental allies.

The pairing of disease and medicine is an attempt to give a utilitarian direction to a universal environmental condition. Some things change us by our assimilation of them in our chemistry; some things change us by the senses, i.e., how we feel them and feel ourselves in their context. Conventionally, the latter are mental, the former are physical; but the organism is an integrated whole and does not really distinguish between these. Our minds may, intellectually, but our bodies do not read the world that way.

Mind/body is itself a misleading way to view reality, but modern rationality is such that we can hardly escape the dichotomy. For centuries now, mainstream science has attempted to train its best minds to perceive phenomena objectively and derive their characteristics separate of man's internal being. We thus come to think of ourselves as dead matter which has life in it or as carbon flesh activated and maintained by a genetic code. We neglect a whole category of information that floods us from the entity that is both mind and body. Yet it is exactly that information which forms the background of our lives, our existences. We take it for granted because it is omnipresent, and we prefer to focus on the foreground of thoughts and actions. We pretend that our thoughts give us intentions which our bodies carry out. Modern definitions of pleasure emerge in this way, so it is no wonder that modern definitions of health have the same sources. In a sense, we live a life which is abstracted from the actual life that lives us. We have no language for the deep mind/body pool that we are, so we borrow language from either mind or body to explain systemic changes.

The current fashion of psychosomatic medicine tends to focus on specific episodes of mental/physical feedback rather than the prior simultaneity of all things mental and physical. It is a model, not the real situation.

Currently, there is a great recognition in America that we are mind-obsessed and mind-enslaved; with it comes an attempt to recover our lost bodies. But then we take back from the false mind/body dichotomy exactly the wrong "body." We choose a physical slave, who does our work, has our pleasure, and keeps healthy for us, which confirms the mental giant. Note the current popularity of physical exercise and jogging. Some people have penetrated these external activities and come to the inner meaning and integration of self. The great majority, though, have treated their bodies like a date picked up at the singles bar, and they hustle it, punish it, and try to make it give them things they want. Inevitably, this leads to the same disappointment with which it began.[1]

Our bodies themselves do not distinguish between mental and physical; they have a self-knowledge, even a wisdom, that precedes and combines both. If our bodies do not distinguish, diseases certainly do not. And medicine itself can make only shallow psychosomatic assumptions. Any substance assimilated changes an organism both physically and mentally. Intention does not affect this. The doctor treating our illness is merely another point of contact with the environment. Whatever he does, he cannot convince the body— *the uneducated intelligence of the body*—that he means well or badly, that he means, in fact, anything other than what anything else means. And the psychiatrist certainly cannot convince the body by convincing the mind. So he cannot convince the mind either. Meditation may change mental states, but it does so by using the neurophysiological basis of thought; it trains consciousness, but does not attempt to convince consciousness.

The disciples of the new medicine see sickness as the movement of the whole organism toward integration through self-exploration. We contain the seeds of sickness at birth. They are nurtured in our mind/body. They feed us, limit us, expand us; they make change inevitable. Even as we eliminate the symptoms of specific illnesses, we cannot eliminate illness itself, for it is an integral part of who we are and a nucleus of our very personalities. Sigmund Freud stated this as a virtual "first law of life," but he *seemed* to mean psychological illness only. By now we recognize that in his psychology, he wrote the laws of the body too and that the body is the missing reservoir of the so-called unconscious mind. This is why his dynamics of unconscious process are so important to holistic health and phenomenological philosophy: both of these are based on a recovery of mind/body unity and, with it, the *experience* of the organism rather than its thoughts or its actions.

Perfect health is a chimera. We have no idea of how we would feel without illness. What we feel, as mind/body, is a large blur made up of health, illness, external matter, internal consciousness, into which we project our egos, our hopes and fears and plans, our sense of being; it is from this that we derive our "experience." There is a common misunderstanding of health as not feeling anything at all. That is, if we do not feel our bodies, everything is okay; if we begin to feel something, it must be sickness. The tragedy of this unexplored stasis is that we tend to block out feelings and interior body wisdom as well as the seeds of disease. So we misread warning signals because we experience them, even for years, only as vague irritation or numbness. And when we experience deep emotional feeling as physical movement, we block it also, making our emotional lives and relationships thin and sentimental. We choose to feel as little as we can so that we can have our "health" as we understand it.[2] It is no wonder that the "twentieth century" was ushered in by the psychological sciences and that it has since been visited by a great variety of self-proclaimed psychosomatic and religious therapies. In our obsession with psychological causation, we are not any more able to distinguish between the so-called mental and physical than our "unpsychological" forebears. This is at least in part because we have taken the split too seriously and tried to apply it with naïve or total faith. The psychosomatic explanation is not meaningless, simply limited in its application.

Suddenly or gradually we are sick. We may not even recognize a change at first, but ultimately the illness disrupts our plans and takes priority. That is how we seem to experience it. However, long before a positive symptomology penetrates awareness, the disease is also pres-

ent, making those very plans, working as an inextricable part of the
over-all personality.

On the mental level there may be conflicts that announce the disease before there is anything conventional medicine can treat. The
body bubbles with contradictions and the mind chatters ceaselessly,
agreeing and disagreeing. The society and the environment have imposed an intolerable burden on the internal processes of the self, and
conflicts seize the organism's attention, reflecting throughout the
mind/body cosmology whatever definitions it has given them:

I am strong. I am weak. I like my job. I hate every day of it. I
love him. I can't stand being with him. I want to be free. I don't
want to be free. I'm creative. I'm stuck. I want to be with someone. I just have to be alone. Why don't I feel more? It's all too
painful. I must be getting terribly sick. It's all finally coming together for me. I am terrified of death. I want to die. When did
that wonderful feeling of clarity leave me? When did this sickness
begin? Has it always been with me?

As the poet Charles Olson put it: "We live out, until there isn't
any, the argument of our lives."[3]

Most of this conflict appears on a mental level, but if that were its
whole genealogy, the resolution would be simple. The mind is only
the top of the pyramid. The body "thinks" these things too, in its
own way. Because people do not understand that their mental and social conflicts are fundamental and biological, they either pretend to
dismiss them or think to change them too easily by changing their
"mind" about them.[4] The very oscillation between opposites, as
above, reflects and maintains a deeper somatic stasis. For these are
only *seeming* opposites, and their underlying collusion makes up the
total environment in which many people live. Some may become
physically ill with known and named diseases; others live and die in
the obscurity of these opposing thoughts. For a medicine concerned
with human freedom and potential, these outcomes are identical.
There is no difference between a visibly pathological death and an
uncontacted blank life.

The moment we start treating health and disease as concrete entities subject to technical remediation, we have lost the meaning of an
integrated system. Disease may be reflected in pathology and tissue
damage, but it is also the place where all other crises and necessities
of the organism come together. It is the most intimate writing of the

turbulence and changes of life on the single bodies and collective body of the biosphere. Nothing else, except maybe dream or vision, forces the organism to reconcile itself instantaneously with the devastating pagan powers of which it is made. The major religions of both the East and West teach this same doctrine as revelation through suffering.

When an individual becomes sick, he is tugged toward the reality of his biological and social existence. The disease is required either because of his genetic destiny, his biological and epidemiological relationship to other organisms, or his psychological and social adjustment to his cultural environment. In this sense, disease cannot be accidental or random, even when it seems it is. As an old Roman proverb states, *Fata volentem ducunt, trahunt nolentem* (Whoever is willing the Fates will lead, the unwilling they will drag along).

We are surrounded by a flagrancy that is like disease: industrial waste; nuclear bombs; growth economy; left- and right-wing dictatorships; political uses of torture; pornography; sadomasochism; crime waves, from the streets to the corporations and governments. All of these crises recur again in our individual bodies and their response and adjustment to them. We respond to their existence in the only way we can—by *our* existence. We and they (more deeply) are products of the same world order. As we evade responsibility for them consciously, we are still unconsciously and somatically implicated in their over-all complexity. Diseases truly arise from them, but they and those diseases share an origin in the rhythm of our civilization.

Scientific medicine cannot alter this basic condition; it can add only its own complexity of drugs and interpretations to the complexities already in the situation. For the person born into an industrialized Western nation, this complexity begins to organize itself at birth, and from the manner of birth, and is thoroughly integrated by the age of consciousness. All of us who have been raised in this system already have the system as an environment by the time we start to choose our doctors and report our symptoms. Even when we adopt new and unusual medicines, we have our condition as context.

This is an evasive subtlety, and I will tighten our hold on it here a step more at the risk of losing it.

We give our problems names, as we give diseases and medicines names, but they exist in reality despite their names. In one decade China is the evil enemy of the United States. In the following decade, it may express, for many, a utopian image of the world's future. But China remains as a real entity despite these images; that real entity is also engaged with these images at various levels of collective consciousness and unconsciousness.[5] Disease has its own existence too. We have various concrete images of it, and they exist as names. The images are real and the disease is real, but in different ways, and they continue to interact and produce further varieties of approximate disease categories.

Orthodox medicine freezes a set of these images and proceeds to work on it, though other images, other "diseases," continue to exist. It is aware of these discrepancies, but most individual doctors have no leisure in which to examine them. They are satisfied to be technicians and cure what they can. Even if we leave the deep metaphysics of disease out of this discussion for the moment, we are left with the phenomenon that probably more than half of the problems people bring to doctors are human and social problems that are expressed in aches, discomforts, and more serious tissue damage. Most doctors do not feel comfortable with these human problems nor are most able to work with them. Some doctors do not even feel they *should* work with them. In any case, the average physician is hopelessly overmatched.

Individual doctors or institutions may respond politically in the absence of a concrete disease image and decide it is social behavior which must be cured. There are only brutal techniques for that.

The real origin of disease is uncertain; it is broadly societal, constitutional, and cosmic. Real things are cured finally by a process, not a particular medicine. Drugs, after all, are only a seeming realization of the fantasy of solving all wrong things at once. But this is impossible anyway. Process healing, on the other hand, avoids ideas and explanations. It works parallel to the condition, in respect of changing symptomology. It does not commit itself to a literal diagnosis even though it may give one in metaphorical language.

We have forgotten what cure is. We have forgotten not because we have forgotten the word "cure," but because the word has lost any concrete applicable meaning. For centuries now, mainstream medicine has existed primarily as theoretical schools of anatomy, pharmacology, and surgery.

The modern physician has inherited a collection of life-saving tools. X-ray machines, microscopes, and computers add a depth and scope to diagnosis and treatment that is awesome in terms of the equipment with which most medicines throughout history have worked. If acupuncture, homoeopathy, or, for that matter, Navaho sand painting had access to these devices, they would be able to use them (certainly homoeopathy has incorporated modern laboratory techniques, and traditional medicine has been merged with Western medicine in China). There is nothing, per se, about the repertoire of modern medical tools and skills that stands against "other" medicines. Innovations may be overspecialized or unneeded in individual circumstances, but they do not *require* an alternative.

When we speak of a modern medicine to which an alternative is proposed, we mean a set of beliefs about what an organism is and what disease is; we also mean a medical system that is a reflection of social, economic, and political goals (and under attack for the same reasons many of these are). The issue is not as simple as the unchecked profitability of surgery and drugs. These are potential corruptions, but even in its most humanitarian application the medical establishment is limited and conditioned by the cultural beliefs and taboos within which it operates. The doctor must stay within the system, and this usually turns out to be more important than his curing of disease. The abandonment of objectivity is so complete and at the same time so subtle that few doctors understand the degree to which *this* is their dilemma.

There are, of course, currently fashionable reasons for being critical of doctors: many put financial gain before the needs of their patients; neglect the poor; try to hide mistakes, even at the risk of a patient's welfare; and, often, are dupes of the pharmaceutical companies, from whom they accept favors. Not all doctors are guilty of these lapses, but most doctors implicitly condone a system in which these things must happen.

Some liberal physicians and social workers become involved in rural health clinics with sliding fee scales and aggressive "outreach programs," or they initiate facsimiles of these in undeveloped countries. The same style of treatment, based on the same philosophy of disease and cure, is made available on a missionary basis. For most of the liberal critics, this is a successful grassroots attack on institutionalized medicine. But then such critics are political in the narrow sense, and they do not see the relationship between the methodology itself and the integral politics of medicine. From a holistic point of view, this "liberalism" is simply a beachhead of the conservative establishment—enlarging its constituency while covering its social

debts at small cost. Global medicine presents the same ultimate ecological problem as global agriculture (with its pesticides) and global
petroleum economy. It is disruptive to short-circuit a complicated
and interconnected system of suffering and meaning. Penicillin and
baby formula may save some lives, but they also may cause irrepara-
ble alienation in a society.

We assume that we know disease by the feel of the internal organs
of our body. But this is not true. The tissue of our sensorium and
brain is not arranged to transmit actual localized sensations from
deep organs. They must first be brought to the surface, as concepts,
as language with one's self, and, finally, as language with the society
and its doctors (who, to the child, are first its parents). With the exception of obvious injuries and hurts, pain is undifferentiated, and
the perception of one's self is dim and global and grows over a long
period of time.[6]

How one feels organic difficulty and classifies it is a culturally
learned form. Taxonomies of diseases and the medicines that ostensibly cure them grow up in conspiracy with each other in a larger and
more complex field of meanings and references than is ever admitted. The creation of supposed "real" diseases is a mutual folly in
which patient, doctor, medical school, and culture have joined over
the ages. It is extremely difficult to match profound organ changes
with visible internal geometries, and both of these with the perception of internal change and the language categories of both sick people and physicians. There are subjective choices all the way down the
line: for the doctor, which organs and geometries to emphasize; for
the patient, which inward discomfort to dignify and act out and in
which way; for the system, which action to relate to which geometry.

Edward Schieffelin, working recently among native peoples of
New Guinea, found that a new disease category, "Evil Spirit Sickness," had come with the missionaries. Local people began to explain all sorts of *different* chronic ailments by this suddenly popular
illness. Social, psychological, and physiological factors were now combined in a new set of meanings, which could be presented to the missionaries for their resolution. As a disease, it demanded a sort of attention that a rebellion would not have, and it brought the natives
and newcomers together in a single diagnosis. Clearly, though, most
of the manifestations of this illness had existed before and were explained in other ways.[7]

Medicine, at times, behaves more like popular philosophy than physical science. The unpredictable and boundlessly creative lexicon of pathology always outduels the fixed categories of science. The words themselves slip: "blood," "virus," "cancer," "schizophrenia," "tonsil," "brain" have different meanings and connotations today than a decade ago and give no indication of stopping here. There is a wild and ineffable quality in disease and the language of anatomy which prevents a universal system. Where ancient plagues have disappeared into historical ledgers, new maladies bud. As medical treatment becomes more complex and profound, diseases toughen and take on unsuspected dimensions. Psychoanalysis seems to have come into being just in time to deal with a virtual plague of mental illness.

The French philosopher and historian Michel Foucault writes: "The exact superposition of the 'body' of the disease and the body of the sick man is no more than a historical, temporary datum. . . . For us, the human body defines, by natural right, the space of origin and of distribution of disease: a space whose lines, volumes, surfaces, and routes are laid down, in accordance with a now familiar geometry, by the anatomical atlas. But this order of the solid, visible body is only one way—in all likelihood neither the first, nor the most fundamental—in which one spatializes disease. There have been, and will be, other distributions of illness."[8]

Medicine's abstract and collective need to identify itself as a technical science dooms it to the little bit of science it has mastered thus far. While physics has a Newtonian core which carries it through most of the difficult operations of urbanized society (the buildings finally stand and the planes take off), medicine suffers, all through its structure, this vagueness of relationship between actual disease, specific organ, quality of being sick, and appropriate cure. Its own solution seems to have been a division of itself into a core area, where most operations are simple and illness is apparently not complicated, and various, almost unlimited, outlying districts, or specializations, where individual physicians are responsible for only one aspect of a dangerous situation. The specialist makes repairs in his own territory, but he often does so without particular regard for the whole structure, either its meaning or health. This may work in engineering, for a bridge across a river, however complex its technology, must finally link two points on a simple surface; it has no other required relevance. For medicine, the equivalent is not true. If it links two points in its own sense of what it is doing, it links many points on other levels of being.

Furthermore, the over-all development of medicine may transform a specialty in a decade, so that when the patient returns, a totally different, equally scientific solution is now offered. It is not that the first operation or medicine was wrong; both the first and the second are right, but the second "right" treatment is the one in present use. Most physicians regard this as a temporary crisis while cleaning house. The nature of the house may be, however, that it can never be cleaned—in which case, correction and revaluation will become the continuous present state of medicine.

In the meantime, a large number of ailments remain incurable. These include both serious life-threatening diseases and a great variety of chronic illnesses that fence-sit between mental and physical. Scientific medicine works to "conquer" both "incurables," perhaps the former more heroically, but both in the sense that they are violations of its completeness. Psychiatry and internal medicine work to assign the chronic diseases to categories so that cures can be developed.

A second difficulty is that a surprisingly large number of conditions "heal themselves" or are healed for inexplicable reasons. Sometimes a patient will use an unsanctioned medicine, such as laetrile, prayer, or a remedy chosen homoeopathically. Generally, orthodox medicine holds that these things could not have caused the improvement, so the cure must have been a psychological response to the method of treatment or a change in the person's life that made him want to get better.

Incurable ailments and mysterious cures are not serious cracks in the armor of technological medicine. Doctors themselves will be the first to admit that medicine is working toward a universality and completeness it has not achieved. Many things are badly understood, and many conditions find the doctor helpless, but these do not undo the beneficial effects of medicine. Spontaneous cure has a number of possible explanations, one of which is the unusual self-repair ability of DNA molecules, though we might still question what activates *it*.

More serious than these flaws in orthodox medicine is their suggestion of another one: that sanctioned cures may also work in inexplicable ways. We will return to this hint later in the book.

The real failure of cure in standard medicine is the one we have foreshadowed so far: that although it can intervene successfully in crises and provide a general "urban" methodology, its cures are always partial and discontinuous. It is basically able to make visible changes where there is visible pathology. It does not place those changes in a larger active frame of meaning.

If any kind of standard doctor is unable to help his patient, neither party is necessarily aggrieved by the situation. The patient accepts that his bad luck may have brought him an incurable ailment, either minor or serious. The doctor accepts that all things cannot be done with the present tools and knowledge. Both are Western businessmen and Enlightenment figures, looking to the progress of the future to solve the present lapse in ingenuity. Cryonics is probably the most extreme case of belief in technological progress. Bodies are frozen, to be thawed in future years when solutions may have been found to their ailments. In many ways, this is the *reductio ad absurdum* of treating disease as an isolated mechanical problem. Even if the freezer is kept going and the thawing awakens the patient, a large stretch of imagination in itself, the patient will have given up the meaning and social context of his life in a desperate quest for health and survival.

This may seem like a capricious point of view, especially in the face of the scientific and technological advances of this century. Medicine and science are not supposed to be biased and limited. They are universal objective systems, not only open to criticism but requiring criticism and experiment for their very existence. Without a belief in past scientific progress and the hope for equivalent advances in the future, the late half of the twentieth century becomes a mighty lonely and uncomfortable place to hang out. What else do we have to show as the civilization spawned by the Enlightenment? What other justification do we have for the destruction of native cultures and ecosystems in favor of global consciousness?

But the jury is still out and probably will not return during our lifetimes. Since there may in fact be no resolution, ever, we must take this issue both ways. The Industrial Revolution has improved man's living conditions; over the years, marvelous humanitarian machines and systems have been invented, "tools for change," as latter-day Enlightenment supporters prefer to call them. They include washing machines, gas-driven plows and combine harvesters, power vehicles, video recorders, space satellites, telephones, chain saws, and the like. But something else has not changed at all. We have these machines and more, and we do not *really* know how to use them.

That is, we do not know when we are improving conditions and when we are making them worse. Even more horrifying is, of course, the possibility that all of this technology will ultimately make conditions worse.[9]

Clearly, though, industrial machinery has made short-range contributions and has increased our knowledge dramatically. We live in an artificial placenta. Even our artists and priests have incorporated material from astronomy, archaeology, microbiology, and the rest into their visions. We are the children of industrialism, and, as Gregory Bateson has pointed out, renunciation, at this stage of the game, is not only difficult but impossible.[10] Even our antimaterialist dreams are the products of post-industrial upbringing and education.

Technological medicine itself has been enormously successful; there are key areas in which it is unmatched by any system which has appeared on the planet. It can alter physiological processes quickly, reversing life-threatening deterioration from severe injury and shock. It prolongs life also by neutralizing pathological toxins, removing diseased tissue, and poisoning body-destroying microbes and parasites.

It is able to deal with large concentrated populations, establishing the parameters of collective hygiene and public health, from family and genetic disease to environmental and industrial poisons. For instance, it is able to determine, on a statistical basis, the likelihood of certain diseases arising from exposures to particular chemicals or matings between organisms carrying particular genetic messages. Whole disease classes have been eliminated by prevention and destruction of disease agents.[11]

Standard medicine also serves a large-scale public health function by training people in large groups in an objective and accountable system of knowledge and skills. Adequate medical personnel can be produced from courses, lectures, books, and demonstrations. This large professional corps is needed to treat the vast and growing populace. Doctors must be recruited along with lawyers, engineers, policemen, etc., because the crisis of disease is a major disrupter of society. Modern civilization must provide at least the possibility of relief.

Over the centuries, then, Western culture has developed this system which handles injury, shock, poisoning, spreading pathology, and contagion in a humane and confident manner, which is easily transmitted, and which can reap the benefits of a central evolving technology and science. Nothing else would be reasonable. Certainly nothing else would be politically possible.

If we accept this heritage and remain optimistic about science and, at the same time decry the present scientific-technological decadence, we must finally acknowledge a deep split in the scientific tradition. What we have is only part of science. We can save our vision of a future of objective universal knowledge by proposing that an imposter rules in the name of science and enlightenment. Pure self-critical selfless experiment may still be the goal, but present-day mainstream science can be seen as a partial distortion.

Most scientists would claim that this is impossible. How, they would ask, under the elaborate and neutral scrutiny of the world scientific community, could basic errors have entered the experiment? The answer may be, They could not have. And then the cry for "another" science would come clear as a last gasp of delusion and romanticism. And that would stand, as well, as the epitaph for this whole book.

The other alternative is to consider a series of related critiques here.

Science is not truly science unless it operates from an ecological perspective taking into account the ultimate consequences of its proposals and discoveries. This does not only mean the obvious technological consequences of scientific application (like weapons, pollutants, economies based on nonrenewable resources, etc.); it means the human implications of every pure law and theory (nonspecificity of subatomic particles, expanding universe, random numbers, evolution by mutation, propulsion by reaction, transmission of electrical signals, and so on). How does it change humanity internally to work on these concepts and adapt them by industry? What is the yet-undelivered human meaning of the technology on whose streets and in whose props and vehicles we carry out much of our lives?

Even if one denies the possibility of a universal meaning, we must deal with cultural relativism. Every law and every application comes from a singular individual with a unique cognitive frame in a specific society in space and time. Unless laws and their applications are "corrected" for this provincialism, they will always be ethnocentric and, in some way, self-serving.

Cultural errors are just the beginning. The human perspective is but one interpretation of the universe. Pure objective science is not a human possibility. Our extraordinarily complex mathematics are stepladders through a fraction of infinity. There are out-and-out errors in science too, and they no doubt spell the limits of experimentation. Perceived often as dilemmas and puzzles (such as quantum theory or biological transmutation), their irresolution itself may be another face of the distortion caused by the misapplication of technology to society. DNA, telekinesis tests, quasars, and polluted rivers and seas all come from the same larger system.[12]

Orthodox Western medicine is concerned with the organic causes of disease. Its various medicinal, surgical, and psychological treatments are mechanical responses to demonstrated disease paths. Although a successful treatment may often be continued without clear reason for its success, the overriding tendency of orthodoxy is to reject inexplicable cures and to search for categories of cause that will generate classes and subsets of treatment. The isolated cures of the individual practitioner are meaningless if they cannot be generalized into a universal law of cure, adoptable by other physicians. The laetrile controversy illustrates this point quite dramatically. No matter how many "successful" treatments of cancer occur with this drug, they are meaningless without a generalized explanation for chemical viability. Without this, a doctor cannot be legally and ethically responsible for his own practice.

Seen from one perspective, even orthodox medicine is a patchwork of myriad inconsistent techniques and magical cures. But this patchwork is under continuous mainstream scientific review and criticism. Knowledge of the body comes from centuries of anatomical research. A map of the subvisual world of genes, viruses, and living cells comes from intense microscopic investigation; the behavior of entities in this undisclosed arena is viewed every day by thousands of well-equipped observers. Blood chemistry, hormonal composition, and specific drug action are also under continuous rigorous experiment.

No treatment exists outside this network. The doctor sees his patient as a living example of the collected laws and unfinished experiments. He knows the person's chemistry, the functions of his organs, the statistical likelihood of certain sorts of pathology, the visible and laboratory signs of such pathology, and the most efficient methods of countering a disease, either by chemical change or surgical intervention.

The psychiatric branch of medical science is the same. Aberrant behavior, neurosis, and psychosis are interpreted biomechanically from the obvious connection of brain, nervous system, and bodily fluids and organs. Psychological illness is a more refined version of physical illness. One should not think that psychology is any less mechanical; its "social" and mental causes for disorders are functionally identical to epidemiological and neurological events in somatic medicine. Psychiatrists may behave as though discussion and insight are important factors, and this is a potential methodological difference; but when the chips are down, scientifically, they adopt a conventional reductionist model of biological function.

In fact, the chips have been down recently, and the psychiatric profession has had to explain the poor record of insight therapy. Its collective response has been to adopt even more mechanical solutions to illness, i.e., to move from a psychodynamic interpretation of a chemical model of consciousness to a pure chemicodynamic model. Many psychiatrists argue that depression, anxiety, and schizophrenia, insofar as they are chemical disorders, *cannot* be cured by insight. Individuals may learn to live with their ailments, but the ailments themselves do not improve (even this can be seen as a curious distinction). The new generation of psychiatric experimenters hopes to locate the precise chemical loci of the mental diseases in the context of a burgeoning psychotropic pharmacy, which will then provide the antidotes.

This situation is serious enough for continued "successful" experimentation to lead to the isolation or even supplantation of this whole class of insight practitioners. No doubt the strength of the drug pushers within psychiatry has come about from the failure of traditional psychoanalytic method to provide the promised "cure." The methodology itself may have lacks, but certainly one of the growing problems of insight therapy is the large number of individuals already too disconnected from deeper societal structures of shared meaning to be helped by a system based on verbal interactional application of those structures.

We can summarily say that the thing which is wrong with orthodox medicine is not the system itself, but the way in which it presents itself as the only or most effective way to treat sickness. In some cases, it is, and people owe their lives to it; their lives become, in a sense, a history of their cures, of living beyond their time.

An old doctor in rural Pennsylvania is summoned to an isolated area to treat a boy seemingly on the verge of death. The worried father hovers for the verdict. The doctor is finished with his examination and turns to the father. He looks at him for a moment, then says:

"He'll die. But first he'll recover."[13]

One suspects that many of us are alive on these terms, and that is our cultural destiny. We are the survivors of a one-time enormous childhood mortality rate. Our lives must curiously reflect that fact.

Sometimes orthodox medicine is shockingly provincial. In order to save its reputation, it gives people the illusion it is handling more than it is and that the other methods for getting things done are either primitive, untested, exotic, unscientific, or un-American. Most patients do not require honesty, even in the face of death. It is still, apparently, less terrible to die within the auspices of science and society than, perhaps, to live by the grace of an alien witchcraft. A person cured, or not cured, by his usual physician remains an American in good standing, a citizen of the century that gave him life. A person cured exotically is converted, for the body cannot "deny" the reason for its new health and develops new traits in completion of the treatment.

The Western doctor presents his illusion of objectivity as a truly objective stance. While he may advocate exercise and herbs in the absence of major pathology, he will not persist if he feels something is seriously wrong. He knows that life-style affects health, but he gives it a mere pittance of his attention. It is the fact that doctors most know but can least use, for they treat pathology and disease categories rather than individuals.

Doctors may curse the high malpractice insurance rates, but they have brought them on themselves in part by their disingenuous stance of objectivity. Traditionally, orthodox medicine has used the threat of malpractice as a tactic to keep other medicines from competing. At the same time, it lacks a consistent set of rules and procedures. Ultimately, it must fall into the same legal snare it has set for its competitors. Its motive is economic, not humanitarian.

Orthodox medicine has a standard humanitarian argument: if a patient gets bewitched in the maze of alternative and fantastic treatments, he or she may delay getting competent professional help for a condition that then becomes incurable. What makes this kind of situation so confusing is that sometimes the argument is provincial and self-serving while other times it is an accurate warning against the criminal grandiosity of many of the alternative systems. An almost classic case of the latter was published in a Bay Area magazine in the fall of 1978. A woman from South Africa (interestingly enough, with degrees in mathematics and chemistry) attempted to heal an ostensible eye disease of hers with a combination of iridology, acupuncture, and meditation among a number of northern California practitioners. In her own interpretation, she gained a tremendous amount of support and fulfillment from the healing experiences, which included needle treatments, learning how to make her own poultices and herbal medicines, and generally calling up her own positive "cosmic energy" to fight the disorder. But the disorder turned out to be a melanoma which had spread to such a degree during the "holistic health" treatments that chemotherapy and laser treatment were impossible, and she had to have enucleation.[14]

Unquestionably such things happen, but they confirm the complexity of these issues rather than the dire results of using an alternative medicine. Most healers acknowledge what they can handle and what they cannot, and part of taking responsibility for one's own health is learning how to make contact with healers, to examine their work critically, and, by all means, to avoid asking them to carry out the miracle which orthodoxy has failed to. Uncritical, passive reverence is generally a dangerous guise in which to seek cure or enlightenment.

For every patient like the above, there are countless others who have wasted their time and money under an almost lifelong fear of killer diseases and irreversible conditions, attempting to track down a ghost. The price we pay for a professional medicine establishment is a paralyzing fear of deadly maladies and insidious unknown bugs and viruses that truly makes the hospitals into penal institutions. Many people who can afford the attention keep up an absurdly prophylactic guard against disease; even some who cannot afford it do. Their whole lives are built on a false perception of what their bodies should be.

And then we face a present epidemic of iatrogenic (physician-caused) diseases, diseases that are the side effects of treatments for previous diseases. They are usually more serious and incurable than the conditions whose treatment led to them. Psychiatric disorder caused by medical treatment of both physical and mental diseases is another lusty newcomer to the pathological atlas.

So when we grant the medical establishment its due recognition as the planetary first-aid center, and of the future too, we must note as well that it is a hazard and a mirage, a source of pathology, fear, and

the manipulation of people's illnesses for personal profit and confirmation. Much that passes for illness is a message that should
lead into a world that is exciting and filled with lights, colors, sounds,
pleasures, tingling, unconstricted breathing, personal growth, and
startling vision, to which the world of sterile chemicals and operating
tables is a cruel reversal and wasteful joke.

II

The Cultural Basis of the Holistic Cure

Medicine is the institution through which societies deal with mind/body relationships and their ramifications. In any culture, the medical establishment "establishes" customs of belief and treatment as the political establishment evolves laws and an economic establishment determines the basis of exchange. Through the medical establishment, birth, disease, and death are brought into a collective cultural security. People are born into the same "world," are threatened by the same germs or spirits, aspire to the same "*mens sana in corpore sano*," and cease to live when that "same life" ends.

Sharing definitions of experience is what psychodynamically holds a culture together. If political experiences were not comparable, there would be no courts or parameters of justice. If economic experiences were not comparable, it would be impossible to tell the difference between rightful ownership and theft. Sanity and health are, likewise, a legality and an accreditation.

Most people accept their culture's medicine, as they accept its money, its schools, and its recreation. Everyone knows, in every society, that some things do not get cured; but this failure is understood in the same way the society itself is understood. The citizens await a "breakthrough" in medical science or in human rights legislation or they await a revelation or visitation. When the "breakthrough" comes, it is often disappointing. The incurable condition is now treatable, but other things are still incurable. If the citizens become dissatisfied with the whole political and economic system, governments topple. This is what it means to have "nonnegotiable demands" that also cannot be met. Either the revolution is crushed, the individual destroyed, or the order itself must change. Revolutionary healing systems also make nonnegotiable demands.

By the time a person in our culture decides to be a doctor, he has been initiated into the same system as an electrician, an executive, and an academic philosopher. The hospital is also a jail, a school, a factory, a resort hotel. Even from the outside these things do not look that different from each other. They may have different confinements and different degrees of strictness, but they are sustained by the same general sense of what kinds of things go wrong, what must be done to correct them, and what kinds of things are right and pleasurable. It is no wonder that people can fear the hospital as if under a life (or death) sentence and seek jail, unconsciously, by committing crimes when they are sick. The culture sets the definitions, but the acts are pure and prior to definition. The penal psychiatrist might as well draw straws as try to tell the criminally insane from the legally punishable. In the end, they are both punishable, they are both treatable. A luxurious room in a hotel on the beach may be more pleasurable than either a hospital room or a jail cell, but its occupant may be just as trapped by his sense of getting better and happier. One would prefer not to be in prison, but from the perspective of a whole life in the cosmos, numbness, illness, lack of freedom, and synthetic pleasure overlap, no matter how they are culturally defined.

Medicine is an impossible category to apply cross-culturally. The very name "medicine man" challenges any comparability of meaning. In primitive and tribal societies, the most common on this planet throughout the history of man, there is no medicine in the terms of Western medicine, but then there is no native economics, native politics, or native religion either in the terms of Western conceptions of these things.

A people exists not in categories and professions but in the homogeneous reality of customs, ideas, artifacts, and geophysical space. Medical procedure is originally and contemporarily integrated with the rest of secular and sacred life; it overlaps with prayer, farming, marriage, war, taboo, etc. Our own professional medicine is imbedded in the same way. We have gradually, in the evolution of complex stratified society, abstracted occupations from primary social structures and institutionalized them as formal systems with their own rules. By contrast, the native doctor never leaves or enters his office; he is always there, and he is never there. In fact, he is a citizen, not a doctor, even when he treats illness. He is a doctor only by the active process of healing. The Western doctor is a doctor by decree and judicial license; it is society he never leaves or enters, but society is not coterminous with his medicine.

The social and religious issues of Western medicine are rarely expressed in medical terms. They exist instead implicitly, in the treatment. In tribal societies, medical language is social language addressed to a specific ritual.

Our own medical mythology is filled with images and ikons: authority, consistency, technoprogress. We trust remedies whose names and constituents we rarely understand and which are as esoteric as any herbal astrology. We trust the mysterious bottle of the industrial hospital because we accept the general system of industry and socioeconomics. In taking the medicine, we confirm a chain of meanings: how the medicine feels and how we are supposed to feel is how the society feels to us. We assume that this is also the objective meaning of the medicine, just as we assumed that the preceding ailment and succeeding health have objective meanings. Our mask is the illusion that we can be free of mythological and internalizing ramifications and that we take the medicine and the therapeutics clean, as machines. No doubt this is because we have images of our bodies as machines.*

The simplest human societies[1] are organized as hunting bands and do not differ much, in functional ecological terms, from higher primate bands. In Africa baboon troops are of shifting size, with anywhere from nine to 185 members, though several troops often mix at waterholes. The diet of these creatures is mostly vegetable, but they also capture young hares, small deer, nestling birds, and insects. Each troop operates in an area of three to fifteen square miles, with a more tightly defended core territory. From outside this core to the boundaries, there is relatively little tension and some willing exchange of

---

* Some medicines are universal remedies, particularly in the realm of botanicals, and we should allow for these without letting it confuse the cultural issues behind medical treatment. When Jacques Cartier and his men arrived in Quebec in 1535 with scurvy, it did not require an Algonquian ceremony for them to be cured by white cedar bark from the local apothecary. Algonquian medicine as a whole, though, does not rest on this event.

members. The troop itself is organized in a strict dominance hierarchy such that all males, and perhaps the females too, stand in an order of precedence to each other. Animals know where they stand, not only in relationship to other animals, but in space as they move and feed in characteristic formation with the leaders in their center. Apparently group organization is the key to survival for onetime tree dwellers outside the protection of the forest. One should not imagine insectlike rigidity and sexual-biological destiny. The troop is held together by a social principle, not blind instinct. We should know, for we remain loosely in such a troop. It little matters if one believes in evolution of man from the apes. Either we remain them or have become them.

Bushmen bands in Africa are organized into shifting territories around waterholes with a defended core and shared hunting and gathering space with other groups. The head male's position is passed on patrilineally (along a male line of males); although he ostensibly owns all the resources, he cannot deny access to them to any member. A nuclear family is built around two adults who make up an economic and sexual unit. The men hunt (the first large kill is qualification for marriage). Women gather small animals, nuts, beans, and wild plants; they also cook and take primary responsibility for the children. Since marriage is not permissible within the nuclear family, two groups must always be bound in an intermarrying chain (one band could hardly generate enough families to prevent incest). Any member regularly has uncles, nephews, and in-laws in surrounding groups. As these bands move by season through different territories (based on the ripening of mangetti nuts and tsi beans and the movement of game), materials are shared and gifts are exchanged. The migratory pattern works against material accumulation. The men carry only weapons and meat; the women load ostrich eggs with water and food and sling on the youngest children.

Plains living frees the arms to make tools, which free the jaw, which frees the skull allometrically for the brain, which requires more synapses and cells anyway to invent tools and organize complex social life. Tools allow the strategic killing of larger game, which produces meat to share and the requirement of storage and transport. The young and the old can now be fed and cared for on a social basis and can contribute to the larger group. Simple survival becomes a web of responsibility based entirely on reciprocal rights and obligations of kin. Blood ties map a figure in space and time, and beyond time, that requires an extremely complex symbolic terminology, backed, often, by a mythic cosmology. After all, kinship does not originate from thought full-blown as a practical and logical system of organization.

This symbolic system distinguishes human from ape society. Our description of its emergence is purposely condensed, for its impact afterwards is what concerns us in this book. It is the web in which all future webs are caught. The first strands are there from the beginning. We continue to think them, though we also have come to think bigger things, more cosmic things, *with* them, so we have forgotten their existence. The first doctors are barely yet apes, and their healing will say that. Our healing will contain their healing embryonically.

We tend to look at groups like the Bushmen from the outside, where we are. We see a fairly simple grid of families bound into local groups, autonomous local groups allied in a society. From within, though, it is a shifting floating space requiring all the wit and deviousness of ritual symbolism to hold it together. The groups move, change, fuse, split, but the symbols do not vanish. They take on a weight that transcends their original meaning, except insofar as that meaning was biological and social survival.

Band society persists in sparsely populated areas of the world, especially in deserts and jungles, but wherever agriculture was developed, a more complicated tribal level of organization emerged along with it. With agriculture, there is new population density, and people become organized in different ways. Occasionally, descent is taken through the female line to keep a domestic continuity of gardeners. Economic, political, and religious institutions are more complicated, and, although there are no corporate entities outside the framework of kin, the roles of doctor, priest, smith, war chief, etc., begin to emerge. Everyone is equal in terms of access to critical goods and judicial rights, but there are titled offices, hereditary societies, and elected councils.

In Western civilization, economics is a game in which there are winners and losers: the players, the citizens, compete for limited desirable goods. Economic survival is the real activity of which gambling itself is an imitative game. In tribal society, life cannot be left to contest and competition. Cooperation and exchange are crucial to group as well as individual survival. Winners make losers, and losers do not make a peaceful social community. Gift giving is an ancient serious custom. The gift giver expects an equal or better gift in the future, but that is not a requirement of the deal itself. It is a real passage of items among people. It is not a game, and it does not generate wealth, only process. Since trading is always of incommensurate items, it is by definition unequal; native society ignores the inequality and puts the weight on the continuation of trade.

The ongoing exchange stimulates kinship ties and softens boundaries. It keeps goods moving between regions of different resources and seasonal harvests. Irregular abundance is shared. What seems to be a primitive economics is simply a system of goods transfer and symbolic social activity, noneconomic, or at least nonmaximizing.

The segments of the society are stable, and the coherence of the larger group is maintained by the segments alone, there being no outside systems or higher authorities, except mythological. Members of different families ultimately trace descent from a common ancestor; a number of these lineages then converge at an even more remote ancestor, until, at the highest and most widespread level of contemporary alliance, they have not a real ancestor but a totem being or animal. These lineages, with their marriage-inherited members, have become clans, and the clans form communities. There is no formal church and no elected government. Power is earned charismatically, or it is passed down in clubs. Leadership evaporates when a particular military crisis or ceremony ends.

The segments are the polity, the marketplace, the army, the church, the hospital, the corporate ownership, the maintenance crew, the initiates of the ceremonies, and the source of all ethical and political sanction. They form an outer wall of reality.

The segments also generate a profound internal geometry where abstract science begins.[2] Social thought cannot maintain all its own subtleties and transformations, so it subtly blends them with daily perception and vision into mythological thought. The origin of the universe merges into the origin of the web itself, which is the limits of society and being. The creation of all things—sun, moon, plants, stars, animals, diseases—comes together with the emergence of the segments, so that each gets its identity from the others and they come to share an identity in daily social life. After all, since the boundaries cannot be transcended, thought becomes mythological as it becomes remote, but it does not stop being social in the sense that "social" is the whole possibility of the emergence of man in durable groups. Tools, methods of farming, boatbuilding, healing, and all other activities express the societal reality of which they are an extension. This may be as simple as the Sun inventing a medicine stick at the same time that He is the founder and father of the Hopi Sun Clan, or it may come from deep within the properties of the web and its symbols. Every curative herb has a cultural and linguistic identity inseparable from its medicinal qualities. Every healing ceremony occurs within the prior ceremony, the big one, in which man and his world come into being, hewed from the timelessness of raw nature. A medicine of prayer sticks and sand paintings and chanting is *both* coterminous with and ancestral to a medicine of antibiotics and serums. Scientific institutionalization has changed the outward reality of medicine, the problems to which it addresses itself and the solutions it offers, but it has not touched the deep core of generative symbols from which medicine emerged. Since ancestry cannot be changed, it must be experienced in contemporary terms. One of the built-in frustrations of cultural evolution is that peoples must always look backward to an original and unknown moment of unity that can never recur.

The new holistic health movement is nostalgic in just that way and, perhaps, with its added insights from modern science, even improves on some ancient techniques. But the prior holism has a thoroughness we lack, short of re-creating such communities, each one identical, from within, to the universe. And it is impossible to do that now, knowing what we do. Our efforts to return to tribalism and nature are important, but they will always be some other thing.

It is no wonder that Indians, Africans, and other aborigines do not show the enthusiasm for harmony and holism one finds in the Western counterculture. They do not know any other world.

There are, of course, also detriments to primitive holistic medicine. The doctor cannot transplant hearts; he cannot intervene successfully in many crisis situations—for instance, where serious infection has set in. Many curable illnesses are terminal in his society. The Western doctor has tools with which to prolong life and escape crises, tools which could have come from nowhere else but the Pleistocene and early farming communities and which have emerged from the symbolic web along with man himself. But what he has lost is the original context and meaning of those tools, and, hence, of life itself.

The native medicine man does not and cannot work in simply the context of the disease. His history and heritage do not give him a technology for isolating diseases, and his ethics teach him the danger of isolated consequences. He has little interest in the abstract prolongation of life; he prolongs life in the act of restoring balance.

His skill is in effecting an *actual* and total cure. He takes the patient out of dysfunction back into society, and both are changed by the experience. We are truly ignorant of how such miracle cures are done. We are also ignorant of the degree to which Western medicine returns its cured patients to society in a physically and psychologically unintegrated way. A native doctor, if he could understand the mechanics, would view these cures as partial, mainly because they deal with isolated pathology and apparent cause. However, Western society as a whole operates on a quick and external enough level for the victims not to be required to change in any deep way that exposes the shallowness of the cure. They ignore the message of alienation of which the illness is an embodiment. They can still drive their cars to work and watch TV at night. The edge is taken off the uncomfortable pathology, but the real disease is the life-style, of which they will die in the end anyway. Even such a death is not as serious a condemnation of this hygiene as the fact that they will live it until they die of it, and they will not get a chance to explore what they might otherwise be.

It took the universe working all the time until our birth to produce us, each of us, and our uniqueness. Native medicine does not think in this way, but shamans somehow act with an equivalent profound sense of the cosmic web. It takes the universe working all the time until our disease to bring it into being too; such disease cannot be dismissed without a deep readjustment. Life can never be made the same as it was before. The patient of the medicine man gets less symptomatic relief, but then he is involved in an initiation rather than in a repair.

In light of this, it is important to look again at the Western export of a universal health system. In areas where infectious diseases thrive and the infant mortality rate is high, the new method makes a miraculous debut—like gunpowder. Just as the master of martial arts can be shot by a pistol, so can the shaman be replaced, in individual instances, by antibiotics. But both technologies are tricks, and once the tricks are familiar, the persistent problems of the society resurface, complexified by the addition of these tools. By isolating medicine, we get the effects of an isolated medicine.

Integrated native medicine is not medicine by scientific standards, for it has "superstitious" and "spiritual" elements. But since it is the core as well as the forerunner of technology and science, we gain little insight by considering it only the primitive historical version. It is a system with different goals and a different meaning. The native doctor works on the overall framework of the person's life and identity, the collection of events and lore locating that person in his culture and among the artifacts of creation. All crises and necessities come together in one symbolic context, ethnomedically condensed by myth and symbols, summarized in a disease and transformed by it into the individual organism.

This disease was never an isolated condition from which the sick person could be extricated. It was his lot, personally and socially. It was also his opportunity.

In much of the world, spiritual development, not personal attainment, is the reason for living. But this is not "spiritual" in the civilized sense; it is not "religious" or "mystical." It is "spiritual" as in "power": power by the agency of cosmic nature through one's own nature. Accumulating power is as common an activity in primitive society as shopping in the United States. Agriculture is power; war is power; marriage is power; transaction is power. That is, each of these things has a spiritual component that is dangerous but harnessable.

And we must not forget: the native Californian Pomo and Miwok called them "doctors"—those who dressed up in bear and panther costumes and hid out in the woods, ambushing and killing people. Doctors! Because of their power. Because they got so good they could mimic even minor details of the behavior of the animals they "were." The bear doctor in the wild was virtually indistinguishable from the wild bear, and his bearskin left equivalent claw marks in his victim.[3]

We see war, brutality, and torture—ritualized and unnecessary. They see epic spiritual events. Among the Plains Indians, war and thievery may be indistinguishable from medicine. The excruciating torture of war captives, described with horror by early European observers, is identical in many of its aspects to the training of a physician. Those who survive or escape have powerful medicines for their travail. They are now doctors, or, if not doctors, controllers of rain and storms, or enchanters—for all these powers derive from the same sources. In their world, spiritual initiation is as primal as the sun rising in the morning and the wind through the grasses.

III

The Origin of Medicine: The Anthropological and Historical Fallacy

Self-healing is an instinct, and rudimentary forms of it exist even among the animals: the cat chews grass and then vomits, the deer licks the dew from flowers.* "A snake which gets wounded heals itself," writes Paracelsus. "If now this is done by the snake, do not be astonished for you are the snake's son. Your father does it, and you inherit his capacity, and therefore you, in a brutish sense, are also a doctor."[1] We are doctors almost before we are beings. Our cells know; they stand as magical sages and midwives at our birth, doing the impossible from matter.

Among early and primitive peoples there is an intuition of wisdom from the forgotten past. Somehow, once, we were in direct touch with a great power. What was it? Today we have mostly science fiction suggestions. Alien beings from another world? Different dimensions of this planetary location? Ourselves in ancient primal forms? Before we were men? The Carrier Indians of British Columbia told the anthropologist Diamond Jenness:

"We know what the animals do, what are the needs of the beaver, the bear, the salmon, and other creatures, because long ago men married them and acquired this knowledge from their animal wives. Today the priests say we lie, but we know better. The white man has

---

* Fresh dew from the different herbs and grasses is still prized as an elixir. It was the inspiration for Edward Bach's early twentieth-century remedies made from flowers in Wales.

been only a short time in this country and knows very little about the animals; we have lived here thousands of years and were taught long ago by the animals themselves. The white man writes everything down in a book so that it will not be forgotten; but our ancestors married the animals, learned all their ways, and passed on the knowledge from one generation to another."[2]

The literal truth of this matter is unimportant, for there may not be a literal truth. Great wisdoms develop their own expressions. The insistence of so many Indian groups that they were originally animals or married to animals must reveal more than it hides. Certainly it describes an intimacy and experiential wisdom to which we have lost access.

Long before we came, in our popular culture, to the curious assumption that the newer is always better and the more progressive is the more accurate, we held the opposite view: that ancient things were powerful and true in ways that could never be again. Brute knowledge was firsthand knowledge of creation. The way in which things were originally made and still hold together is the best account we have of their agency and origin. And what could be a more appropriate medicine than the agency that once created all things: animals, matter, man, diseases, flowers, stars, worlds. Lacking that skill, we are stiff robot doctors attempting to work on petals and threads of light.

Paracelsus again: "[Do] not be astonished that the snake knows medicine. She has had it for a longer time than you, and you have it from her; for you are made of the matter of brutish nature, and therefore both of you are equal."[3]

Far and away the most common source of medicinal knowledge on this planet is dream and vision. Native doctors are empirical, but the data they test do not come from the conscious scientific mind. They come raw from nature and vision and are interpreted by mythology and totemism.

Modern Western medical research is done in a laboratory; the mind of the scientist, represented by his own trained analytic mind, is the only connection between person and experiment. He may, in the sense it is usually meant, have other things "on his mind." More profoundly, he may be alienated from the experiment, his devotion to science notwithstanding. Alienation need not be some monstrous exercise of distance; it can also be a subtle distraction. He may think, "This experiment isn't me; it's chemicals, it's rats; I don't care whether they live or die; I don't even have this disease."

The sense that he may be working toward a cure that will someday be used on him or someone he knows probably has no somatic urgency. It may interest him mentally, but the *actual* quality of his drive is not harnessed to the research. The history of science and its operational categories stand in the way. His body itself is irrelevant, except as a laboratory tool. Rats or guinea pigs may replace it insofar as "bodies" are needed. And his relationship to these intermediary animals is neither intimate nor benevolent. His real presence in the experiment is professional, with all that that means socially and economically. The work he does in an abstraction from the immediate event in which he is involved. The medicine is a further derivative of that.

Early human experimenters tried instead to get back inside nature so they could hear her original voice. As doctors, they cured illness as subjective links between the patient and nature (including, within nature, the nature of the sick person, of course). The doctor was an initiate, often a self-initiate, in a system in which he tried to initiate his patients. Psychoanalysis picks up the echo of this. The native doctor also healed by the actual health emanating from his own being. That health was maintained by his visions and "experiments" and his successful interactions with patients. Psychoanalysis picks up this echo too.

We must not be misled by the primitivity of native medicine. Wisdom is there; experiment is there; only the awakened objective mind is not. And the universal value of that mind is hardly beyond dispute.

"I had a powerful dream," says the Delaware Indian doctor. "It was a clear day, a beautiful day. The sky was bluer than I have ever seen it. There were white birds flying directly at me. Then I awoke."[4]

This is the first stage in an opposite type of medical research. The dream suggests a direction worth following. The doctor can either wait for another dream or test it right away. If the day is good, he may drop his plans and go immediately into the wilderness: "Office hours canceled. I'm doing four days of research out of town."

He must now get *inside* nature. He seeks the place—where the sky is blue and clear and the birds are flying *at* him. Unless he pursues it and takes it seriously, the dream is forgotten and is merely a pleasant interlude in a busy week. If he ignores it, perhaps it will return, slightly changed, but he will have the same decision to make again. There could be no clearer statement of different cultural relevances. We postpone the dream until past our lifetimes. We are always busy at other things. The native doctor must also postpone objective scientific thought until beyond his lifetime and the lifetime of his culture.

The Indian assumes that a dream's choice of him indicates a true relationship and that his research will succeed only along the lines of his own inner nature, which determined the affinity. The research scientist has no use for such a dream, or any like divination. His responsibility is to clear his mind of just such affinities and to pick up the thread in an external predetermined grid. The significant connection already exists and has nothing to do with him; he must only recognize it. But he is not a unique receptor. If he doesn't find the serum, someone else will.

There *are* documented cases of scientists discovering things in dreams (a priest holding tablets with the translation of unknown Babylonian) or visions (Friedrich Kekulé seeing the chemical bonds of the benzene ring arise as a serpent biting its tail in the fire and James Watson getting insight into the DNA helix from transposed images of a Hedy Lamarr movie).[5] These confirm the unexpected power of that mode, but they do not lead the mainstream to a dream methodology.

The native physician is well trained. It is not a matter of a super vision, some luck, and a little trickery. Medical knowledge from visions is a treacherous business; there *is* a right way to do things. We may question "how" the "right way" could possibly ensure the success of the experiment—what do birds know about healing? And even if they knew, what could they possibly say? And how would we understand it? And who's to say what's good for them is good for us?—but we have little experience in the matter. We do not play the game, and the sense of the Western scientist has traditionally been that it is a game not worth playing. But this cannot really count, since he is judging it by the rules of his own game, which is all he plays.

The subjective experiment is a serious business. The anthropological literature begins to give us a sense of its beauty and power as well as its danger. Among the Jívaro Indians of the Ecuadorian Amazon Basin, a boy may begin to seek his soul at the age of six. He does not get one simply by being born, and he must, at all costs, avoid dying without one. Although this is not strictly a medical quest, it is a quest for those powers of which healing medicine is one. According to Michael Harner:

"If the *arutam* (soul) seeker is fortunate, he will awaken at about midnight to find the stars gone from the sky, the earth trembling, and a great wind felling the trees of the forest amid thunder and lightning. To keep from being blown down, he grasps a tree trunk and awaits the *arutam*. Shortly the *arutam* appears from the depths of the forest, often in the form of a pair of large creatures. The particular animal forms can vary considerably, but some of the most common *arutam* include a pair of giant jaguars fighting one another as they roll over and over towards the vision seeker, or two anacondas doing the same. Often the vision may simply be a single huge disembodied human head or a ball of fire drifting through the forest toward the *arutam* seeker. When the apparition arrives to within twenty or thirty feet, the Jívaro must run forward and touch it, either with a small stick or his hand. . . . It instantly explodes like dynamite and disappears.

"After nightfall, the soul of the same *arutam* he touched comes to him as he dreams. His dream visitor is in the form of an old Jívaro man who says to him, 'I am your ancestor. Just as I have lived a long time, so will you. Just as I have killed many times, so will you.' Without another word the old man disappears and immediately the *arutam* soul of this unknown ancestor enters the body of the dreamer, where it is lodged in his chest."[6]

The Crow doctor of the Great Plains prepares for *his* vision quest with various deep baths.[7] He scrubs his flesh, then smokes his pores and brain with burning pine needles. Thus cleansed, he does not eat anymore. He chooses the place. It is atop a high hill or mountain. Or on the barren windy prairie. Wearing his buffalo robe smeared with clay, he lies on a mound of rocks three feet high, oriented east and west. In order to hasten a vision, or if a vision does not come during the first couple of days and he is anxious, he may torture himself— dig lines into his arms or chest—cut off a fingertip. It is not done lightly, and it is a testament to the seriousness of the occasion. We may even have a distant memory of the formula: the greater the sacrifice (i.e., the deeper into one's self it goes), the more powerful the medicine.

The quester lies there, hungry, exposed, in pain, meditating and praying to the supernatural beings of the world "Without Fires."

Here the drive and the event are identical, equivalent. Research is conducted inside phenomena. The scientist presents his own body. He is not sick, but he is now suffering. By his life as a Crow and his training in mythology, he is prepared for wisdom. An animal appears, in creature or human form (if human, with animal robes indicating species); it speaks. Perhaps in words. Perhaps by actions and signs . . .

"A chicken hawk flew at me, landed as a man, and then did a dance. His enemies surrounded him, but they could not touch him. Then he became a hawk and took off back into the sky."

"I was lying there for three days when a jackrabbit came toward me. I looked again and it changed into a man. He was wearing a wolf's skin on his shoulders. The wolf's head was red and shone in the sunlight. The wolf's body was painted with yellow stripes, and its tail was a bunch of grouse feathers with a jackrabbit tail. It sang two songs in succession, ending each with a wolf howl. Then it showed me how to make a suit like that."

"After five days, I saw an elk in the water. But it walked up to me and changed into a man wearing an elkskin robe and carrying a bone whistle. He turned in all the directions, first to the north, blowing his whistle so that lightning seemed to shoot out of it, singing songs. Each time hundreds of animals, all the females of the different species, walked toward him from the direction to which he was blowing. He said: 'I am the medicine man of the wilderness. Go home and make such a robe. Sing these songs and whistle as I have. The girl you love cannot refuse you.' Then he sang another song, and a thunderstorm brewed right up. Lightning sprang into the sky, and I was soaked with rain."

From the first two visions, war powers came. From the third, a love charm was invented and a man was conferred with powers of making rain. He was middle-aged and had been spurned by a young woman, so he went to the mountain, fasted, received the elk vision, then successfully wooed her, and lived to the age of one hundred as a rainmaker. Out of this so-called mid-life crisis came a new career.

Slippery Eyes's healing medicine was presented in a reptile vision. After fasting unrewarded for three days, he wanted to give up. But he had suffered from smallpox and his face was so horribly pitted people had difficulty looking at him. A new direction was essential. On the fourth night he was called to a spring by a voice. The water turned into a tipi, and he entered to find snakes living there. The largest was a male, with a big eye in the center of its head and a horn. One of the others told Slippery Eyes that this one was the doctor and had taken pity on him. Then they all changed into humans, and a real human was carried in on a buffalo-hide stretcher. He was very sick, but the snakes cured him, teaching Slippery Eyes their techniques. Then the chief led him to another tipi, which was his house (also previously a spring). It was a magnificent dwelling, shingled with furs and jewels. The snakes treated him there, removing most of the pockmarks.

After this episode, Slippery Eyes became a successful doctor, and he continued his relationship with the snakes; they often came to talk with him, and he would pet and hold them and no doubt go over "new" (meaning "old") medical techniques.

Vision quest is the primary source of medical and magical knowledge, but the information is certainly not self-evident or literal as given. It comes under esoteric circumstances and must be brought into daily life.

Some features may be obvious: make a medicine from this plant, prepare a robe like mine, sing this song over this sick person, I will teach you the song. The supplicant must remember what he sees and hears, but he comes prepared. His whole life and career hangs in the balance, and his discipline is rigorous.

The experiment is not "written down"; these are preliterate peoples. It is preserved, instead, in a far more indelible language, in song and in a medicine bundle. There is a moment of insight, the moment when all nature, as it were, falls from its visible aspect and shows a feature of hidden artistry. The medicine man does not re-enact the vision. His powers come from having received it. He records the symbolic and mythological cues in the materials of the bundle. The bundle is then a resource in itself. He can add details of future visions to it; he can record his actual doctoring experiences; and he can pass it on as a formulated medicine to someone who did not have the vision. The code is consistent and vernacular, no matter how wild and exotic its source. Several generations after the vision, the medicine bundle is an objective technique of sorts. It has songs, herbs, charms, stories, all keyed to the original revelation and added to by those who have used the medicine.

William Wildschut writes: "The contents of the medicine bundles comprised symbolic representations of the supernatural beings and forces seen in the owner's dream or vision. Together with the owner they formed a clan. The chief of this clan, the principal supernatural responsible for the vision, is represented in each bundle. With it are included its helpers or servants who assist in guarding the life of the owner. The vision may also have been seen wearing distinctive facial or body painting. If so, different paints were included in the bundle. If a certain kind of necklace was worn by a supernatural visitant, a close copy of it was made and placed in the bundle."[8]

A bundle might include feathers, beads, skeletons of animals, a snakeskin, a wolf pelt, stones, shells, dried plants, etc. Since its elements are "words" and have no required potency in and of themselves, there is no reason why anything might not be in a bundle. The bundle itself correlates the relationships of power at a given eternal moment. As transitional power changes, the bundle is revised, translated for historical time. Later Crow medicine codes include old rusty guns, matches, lanterns, and other European "junk." The Indian interest in trinkets parallels, on a different level, the alchemist's interest in old books. The later white man's mockery that an Indian attached so much meaning to a trinket or feather that he might trade half a dozen good horses for it makes sense only by comparison with rare books or the delicate trinkets of the laboratory, which would be equally valueless to the Crow. A Crow's precious experience precedes the trinket, and its value is finally immaterial. The value of the microscope, after all, is that *it* is the source of new experience. The Crow has already had the experience and seeks interpretation.

A certain vast compendium of knowledge has been collected by native scientists from the beginning of time, in songs, myths, and practical instructions and in the various codes of sand paintings, medicine bundles, garden designs, plant species, and even, it appears, astrological botanies and zoologies of bone, parchment, and stone from periods deep within the Ice Age.[9]

The principles of assembling a medicine bundle or conceptualizing the choreography of a healing ceremony are as complex in their own way as any mathematics or physics. They may lack detailed quantified information, knowledge of microstructure, and a technology of information retrieval, but none of these affect their precision of observation and its compilation into working systems.

"Native classifications," writes Claude Lévi-Strauss, "are not only methodical and based on carefully built up theoretical knowledge. They are also at times comparable, from a formal point of view, to those still in use in zoology and botany."[10]

When he called it "the savage mind" (in his book title), he meant, in the end, to include our mind as well—the human mind in all of its cultures and conditions. He meant: the mind itself is savage—not "the mind of the savage."

Once we accept that native science's basic commitment is to a world we no longer inhabit, we can understand both its toughness and delicacy. We may doubt that the Indians actually had animal wives, but the length of time they spent noticing plants, animals, clouds, stones, spirit things, and their associations is beyond dispute. Field scientists have learned regional taxonomies from natives that have gone beyond the number of species reported or even suspected.

The Pinatubo Negritos of the Philippines report something in the neighborhood of 15 species of bats according to living habits—for instance, one that inhabits the dry palm leaves, another that lives on the underside of the leaves of the wild banana tree, another in bamboo clumps, another in dark thickets, etc. This same people classifies 450 species of plants, 75 species of birds, and even 20 species of ants. The Negritos also have more than 50 different types of arrows and can identify, from childhood, the kind and "sex" of tree from the smell, hardness, and appearance of a small fragment of wood. They are also thoroughly acquainted with the behavior and sexual differences of fish and shellfish.[11]

Primitive peoples have had vast gardens, have hunted creatures ranging from insects to mammoths, and have invented the whole technology we inherit, from agriculture and metallurgy to marriage and the family. With our present limitations, we could not reinvent these things. And we do not have to reinvent them. Primitive man has given them to us, and they will always be fundamental, as he is.

Who else could have taken a tropical grass from the jungles of South America with no particular distinguishing characteristics and nursed from it countless varieties of corn—ornamental and popping corn, grain corn, medicinal corn, magical corn—and adapted it, by way of Mesoamerica, to virtually every climate short of the polar in

North and South America? Gardens of this tamed grass, cultivated locus by locus without any genetic knowledge, covered pre-Columbian Mexico and extended clear out over the Penobscot River and the Gulf of St. Lawrence to Nova Scotia, equally west and north across the Mississippi and the Sierras.[12]

Two unexamined concepts stand in the way of our understanding the importance and scope of native medicine: our ethnic chauvinism and our temporal chauvinism (or modernism). These may be identical problems, but the former is generally considered the province of anthropology and the latter of history. We will attempt to examine them simultaneously, for they conspire to give us a false sense of primitivity as a condition we have escaped.

If we take, roughly, four million years as the length of time for the human species (and even that figure will probably be conservative by the time most people read this), that makes the last three thousand years, the years to which we relate as comprising most of known historical time, less than one tenth of one per cent of human history. Four million years is 40,000 centuries; it is 160,000 generations. Although all of those centuries were "stagnant" in comparison to even the last hundred years, they are still centuries of human thought, economic transactions, healing, scientific speculation, love, grief, warfare, and communion with supernatural beings. They were technologically stagnant, but they were not phenomenologically stagnant.[13]

Medicine was probably practiced in each of these generations and by all of the cultures on the planet, but we pick up the history in the last of these thousands of ancient worlds which lead to our single modern time. By then it is too late for us to talk about origins, so instead we reconstruct ancient and classical medical thought and hypothesize the rest from primitive cultures still in existence. For most uses, this is an acceptable approximation, and, even if it were not, it could hardly be improved upon except by hypothetical surmises. We will explore those later in a different light.

Things began in the remote and infinite past (for all practical purposes, the origin of language is as remote from us as the origin of the universe itself). When we try to re-create the past, we run into two basic difficulties: (1) we have no firsthand account of the events—no one is presently alive who was alive at the dawn of time; and (2) the nature of our understanding is probably totally different from the way in which things happened—so that even should a marvelous event suddenly place us at the dawn of matter itself or even man, we would not know what we were seeing and we would have no way of communicating it in concrete specific terms. Of course, the second difficulty exists in the present also and is really the difficulty of understanding anything in an alien context. Members of the same family do not see eye to eye, so what possible insight could we have into the mind of prehistoric man?

While this may appear obvious, it is important to understand that our removal from original things is not just a removal by vast amounts of simple time, millions and millions, or billions and billions, of years. The epochs of nature contain different phenomena, and, though universal physical laws hold from one end of creation to another, those universal physical laws are basically unknown. Newton, Darwin, Einstein, Heisenberg simply offer interpretations of them in the context of one particular culture's view of nature. Their theories are not themselves the "universal physical laws."

Anthropologists tend to simplify origins and work toward a theory of human behavior and culture at the expense of a record of real human peoples living their lives in the different places and different times of the Earth. The specific informants are made into general social cases, not because the researcher did not care about their individuality but because he had a hopeless job on his hands that could only have been solved by generalization. As a result, something valuable, in truth, was recovered, but something even more valuable was lost. Medicine was a major victim.

There is also a tendency to equate prehistoric medicine with contemporary tribal medicine and, at the same time, to define tribal medicine, on the supposed evidence of firsthand viewing, as primitive first aid mixed with magic. One history, fairly typically, claims that in primitive societies, a sick person was deserted "as a menace to the community . . . and left to die; or to recover on his own, if he was lucky."[14] This kind of fictive narrative is convincing and reasonable, but we must ourselves realize that the deserted victim is either a single undocumented episode that the author has generalized into a custom or an out-of-context fragment of a larger system. It says absolutely nothing about primitive medicine.

Victor Turner's writings on African religion, especially of the Ndembu Lunda of Zambia, are much admired in liberal academic circles. He is considered one of the more sympathetic observers. Generally, he is, but not in matters of medicine, i.e., of practical science.

He concludes that "medicine is given to humor rather than to cure" and that "a rich and elaborate system of ritual and magical beliefs and practices provides a set of explanations for sickness and death and gives people a false sense of confidence that they have the means of coping with disease." Why do such beliefs persist? he wonders. And his answer is that "they are part of a religious system which itself constitutes an explanation of the universe and guarantees the norms and values on which orderly social arrangements rest."[15] In other words, they are stuck with their medicine because they are stuck with the symbols which back it up and which their survival has come to require. The author goes on to prescribe a big dose of Western medicine and an extension of Western-type hospital facilities.

So much for African medicine. There's nothing happening but hocus-pocus, delusion, and placebo. And this from a person who knows more about the subject than the author of this book and 99.9 per cent of his readers. Knowledge, it appears, doesn't make the difference.

We must do away with our illusion of diseased and miserable native society, which is correct to no greater or lesser degree (though in a totally different way) than our illusion of diseased and miserable industrial society. The longevity we value, which our medicine has seemingly won for us, may be a false one, especially since it is a longevity in an industrial society which steals years and years of life by labor alone. Our medicine has given us a statistical longevity only, which our machines and bureaucracies have then taken back. The primitive mortality rate is also only a statistical mortality rate; it says nothing of the lives or real possibilities of individuals. Furthermore, diseased native society is at least in part a result of the colonial invasion, which brought not only new diseases but destroyed much of the existential fabric of native cultural life.

We are talking about 160,000 generations of medicines, during some of which there may have been tens of thousands of different medical traditions practiced on the Earth. If medicine were only the progressive development of more systematized technological coda, then we might be justified in oversimplifying and dealing briefly with native medicine. But if medicine is the art of healing, these other traditions are comparable. Unless we accept, from the beginning, that they are successful, complex medicines, then we cannot proceed with any clarity into the muddle that anthropology and history have left us. That there are corrupt and superstitious native systems also—

indeed, corrupt and superstitious elements in all systems—is obvious; to emphasize it would be to harp on the familiar. We do not describe science by its frauds and errors. Every human being has lived in the midst of contradictions and insoluble riddles, which work their way into every system—since no system is perfect or permanent —and they represent, as illness itself in the body, the movement of life through a changing universe.

The man wrongly killed by poison in an African witchcraft trial is an innocent victim of imperfect science. So is the worker in the factory who comes down with environmental cancer, or the political prisoners in totalitarian states, or the soldiers killed in wars of their times.

Because of the global spread of our culture and its accompanying industrialism, we tend to assume that the actual spread of information and real scientific knowledge also takes place. We forget that each individual culture, like each individual, can have only one existential reality. Information is limitless. When a culture builds machines to ferret out and increase its information, it does not change the reality. That goes as deep as the world goes, and as deep as human beings go for living in the world. The Navaho and Australian Aborigine have the same amount of real information as we do; they go as far into meaning, but not on the basis of industrial achievements or global spread and certainly not on the basis of number of members. They are as deep and real as we are on the basis of their singular and discrete profundity and their ability to hold even one advocate, _even one_, in a way that is fundamental. It requires not massive government, world exploration, nor knowledge about cell growth and the actual composition of stars. It requires essential understanding of the internal qualitative facts of existence and the ability to perceive all phenomena in an integrated system. The native reality is as real as the Western orthodox reality. The anthropologist or historian, for all their access to dozens of different cultures, do not really have any more access to information than any one inhabitant of any one of those cultures.[16]

But the early anthropologists, like James Frazer and Bronislaw Malinowski, saw tribal man as primitive and naïve. _La pensée sauvage_ was a sentence, condemning him to the jungles of human thought. The societies had a rough look to them, and these anthropologists were not inclined to observe beyond their initial judgments, though they reported much from within them. In a sense, ethnological bias about native peoples was established over centuries of European self-congratulation for getting out of their own Dark Ages.

In the last fifty years that prejudice has all but turned around. General anthropology has discovered, or rediscovered, institutions of tribal society that equal and even dwarf those of civilization. These range from practical skills of hunting, toolmaking, cooking, etc., to systems of resource exchange, peaceable marriage between small groups, and cosmic philosophy. In the last twenty or thirty years, some anthropologists (notably in the tradition arising from Leslie White and including Marshall Sahlins and Elman Service) have made a working distinction between technological evolution, in which larger amounts of energy are harnessed by a society, and basic cultural coherence, which has no intercausal relationship with increasing amounts of accessible energy. Agricultural societies release and use more energy than hunting bands, and industrial societies use exponentially more energy than even large agrarian civilizations. The precision and refinement of craft and thought and justice have nothing at all to do with this technological development.

Re-evaluating the native physician is difficult for a number of reasons, not the least of which is the gap between healing as an art and medicine as a science. However, Sahlins' later work on the economics of primitive peoples gives us a model for comparison. Malnutrition is the condition most often assigned, along with disease, to primitive societies. Even enlightened anthropologists have described their situations as brutal, with ceaseless backbreaking labor the absolute lot of most humans unfortunate enough to have been born before or outside the modern era. Sahlins lists catch phrases of the average anthropological opinion of primitive societies: " 'Mere subsistence economy,' 'limited leisure save in exceptional circumstances,' 'incessant quest for food,' 'meagre and relatively unreliable natural resources,' 'absence of an economic surplus,' 'maximum energy from a maximum number of people.' "[17]

It turns out that these opinions are mostly a mixture of exaggeration and misinformation. Primitives work relatively short hours, live in a limited abundance of resources whose cycles of replenishment they rarely exceed, and share easily without the disruption of formal institutions for maximizing wealth.

No doubt, anthropologists looked at the absolute material poverty of natives and deduced from that an unhappiness and suffering that were probably more projection than observation. These same primitive peoples have a low standard of living and few requirements, but, as Sahlins put it, *"they are not poor.* Poverty is not a certain small amount of goods, nor is it just a relation between means and ends; above all it is a relation between people. Poverty is a social status. As such it is the invention of civilization."[18]

Poverty, it turns out, is more our birthright than theirs. We are the ones who live in a market-industrial system that institutes false scarcity "in a manner completely unparalleled and to a degree nowhere else approximated."[19] It is our world in which "every acquisition is simultaneously a deprivation . . . a foregoing of something else, in general only marginally less desirable, and in some particulars more desirable, that could have been had instead."[20] Now is the time when almost half the population of the planet goes hungry—*"this* is the era of hunger unprecedented."[21]

We have actually projected the wolf who is at our own door onto primitive peoples who, we believe, could not have existed in a more peaceful and better-fed society. Says Sahlins: "That sentence of 'life at hard labor' was passed uniquely upon us. . . . And it is precisely from this anxious vantage that we look back upon hunters. . . . if modern man, with all his technological advantages, still hasn't got the wherewithal, what chance has this naked savage with his puny bow and arrow? Having equipped the hunter with bourgeois impulses and palaeolithic tools, we judge his situation hopeless in advance."[22]

Sahlins' title, *Stone Age Economics,* perhaps not accidentally echoes Lévi-Strauss's *The Savage Mind.* It also suggests an alternative title for this book: *Stone Age Medicine.* Either one, Stone Age Economics or Stone Age Medicine, is what we point toward in the future—post-Marxist, post-capitalist—in our imagination of small cooperative communities. But it is also something we have left behind. We have improved the means of production and freed culture partially from environmental control, but we have laid waste regional agriculture, the art of healing, and subsistence economics. We have, in Sahlins' terms, "enriched" ourselves while "impoverishing" ourselves. We have increased anxiety and poverty in exactly the way we have increased information and wealth, without deepening the profundity of our awareness. We have reached a point where our industrial wizardry is aghast at our social and humanitarian barbarism. Are we, in fact, healthier and wealthier today? Do we even understand what we have given up, let alone what we have gained?

Perhaps the single most shocking event on this planet during the last five hundred years has been, relatively speaking, overlooked. Because the remnants of native technology are still available for viewing and scientific report and because there remain a few practitioners trained in local traditions (and because our very fragmentary literature on these subjects is itself vast and unmanageable in a lifetime), we retain the illusion of an accessible primitive world. In fact, most anthropology, even that of the nineteenth and early twentieth centuries and certainly that of later decades, has come far too late for accurate accounts. And, besides, it was already far too late right from the beginning. The Western world was a blundering child with powerful tools when it stumbled upon the planet. Spain sent her criminals to the New World, to meet with philosophers, medicine men, and priests. And the scientists that followed were concerned more often with preserving the dignity and superiority of their sciences than with having a dialogue with equals.

It is for this reason that Carlos Castaneda's account of his training with the Yaqui shaman Don Juan Matus in Mexico had such a stunning effect, especially outside of anthropological circles.[23] Castaneda gave his readers what they had been looking to anthropology for, with disappointment: an account of the native's experience of his own magic and visions. There is no technique described in these books that was not already thoroughly documented in anthropological literature. In fact, all of it had already appeared in the anthropological literature of just North America. Vision quest: we've gone over that earlier in this chapter. Talking to animals: we could fill a library with accounts of Indians talking to animals, animals seeking Indians. Drugs: a regular feature of native American society. Appearing and disappearing: shamans the world over cultivate this ability. Waking one's self within dream: the Crow, among others, do this. Engaging in magical war on the desert, in the wilderness: anthropologists have always acknowledged that Indians were committed to hallucinating their inherited totemic symbols. Castaneda reported only these well-known things—nothing outstanding or shocking. Yet there *is* something shocking about his account, both in what it says and what it suggests about all the others.

Castaneda reports that, from within, the system is very different than it seems from without. Notably it is vaster and more complete, not only than it would appear from previous accounts but also than the whole of Western philosophy and science. Don Juan is not specifically a doctor of disease, but, in light of his training and activity as described in the narrative, we must consider him a healer above all. He is, also, a doctor. He is a practitioner of universal shamanism, thus of medicine, which is one of its branches.

Carlos comes to Don Juan in order to be trained in his Yaqui Indian system of occult knowledge. His initial intention is not to become a Yaqui shaman but to go through some aspects of the teaching so that he can write a traditional, descriptive account. By the very premise of his inquiry, Carlos is already miles ahead of most anthropological observers, who are content to watch from outside and record what they see.

All of his initial questions and activities are consonant with his specific professional goal. He speaks to Don Juan as though they are both reasonable intelligent people. Carlos will go on being an anthropologist; Don Juan will go on being a shaman; and neither will think less of the other for his culturally determined preference. This is roughly how Carlos Castaneda portrays himself: a liberal anthropologist, sympathetic to Indian mythology.

For various reasons, Don Juan does not accept these terms. When Carlos offers him money as an informant, Don Juan says that he requires only Carlos' time. He then proceeds to initiate him into his own system. He does not describe or explain what is happening, at least not in the polite language of scientific cause and effect. Carlos finds himself in a world that is miraculous and terrifying. Drugs are involved, but there are things that cannot be explained away as hallucination. Carlos speaks to lizards, moths, cacti; he meets spirits; not only do they disappear and reappear, but he does too, along with them. The usual anthropological account says that Indians are extremely close to the animals and that sorcerers often take on the form and character of animals. Even the best accounts, ones which do not mock or deny what natives tell them, suggest that there is some other familiar explanation for these occurrences, and that the answer lies in mythology, trickery, social pressure, and cultural convention. Carlos says: *I* talked to the lizards, they talked to me; *I* was a crow, *I* flew. Anthropologists report that shamans construct their doubles. Carlos says that he talked to both the sorcerer and his double, and they were the same—and also different.

Carlos continuously questions Don Juan: Are these things real? Did they happen? Or is it only in my mind? He asks: Would my friends have seen me flying like a crow? Don Juan answers: If they knew how to look.

The implication is that if they knew how to look, they would have seen a crow, not Carlos, but would have recognized that crow as Carlos.

The matter becomes only more serious, or, as Don Juan puts it, "It is no picnic." The tricks alone would not be enough to hold Carlos' or our interest, but then the tricks alone would not have been worth the trouble of inventing. The reason for this fantastic initiation is that, without it, one lives in a lesser, painful, meaningless world. Carlos is not only awestruck by the remarkable visions; he is devastated by the shallowness of his world. As an anthropologist, he reports not on the poverty and misery of this primitive society, but on the richness and beauty of a life lived within its magic. *He* is deprived, naïve, and cosmically insignificant. Don Juan towers above him in a creation that seems so much more worth inhabiting. The science, the rationale that Carlos clings to, primarily to keep from losing his identity and sanity altogether, is a useless virtue in Don Juan's world. Only a small fraction of things are explained by reason. The rock in the desert is a rock by convention only, but that is not its most interesting or useful attribute. The physical body is not a firm substance at all, but a bundle of fluid, luminous fibers.

At first Carlos sets his sense of continuity against Don Juan's world of unpredictability and surprise. In addition, the physical base is necessary to have any understanding of phenomena, he insists. How can the doctor cure without a real person to treat? Don Juan never deigns to debate at this level. Instead, he asks Carlos what he has from his rigid continuity: Does he have power? Does he have happiness? Does he have anything more than his goods and a rigid sense of personal history?

It is important to see that Carlos is overwhelmed not by a parapsychological experiment or a trick; he is stunned because Don Juan has proven to him the emptiness of his own life. The tricks are important not because they work, but because they are "real," in some totally other way; they are clues to a world in which Carlos' life might have new meaning. This is the critical issue in healing and will remain so throughout this book. The ostensible diseases and their accompanying (posited) cures are not the key to a science of planet medicine. Real medicine gives freedom, power, and happiness. It ignores disease-as-an-object. Likewise, Don Juan ignores Carlos' objections; they are simply *his* disease. He ignores the science of continuity which "proves" him impossible because that science is a boring and restricted way in which to live a life. The *life* is important, not imposed explanations. It establishes its own meaning through being lived. Phenomena are important as the life interacts with them, but they have no abstract significance. Don Juan tells Carlos:

"For you the world is weird because if you're not bored with it you're at odds with it. For me the world is weird because it is stupendous, awesome, mysterious, unfathomable; my interest has been to convince you that you must assume responsibility for being here, in this marvelous world, in this marvelous desert, in this marvelous time. I wanted to convince you that you must learn to make every act count, since you are going to be here for only a short while, in fact, too short for witnessing all the marvels of it."[24]

From the Western *scientific* point of view, this is an outrageous proposition. Sociologists can admit side benefits from herbal, massage, or ritual, but they do not endorse the underlying premise of the medicine. They may think that their praise is sufficient for a primitive, but the shaman is, of course, Don Juan's brother in arms.

Medicines from dreams, somatic resurrection, psychic vision into the disease body, voices from clouds and cacti, magical darts, supernatural visitations—all of these are described with faint heart and withheld enthusiasm by even the most sympathetic observers. One gets the sense that our ethnographic witnesses feel they have been told something childish, something queer. Their ethnological and scientific responsibility is to report it maturely and explain it, but their language betrays them. They credit the savage mind with a dazzling display before its naïve constituency or a psychedelic transcendence of normal reality. For instance, Lévi-Strauss grants the complexity of this mind, but at the expense of microbiological accuracy. Native peoples are brilliant "psychologists" and plant "geneticists," but not spirit healers.

Castaneda's work is a breakthrough, for it reveals the inner ceremony. He comes late in history to an almost vanished people, but he reports something that was almost totally missed for centuries. We ourselves must approach the native medicine that anthropology gives us with our attention beneath its accountable surface. It is its own culture's version of the external features of another event. Almost from the beginning, previous accounts of native medicine set the boundaries and terms for later investigators. Later investigators were almost always true to anthropological tradition rather than to the "weirdness." Of each ceremony and healing event we now have only the outlines; we do not know what actually happened inside. And the outlines and external descriptions themselves were culled at a time when the culture existed in an extreme, almost terminal doubt as to its own validity and the validity of its traditions. This is the famous precondition for anthropology; it comes when the moment has already passed. Even individual informants who cling stubbornly to the old and traditional are already born into a world of invaders that must be explained and integrated into their cosmology—invaders who have power, unimaginable power, even though they deny and violate the deities and the sacred law.

In 1523 the Aztec priest replied to the emissaries of Pope Hadrian VI and Emperor Charles V, as translated in verse: "You say/that we don't know/the Omneity, of heaven and earth/you say that our gods are not original/That's news to us/and it drives us crazy/it's a shock and a scandal/for our ancestors came to earth/and they spoke quite differently/they gave the law to us/and they believed/they served and they taught/honour among gods/they taught the whole service."[25]

We must certainly do away with the fantasy that we have access to a true native medicine tradition. As with economics, our illusion of fullness dooms us to find only hunger and disease where there is not the same kind of fullness. Our "purchase" lies in kind with the famous joke about Manhattan being bought from the Indians by the Dutch for sixty guilders, when "in the eyes of these same Delawares the currency was the symbol not the value equivalent of the relinquishment of their hereditary rights to the land as well as its products . . . a symbol over which they transferred their good-will and spiritual power over forces dormant in the land."[26]

Not only must we do away with the illusion of access to native medicine, but, with it, we must do away with the illusion that recovery of lost traditions is our main hope. Recovery is no longer possible. These alien systems are hidden by nature and time, and their final obscurity is their seeming to stand in clear, understandable English or some other Western language, which makes them even less accessible by making them superficially close. We are members of a scientific Western society, and that is what we must live out; our greed will not give us back what we have already forfeited via the deeds of Hernando Cortez or our purchase of Manhattan. Castaneda comes closest to recovery, and even he leads to another point and another problem, as we shall see. In the terms of our scientific society and its modes of inquiry, we can begin to move toward new native traditions and new discrete regional varieties of craft and knowledge. It is that movement that can be informed by the last relics of a dying order. Having lost Creek and Australian Aboriginal medicines, we must reinvent them, from "memory," as something else.

Reinvention takes into account who we are, the reality of our own circumstance rather than the misleading neutrality of reconstruction. We, as people, as a culture, are in crisis and face real paradoxes and terrors. To pretend that our aim is now to set up a museum of extinct practices and peoples is as dishonest as it would be wasteful if it were true. We do not have the time or the resources. The fact that, by our presence here, we are the true descendants of Miles Standish and Cortez will not allow us to be innocent keepers of archives, but it also does not prevent us from going ahead into our own history. For many Africans, American Indians, Australian Aborigines, the problem is the same; the ancient wisdom is gone and they struggle, along with Europeans, to make something that will sustain them now.

There is a further paradox in the Castaneda lore. Anthropologists have come, more and more, to suspect that the tales of Don Juan are fiction. At this point, a substantial proportion of the scientific community refuses to admit them as ethnographic evidence. They cannot be cited, as I have cited them here, as evidence for anything real. This verdict only seemingly restores law and order to shamanism and healing. In fact, once the anthropological judges admit they have been fooled by a fiction posing as ethnographic description, they have opened Pandora's box, for how can any report of another culture be verified? That there is a peculiar crisis with Castaneda is indisputable, but it has hardly yet been resolved. It has no more been proven that the works are fiction than it was previously demonstrated that they were fact. It is not impossible that they are a mythologized or esoteric account of an initiation. It is also possible that the narrator entered a realm in which he himself was unable to distinguish between hallucination and objective experience. There is no explicit way for any subsequent anthropologist to "find" Don Juan Matus and confirm or refute the events.

Freeing a murderer on the basis of "diminished capacity" does not undo the killing nor does it prevent further killings. Likewise, anthropology cannot "go back on" Castaneda without opening the whole field to a fundamental crisis of meaning. It is already open to that, and the haggling over Castaneda's fieldwork has brought it to the forefront. Different systems of meaning exist out there in real space. Don Juan cannot be disproven, though, for some in committee, he may be postponed. If he is not the shaman to show the West the disparity of meaning and reality on this planet, another will take his place in time. Castaneda either *had* the experience (and is no longer interested in convincing us of that because the "fieldwork" became more of an initiation than the academic defense it originally served) or he has a profound intuition of what that experience is like and has given it to us as a sort of parable. For our purposes, in raising questions of meaning in cross-cultural contexts, either resolution, or another more esoteric one, is acceptable.

The theosophist Owen Barfield wrote: "The interior is anterior."[27] That is, the primal complexity of the earliest systems (whether of matter itself, or of thought, or of language), as well as the specific transformations and evolutions of their fabric over thousands and millions of years, are contained entirely in the present system in some other form. The various continuities, of matter and energy, of DNA, of cultural tradition, insure that ancient modes are locked into current modes. They are contained there not at the surface or by simple parallel. They are contained in depth. Looking inside ourselves, into the flux of mind and matter that we are, we can perceive the sum of remote influences of which we are the result. As they are anterior to us in time and space, they become interior to our physical and psychic composition.

This book begins by establishing the rightful position of "old" medicines, but it is about "the new medicine." This apparent contradiction masks a unity which modern culture, obsessed with progress, has tried to dualize. In fact, the "new age" seers, Castaneda among them, are at the same time "recoverers," reinventors of ancient wisdom. Our intelligence *is* a collection of all that has gone before us. Certainly philosophy looks inward for basic laws of nature, and science and mathematics are as much reflections of the mind as they are replicas of some outer world. Religion and mythology re-create origins in the hope that our depth as beings will cover for the loss of information and thinning out of creative intensity over time.

Although many of the holistic medicines abjure concrete etiology of disease they are very much interested in the way the sick person conceives of the coming of the disease. "How I came to be sick," whether or not it is the real story, is itself part of the illness. The doctor is usually not even satisfied with a sick person's account as mythology; he demands a present redynamization of the disease on the assumption that the causes are still locked in the person's system, although not in the way they were at the time of his becoming sick. There is no true history anymore, either of self or of cosmos. The stars shining in the heavens are those whose light reaches us *now*, as this fire burns in the city and wind blows through the oak leaves. The thoughts we are having now are the thoughts that will enable us to understand who we are and how we became this.

The poet and lay physician Theodore Enslin writes: "Things are what they are, and no amount of worry over 'primal causes' will change what they are at the moment of perception. There is a direct link here between a consideration of the totality of symptoms at a given moment, and treating *them*, rather than an unreal idea of disease. . . ."[28]

We can imitate this process in making a book about it. Along with our reconstruction of the origins of medicine, and our sympathy for mythological and quasi-historical sequences, we can re-create, in a dynamic manner that suits this present moment in history and in this author's history, the source of medicine on this planet. And the book itself will be passed along as our case to some other "doctor," a record of the incurable condition we lived.

It will also be an account, paradoxically, of the beginning of our attempt to get well. As long as the book follows the mystery, true to its course but not pretending to resolve it, it will suggest the unknown cures to which we are coming, at least insofar as such things could exist. The alternative would be an external summary of the healing going on, and an attempt to name our disease and dilemma and place the blame on us for it. That would be a book about something happening elsewhere. And we would be working under the assumption that publishing, anthropology, writing, and Manhattan Island were more important than the silent occasion of healing in the world.

IV

The Distribution of Healing Complexes on the Earth

The distribution of healing systems is an enigmatic topic for an age in which we know both too much and too little. We are either overwhelmed with details which are connected to each other only by random methods of categorization or we have easy generalizations which lack any meaningful application. The only useful tack, short of an exhaustive compendium, is to be daring with the images we have, avoiding the more common truisms.

We are trapped between the globalism which gives us our partial knowledge of a variety of techniques and the regional intelligences which are immune to full translation. Both must be dealt with in any sort of medicinal map making. There are universal facts and skills which arise from the human condition. All medicines, when-ever and wherever occurring, have a native origin. This unity lies at the basis of the current attempts to achieve cross-cultural holistic healing. It is why medicines can be shared at all, despite cultural differences.

World medicine shows both idiosyncrasies and widespread symme-tries. Any system has unique items, and these are the ones most often lost in the translation, unless they are concrete artifacts or techniques which are tough enough to stand outside cultural context. Many geographical patterns, especially transoceanic ones, reflect un-derlying migrations, trade, or cultural contact.

In order to understand contemporary issues in healing, we must keep in mind the sources, at least as we know them. Some methods are extremely ancient and persist in every culture of our global melting pot. Some things we have learned anew, either from the aborigines in areas the Western world has resettled or from other Eurasian civilizations throughout millennia of contact. There are other issues and techniques that are idiosyncratically Western, but for which we have borrowed new primitive or oriental images. The images should not be confused with the actualities. We must also respect the difference between medicines which have developed purely within oral traditions (even if recorded later) and those which are clearly the product of generations of written transmission and scholarship. This is a distinction which applies as certainly to ancient Asia and the Middle East as to the modern world of Western science and anthropology.

Our atlas will be brief and intuitive. One hopes it can stand as a token for the real research that needs to be done.

Many healing techniques are so basic that they have arisen independently around the world. Certainly, pharmacy is a concomitant of the simplest human systems of thought and a regular by-product of food gathering. Lévi-Strauss has suggested that fish poisoning in the jungle pools of South America may be the missing link between plant gathering and plant cultivation: *timbó*, the vegetable fish poison, is mythologically related to watermelons, an agricultural product, and honey, which is the product of insect husbandry. *Timbó* may not be medicine, but it is certainly pharmacy—pharmacy linked to hunting and pharmacy in transition to domestic botany.[1] Arrow poison may be a similar bridge.

Massage and incision seem to occur spontaneously from a raw kinesthesia of health and illness. These activities may then be symbolized and ritualized differently, depending on the system of thought into which they are incorporated.

The emphasis on witchcraft and spirit-caused illness is strongest in the Southern Hemisphere. In most areas of Africa, witchcraft and voodoo appear to be the favorite treatments. This "information" may also come from the fact that British anthropologists in Africa, our main sources, focused heavily on political structure and power relations within society—hence their enthusiasm for voodoo ostracisms and magical wars. They may well have overlooked pharmaceutical components of native medicine. American anthropologists, on the other hand, followed in the trail of Lewis and Clark as explorers in the American Northwest and tended to collect any information they could get on local Indian customs with the result that the North American herbal is extraordinarily rich.

In both Africa and North America, witchcraft and herbalism exist side by side, often with different specialists. Frequently, the rule of thumb is to give medicines until it is clear the disease is due to psychic or supernatural interference; then treat by magic. In Africa, there is a tendency to relate disease, judgment, and voodoo in a single complex. North America, on the other hand, is dominated by elaborate healing ceremonies, often in conjunction with seasonal changes. Medicines made during these ceremonies are distributed to members of the group for later use. A similar type of ceremony exists in Bali, suggesting a greater Pacific range for this treatment.

Shamanism, with the sucking out of the disease object, is a major activity throughout the Southern Hemisphere, including South America, the Atlantic and Pacific archipelagoes, and Australia. Sucking is also practiced on the northwest coast of North America where there is a late palaeolithic Asian influence. Trance healing and shamanism are especially widespread in South America. Numerous authors have suggested aboriginal African and Pacific influences in this region, attempting to back up their claim of cultural contacts with the related genetics of cultigens. This kind of Stone Age globalism is frowned upon by professional anthropology, but it is interesting to entertain the image of a Southern Hemisphere fraternity of shamans. In later times, via the post-contact slave ships, West African voodoo was imported to the New World, and hybrid forms of shamanic cure and crises of possession arose. In fact, transatlantic voodoo has gained a certain Third World prestige, implying the soul tie between the Caribbean Islands and mainland and the ancient motherland. Voodoo societies are now becoming international affairs.

South America is certainly the planetary center of hallucinogenic medicine, both in the treatment of disease and the training of physicians. Although there is no comprehensive study of this, some observers claim there is no *non*hallucinogenic pharmacy in South America. Perhaps this tradition found its university in the remote jungle civilizations of Bolivia, Ecuador, and Brazil and was exported, in times and ways obscure to us, to the later farming and military cultures of Mexico, Guatemala, and Peru.[2]

As we move from Africa eastward across the Indian Ocean, witchcraft changes from primarily psychic to primarily supernatural (in Australia). In Africa, the source of an illness is usually another "doctor," trained perhaps in the dark half of the healing arts or at least disposed to practice them; the cure is a defeat of this interfering power. In Australia, there are masters of something that resembles voodoo, but the emphasis is on supernatural beings and *their* role in causing disease. Australian supernatural worlds also resemble North American supernatural worlds; both landscapes are profoundly internalized with ancestors and mythological beings in the form of animals, rocks, hills, water holes, etc., with disembodied spirits attached to natural phenomena. Both cultures "dream" in order to transform waking reality. The dreamtime and the ghost dance share a moment on this Earth that must shine like a star through our planetary mythology.

If spirits in Africa seem more involved with vendettas, the American supernatural is like a collage of nature and the Australian supernatural resembles an enormous holy war of ancestors. This is no doubt equally a prejudice of our sources. All gods play music, reside in herbs and ponds, and lead their peoples on aeonic migrations. The vision quest meanwhile, whose moment of brilliance lies in the hemispheres of the New World, is a global phenomenon, a mode of initiation native to the biosphere itself.

Incision, including various modes of inserting needles, scarring flesh, scratching grooves in skin, scraping tissue, cutting of parts of the anatomy, is particularly common in Australia and Asia and is part of the vision quest in North America. In Africa and the Pacific, excluding Australia, massage is more widely reported than incision, and in both the Pacific and Asia, systems of divination, often as elaborate as the solstice rituals of North America, are intimate adjuncts to healing.

The rural systems of native Europe and native Asia have been overshadowed by the medicines of the civilizations that developed there, though many of the ancient techniques have been preserved. It is possible, even likely, that the documented medical system that arose in the West, and, along different lines, in the East, is the same original Eurasian system developed during tens of thousands of years of migration back and forth between the European and Asian limbs of the Old World. The distinction between European and Asian traditions is a relatively new event in the history of the world. Marco Polo's journey to China in the thirteenth century symbolized the breakdown of the barriers of a few thousand years, before which waves of Asian settlers colonized Europe and a smaller number of European groups migrated to Asia.[3]

The elemental systems of Europe, India, and Asia are remarkably similar. Alchemy is a system of thought that spans the entire Old World with regional dialects that tend to confirm a common origin. Acupuncture and homoeopathy suggest each other, but only on the deepest level; their techniques are singularly different.[4] It is a mistake to think that the West was involved in physiology from the beginning and that the East was not. There is a skeleton and cadaver in the closet of the East too, and he appears in all the earliest medical texts. The existence of dozens of kinds of ancient Asian surgical and medical instruments reminds us that technology and science had beginnings there too, but on different terms. In Tibet there are bottle-shaped tools with nipples and holes for diagnosing anal disorders and trumpet-shaped tools for sending medicine through the anus. There are saws, hooks for removing tumors and stones, and three kinds of spoons, shaped, respectively, like a bird's beak, a frog's head, and a grain of barley, for removing pus, water, and tumors from surficial and internal cavities of the body. There is also a variety of pincers and scalpels, the former shaped like a lion's head, a crane's or crow's beak, etc., and the latter like the feather of a sparrow or a sickle.[5]

China has a later tradition of opposition to surgery because it violated the sacred space of the organism, but its medical technology is still the earliest. There are fabulous *reports* of heart transplants from the second century B.C., at least showing an early interest in exploring and altering innards, but, since surgery and anatomy did not fit the Chinese philosophy of healing, it was a historically much later Europe that developed the global system of medical technology.[6]

Meanwhile, the amount of traditional Chinese medicine practiced in the world today is less than might appear at first glance. The People's Republic makes use of the techniques of acupuncture and rural folk medicine, but it has abandoned textually the mythology and the general system behind it. That system is totally lost in China except insofar as traditional Chinese doctors keep it in their practice and heritage or insofar as Mao's China effected, in a certain sense, the twentieth-century industrial transformation of the Chinese sacred books into Western terms.

Our present access to such a wide variety of systems and traditions is also misleading. We have neither the time nor the personal knowl-

edge or training to incorporate these things into our culture. Take
Asian medicine for example. What we have in the United States is a
series of partial, often inaccurate translations of traditional Oriental
medical texts, as well as the actual occurrence of the art of healing as
it has been transmitted in apprenticeship from Asians to Americans,
from Americans to other Americans. Of the texts, the most prominent is the Ilza Veith translation appearing under the English title
The Yellow Emperor's Classic of Internal Medicine.[7] Although extremely complex, symbolic, and put into an unfortunate English,
The Yellow Emperor survives. It survives difficulties of time, space,
and language to propose a clear, incisive, and often terrifying doctrine of the human condition and the absolute basis for life on this
planet. It is not a medical book in our sense of the term. It is, first, a
philosophy of nature and the formation of matter. It is a medical
book because it treats the subject of how man comes into being and
perishes. It presents a medical technology in the context of its investigations of nature.

The premise of *The Yellow Emperor's* cosmology is that nature
originates from the interplay of eternal forces. We never see them,
but everything we see, including our act of seeing, is their effect. The
Chinese text itself is maybe four thousand years old, and the principles it describes are obviously much older. It is no exaggeration to
think of *The Yellow Emperor* as one of our only guides to late Stone
Age medicine. Like other possible Stone Age texts we get through
Egyptian, Scandinavian, and even New World sources, it lives in a
world of unceasing creation, cataclysmic change, and the subjection
of all to a severe and merciless hierarchy of gods and law.

We today arrive here, having eaten foods from all different climates, perhaps oranges from tropical Florida, potatoes from Idaho
and Maine, grain from Kansas and Iowa, pineapples from Hawaii.
We sit in the Medi-American summer or autumn or coastal cities
trying to adapt to an ancient text that formed over hundreds of generations of masters who stayed in one place, without grandiose technology or global pretensions, and observed and recorded and healed.
The real teaching and healing are as remote as the clouds forming
and dissolving palpably in the sky, or as grass on the next mountains,
or as the sun itself, from which the particles of sunlight explode over
every visibility we see. By the time we are old enough to read, we
have already forfeited the wisdom of *The Yellow Emperor.*

But this provinciality does not negate our treatments any more than strict adherence to a set of rules confirms the virtue of a healing methodology. Healing does not exist by permission of names; it exists in fact. Medicine thrusts into nature as it is, with all the local roughness and bias of things. Appropriate treatments are discovered in all cultures, as people are born, inhabit this world, and die. There are many ways to use needles, and there are also many ways to use hands. This is the clarity of folk medicine. No doubt lay peasant doctors flourished throughout traditional China and continue to flourish in many areas of the world.

There is also a substantial American underground folk tradition. Each group of immigrants brought their own home remedies and native techniques, and these mixed and overlapped, especially in poor rural areas and the growing urban slums of the nineteenth century. It was not simply European herbalism, but included a substantial component of African voodoo medicine in the South and, of course, Oriental medicine in the West, both of which continue to be rediscovered today (for instance, in New Orleans and San Francisco). German and English folk medicine are somewhat known quantities, but there was also Spanish, Irish, Scottish, Semitic, Norwegian, Finnish, Eastern European, etc., plus a substantial transmission of native North American medicine, not only from contemporary Indian tribes but also from European herb doctors who studied with Indians or whose fathers or grandfathers had studied with Indians, as well as people of mixed Indian blood, and Central and South Americans who learned other native traditions.

The medicines of China and India have dominated Asia in much the way European medicine dominated the native traditions of Europe and America. Chinese medicine is strongest in Tibet and Vietnam, whereas a mixture of Hindu, Buddhist, Parsi, and Moslem medicine prevails in South and Southeast Asia. Whether there is a Chinese influence in the Pacific, or even in North America, is uncertain, but an intriguing possibility to examine. Does the Australian practice of incision share a Stone Age ancestor with the Chinese practice of acupuncture? Do the trance powers of the Australian shaman come from the same ritual instruction as those of the Tibetan shaman? Both masters gain their power from confronting visions of evil and dangerous spirits. Both learn to create illusions, to vanish and reappear elsewhere. And what about the quartz crystal containing other worldly powers, so dominant in both Africa and Australia? Do the African influences on Australia come later, or is quartz a basic element of some very early Old World healing complex that vanished in most regions but was retained in Africa, parts of North America, and Australia?

The possible connection of Asia and North America was dramatized a few years ago by the visit of the exiled Tibetan karmapa to the Hopi village of Hotevilla. The Buddhist spiritual leader was welcomed by the Indians as a kinsman, also as an ancestor. He and several other Tibetans joined the Hopis in the kiva, the underground religious quarters, to chant together for rain. It had been dry for many months. Superficially, the most remarkable event was the rain that followed. However, the joint participation is what stands out over time. The Hopis and Tibetans "understood" each other in the chants, and the Hopis claimed later that they had lost certain primary elements of their rain chant over the rough intervening years, and that the Tibetans were able to help them back into the vitality and efficacy of their own ceremony.[8] If substantial elements have persisted for a hundred thousand years—and there is no reason why they could not have—we are confirmed in our sense that healing and related artistic and spiritual systems of high integrity have existed and continue to exist outside the framework of history and science. Traditions of curing, chant, evoking, etc., go back to the oldest times and so, like the radio noise of the galactic explosion, are distributed most widely throughout our cultural universe.

The gap between prehistoric medicine and ancient medicine, if we may use these as categories, is like the gap between prehistory and history: artificial and yet substantial. The earliest Western medical codices—Egyptian, Babylonian, and Greek—already suggest a formalization of medical theory and practice quite different than anything we find in present-day native cultures or the archaeology of preliterate Western peoples. The Hippocratic Corpus, assigned by historians to the fourth and fifth centuries B.C., is the usual starting point for Western medicine, and though it is full of magical ideas, it is clearly an early science book, as is *The Yellow Emperor's Classic*.

The separation between these written texts and preliterate medicine is small, almost nonexistent on many points. Both are apparently concerned with pharmacy and the course of disease. Both develop theories of medicine in the context of general theories about nature. Both allow for an active lay practice of medicine, though, with the development of civilized economies, medicine becomes a profession also. The most significant difference is the writing itself, for writing makes for a continuity of biological and chemical speculation from generation to generations, and even cross-culturally, as Persians succeeded Egyptians and Assyrians, and Greeks succeeded all. These early Eurasian civilizations began the documented research into the nature of disease and treatment, and they set the terms and issues which future science then followed.

By contrast, primitive medicine has no center or limits and exists forever in a vast and undifferentiated field. It is in the hands of the shaman and the apothecary, and their cures go back to the beginning of time. We recover this territory, i.e., that such forms existed at all, artificially, in our archaeology and ethnography, as our formal documentation of "mute peoples." These races and tribes are also a well-disguised fiction which is meant to "support us in time from underneath," to explain to us who we are and where we came from. The actual peoples of the past, despite their tombs and bones, are incidental to us now. Science must literally fold back on itself, millennia later, to discover that it has indispensable roots in prehistoric ceremonies and crafts. We are left with a curious paradox: we have forgotten which comes first, primitive medicine or ancient medicine, because we have lived with ancient medicine from our childhood, while we discovered primitive medicine, as it were, just yesterday.

V

The Psychosomatic Dilemma in Western and Native Thought

The mind/body split poses one of the most difficult epistemological and functional problems in medicine. Despite the superficial predilection to classify illnesses as either mental or physical, mental illnesses have central physical components and there is no physical ailment that is not also a mental imbalance of some sort. The disease locus is apparently physical, even in mental disease, but the patient's description of his disease, as well as the scientist's cognition and classification of it, is verbal and mental in its phenomenology.

Logically, then, the cure is also both mental and physical, in *all* disease. Even the most blatantly physical surgery or the densest material dose of a drug has its mental and linguistic components—first in the history of the methodology itself, second in the individual diagnosis, and third in the dynamics of the patient's relationship to the physician and the physician's relationship to the patient. There is also the patient's self-dialogue, on both conscious and unconscious levels, around the disease and the treatment, which is integrated with his psychosomatic response to it.

The body/mind split is central to medicine because it is central to European thought. Matter/spirit is mind/body again; so is matter/energy. Being/language suggests this duality on another axis. As long as a false dichotomy is enforced, the solutions must always be partial.

New Western holistic health models work toward doing away with a body/mind duality, but from a general cosmological standpoint (including the various native medicines of the Earth), their proposed unity is insufficient. What we have assigned to mind and what we have assigned to body, most dramatically in contemporary medicine and its distinction between psychology and physiology, are profound expressions of an over-all cultural boundary. No synthesis can be proposed that does not inherit the limitation as well. Psychosomatic medicines, as well as many holistic health exercises, tend to emphasize the dichotomy they pretend to resolve.

Traditionally, mind includes such things as thoughts, ideas, intentions, visualizations, images, fantasies, and neuroses. Body includes organs, skeletal structure, systems of circulating fluids, kinesthesia, coordination, physical movement, and so on. When all the foregoing are taken as a unit, organs merge with images, fantasies with hormones, intentions with movements in such a way that the systems are interdependent and any particular condition, whether or not an ailment, can be treated on either of its parallel courses, even though there may be satisfactory techniques for only one of them.

In recent years psychiatrists have been abandoning the mental, or insight-trauma-abreaction, approach and replacing it with a drug-based therapy on the assumption that the chemicals of the body take precedent over the thoughts and behavior of the organism. Both approaches emphasize the priority of the split. The idea that a change in chemistry changes also the moods and behavior of the organism has been played to the hilt by drug oriented culture. Psychedelics had their highest appeal in the seeming permeability and simultaneity of body and mind. A profound difficulty followed. By identifying consciousness-changing visions with a chemical change in the sensorium, individuals were trapped in their own definitions of what their inner chemical process was. The visions were the chemicals and were only the chemicals. The potentially vast territories hallucinogens opened up (as in Jívaro vision quest, for instance) were reduced to a cosmic cinema of molecules, cells, and matter unfolding in nature and viewed internally. Western man had his enlarged consciousness, but it was purchased, along with his technology, from a body/mind universe. The Jívaro soul vision, also inspired by hallucinogens (usually *datura*), was never anything less than a penetration of the mainline of cosmic and human destiny. Since the mind/body distinction was not present before the chemicals and the vision, it did not have to dominate their interpretation.

Native medicine does not resolve the mind/body split, or at least *our* mind/body split, because it operates under other forces. When psychoanalytic theory apparently restores to Western medicine the missing psychosomatic element, it does so in a tradition already defined by classical philosophy. Even as we are given an intimation of primordial unconscious powers, we are given a clinical framework in which to apply it. The "unconscious," as psychiatrically defined, includes the things we are and do not know, but, by summarizing them symbolically in a single system, it also continues to keep them out. This is the reason Reichian and Jungian metaphors formed in the Freudian system so early; their originators were trying to make a more authentic, less ethnocentric, unconscious.

Later archetypal psychologists, for instance, saw, in the debris of African and American Indian religion, in European alchemy, and in Oriental philosophy, a reflection of the powerful ancient force of life. They understood that "primitive" peoples lived closer to the meaning of unconscious and primal symbols. Much of the popular literature on mythology, ancient cosmology, and native lore is written on the assumption that we understand them and we "are" them; but we have lost them. "Meaning" and "symbol," however, are Western concepts, and non-Western modes of being have become excuses for psychohistorians, like Mircea Eliade and Joseph Campbell, to carve out new intellectual territory—new territory which expresses the ambition of the West more than the life drama of the native, for it is an ambition to get back to something, to heal ourselves, and to reclaim the internal sense of things now that we have an objective perspective on science and myth.

It is much like the fabled return to nature. Surely we *are* nature. What we go to in the wilderness is our own trained minds. Likewise, what we find in Amerindia is Western symbolic process, a confirmation of Jungian imagery, a treasury of personal images of ecological tranquillity and cosmic harmony. But this is who *we* are, not what *they* are. We must be careful not to seem to steal the religion as we have stolen the land or to claim that we can go back to primary symbolic process in the same way we have pretended to go back to the land. If our visualizations and symbols are to work, they must contain within them exactly those things indigenous to us. We can probably make prettier sand paintings than this, but they won't work.

Phenomena reach us in mind and body, and no doubt in other ways too, but we have no name for them since we consider mind and body a duality comprising a complete system. We would assign those other ways to mind and body also. It is not the Apache "mind," though, by which their whole world and the domain of Earth and Sky was overridden.

The Western mind is psychological and philosophical, composed of primary images and developed ideas. When other things are assigned to this mind, they are either fitted into one of these two categories or considered not *really* to exist. We call the latter either parapsychological or imaginative. The parapsychological comprises a number of possible activities which of course are as paraphysical as they are parapsychological. Telepathy, psychokinesis, astral traveling, future dreaming, and mediumistic trances all involve the mind influencing matter and time in a way that cannot be explained by reality as we know it. The imaginative worlds of music, poetry, expressionist painting, and religious vision are also assigned to mind but in a different way. Psychic phenomena may be scientifically hypothetical, but artistic and spiritual life has no scientific status at all and is usually assigned to an ethnocentric hierarchy of tastes called "aesthetics."

Then what of body? Those who deal professionally with the body —doctors and athletic coaches and physical therapists included—see a functioning unity of organs and systems, of which one, the nervous system, connects mind to the over-all network. Dance is assigned to body and choreography to mind, but a rudimentary description of physical mechanics does not cover the full physiology of the former. Body can be intuitive and imaginative too. Body has resources of creation rivaling mind at its most refined, as in lovemaking and healing. Nothing more centrally expresses the body's creative power than the very fact of its physical existence. The development of a full being from an embryo requires coherence and complexity far more resembling metaphors of mind than of body. Our systems continue to sustain and grow from cell division through a lifetime, even as they retain the ability to cast their seed into other living systems, theoretically to the ends of time itself. Embryology and human growth contain mysteries, mysteries that do not have to be solved for us to embody them, and, by embodying them, to think them without thinking them, to express them, in our analysis of everything else, every moment we live. Beside this deeper mind, the mind of psychology and philosophy is a brief flash of light in an abyss.

Can we speak of movement separate from mind? Can music exist without body? Is telekinesis only the mind pulling? How does the mind even know it exists in order to pull? Is the heart only a pump or was the mediaeval notion of it as the seat of emotions and spirit more appropriate to our human situation? Is meditation the work of the mind or of the body? And healing—is it mindwork or bodywork? If it is both, is it not then neither? For the Apache of the Western Hemisphere and the Aborigine of Australia these problems do not exist. Their science intersects the living entities that make up the world, human and otherwise, in a different plane.

Things which are neither and both are things not in our system. The Jívaro boy and Don Juan both stake their life on a fact that is both mind and body and neither mind nor body, assignable to neither, even by component, as we might assign the impulse behind a dance step to mind and the breathing of meditation to body.

Intelligence is that thing (or name) I will propose for the stuff which embodies all being and through which other entities pass, which most resembles the mind, and which includes most of the components of Western mind. *Spirit* will be its physical counterpart. If both names sound nonphysical, we must remember that they are nonmental too. For coming from our language, they are heir to the mind/body dichotomy, suggesting that we assign to mind (to fantasy and delusion) most of those things whose existence is uncertain.

Although all native medicines have components which translate into our purely physical or purely mental, these same events are integrated in a system of the Intelligence and the Spirit.

The Intelligence is the pure idea or shape of things. It is creation, it is the impulse behind the hunt, the vision quest, it informs a plant of the mode of its own existence, also a stone, or the Moon; it is why atoms and genes seem to be letters in a hidden language, why the embryo grows intelligently, why plants, animals, and stars are arranged in a "philosophy" older than life or man: it does not require Mind in order to be Intelligence. It might also be called "existence," but this word is too neutral, coming as it does from the Latin for "stands," and taking on the sense of a portrait or finished action. Intelligence moves and changes, and that thing which directs its change, however seemingly neutral and accidental and natural, is its Mind—the primary componential Mind, which is also Nature.

The poet Edward Dorn states this in terms of an Apache creation myth: "He is the Sky Man/the agency of the metaphor/the One, who lives above.//He wakes as from a long sleep./He rubs his face & eyes/with both hands, and where/his eyes light, light appears/Everywhere//Above and below/a sea of light."[1]

The Spirit is the physical manifestation of all things—the present shape of hidden impulses and intentions, the body of the planet in process. It includes spirit animals and physical animals, voodoo darts and the arrowlike potency of medicines, ghosts and people, ancestors and relatives, supernatural entities and rivers and mountains and fields. It is where the world most resembles Body, but it is thoroughly endowed with Mind.

Spirit/Intelligence is a false duality also. Just as we develop psychosomatic medicines to express the suspected mind/body unity, native healing and philosophy work toward a unity of something like Intelligence and Spirit. We look at these systems as if they were joining Mind and Body, for they do that too. Our difficulty in understanding them is our traditional difficulty in understanding the unity of Mind and Body as prior, hence irrelevant, to the unity of Intelligence and Spirit. We credit the Indians and Africans, et al., with solving our special problem, and that is truly to damn them with faint praise. They are not interested in our problem, and they perhaps understand us better than we understand them. Intelligence and Spirit are notions totally unfamiliar to us, so we translate them into Mind, and, at best, in rare cases, into Mind/Body. Even if at times we think about native categories expressing them, we do not think *in* them. We translate Cherokee and Bali words into American, but the people do not think of themselves as Cherokee. They are simply "the people." Their world is "the world."

A medicine of Spirit and Intelligence is a medicine of the dynamic process of embodiment and world making, of mind becoming nature, of spirit entering matter. It is the ultimate unity that lies behind the true unity of Mind and Body. This is not the final statement on the situation; it is primarily a suggestion to look more deeply within a dichotomy which influences all our schematizing of healing systems.

Orthodox Western medicine is a particular practice within an objective tradition. Its concreteness is, in fact, its advantage. It is not subject to the same kinds of misuse, fraud, and final court of paradox as native traditional medicine. It deals with specific conditions within specified guidelines. It allows us to have minds and bodies without having to enter the peculiar, weird fiber of creation. We can extrapolate a life from and out of that. We do not have to be Apache or Aborigine, and, from the general outlook that civilized beings have on these cultures, it appears that we do not want to either. All is finally safe as it is. Being an Apache doctor would require being an Apache warrior. Being an Australian doctor in America would mean hunting spirit animals through the outback of the cities. We are well satisfied not to qualify for these adventures. We prefer the life of being governors of the planet, keepers of its history. But we must not pretend to escape the initiation of warriors and, at the same time, lay claim to their great wonders. Taking Apache cosmology and Cherokee medicine in this way is like taking the land but killing its children. We can visit the reservation in mind and body (albeit some barely accomplish that), but we cannot visit the people in Intelligence and Spirit, so we cannot have the treasures. We must find our own treasures on the global marketplace into which time has delivered us.

VI

Practical Ethnomedicine: The Ancient Skills

The previous chapter is an idealization of "planet medicine." It gives a model for understanding the potential sophistication of Stone Age healing, but it does not account for either the actual variety of peoples and environments it purports to represent or the essential primitivity that must go hand in hand with even the most magnificent cosmological refinements. Any ethnomedicine is both an elegant and comprehensive response to social and ecological resources and a patchwork of desperate solutions to an ongoing crisis of health and survival. All systems are technologically limited. Even our own medicines will be judged primitive by those who follow us or perhaps those who visit us from other worlds.

We must not overlook the fact that native medicine contains not only a powerful spiritual attunement we mostly lack but the awkward groping toward tools and principles we have gradually developed over the ages. We must also remember that not all primitives were equally brilliant. Some cultures were more accomplished in the medical arts than others, and, within any culture, some shamans knew their work thoroughly and others dabbled or faked. It is almost as "racist" to consider any aborigine a natural doctor as it is to consider any Afro-American a talented dancer and athlete.

Here, then, we will abandon our utopian overview of the native medical collegium, though we will work back toward it in numerous specific cases. Instead, we will explore the fragments of primitive healing as we have information about them and attempt to find their synchronic and diachronic patterns.

The first and most obvious issue is the division between practical and spiritual medicine. The later and present schism between healing and technological medicine begins in the occupational distinction between faith healers and surgeons, between shamans, medicine men, and voodoo chiefs, on the one hand, and herbalists, wound-dressers, and midwives on the other. On some level, the lineage of healing remains unbroken from the first shamans to Mary Baker Eddy and Oral Roberts; likewise, progressive science, as a tradition, has developed more exact answers to ancient riddles and more appropriate tools for surgery and diagnosis.

The schism is not total. There have been many scientist-healers throughout history—individuals who have cured inspirationally and charismatically and who have also contributed to the practical knowledge of pharmacy and anatomy. Paracelsus, for one, was immersed simultaneously in an ancient priesthood and the nascent experimental sciences of his time.

There are really three different kinds of pragmatic medicines practiced by primitive peoples, and the third is of a somewhat different order than the other two and forms the bridge to spiritual medicine. The two more obvious and intentional kinds are the pharmaceutical and the mechanical.

Pharmaceutical medicine, with its central herbal component, is a universal empirical science. Natural remedies are available to peoples in all habitats. A great variety of sources is used: plants, animals (including fish, insects, and reptiles), rocks and minerals, waters (salt and fresh, surface and subterranean), earths and sands, fossils, and, occasionally, manufactured items. These are administered either as simple substances, as compound substances, or as specially prepared substances. Much of modern pharmacy comes from these ancient remedies, but it is disguised under names of complex compounds and synthetic adaptations. Whether the Western drug industry uses its materials properly (in their compounded and synthesized forms) or whether it has weakened them from ignorance, these remedies were its starting point and are still the staples. Some of them were transmitted directly through the Western tradition, from prehistoric European and Middle Eastern sources; others were picked up from later European contacts with Asian, African, American, Pacific, and Australian peoples. Many of the straightforward ethnobotanical lists for almost every native people that one finds in the library were collected during the nineteenth and early twentieth centuries with either direct or indirect support from pharmaceutical companies.

During the early twentieth century, a new drug industry began to compete with herbalists and botanical doctors and to offer its own medicines. Insofar as we inherit its victory, we are unavoidably misled both as to the degree of traditional remedies in modern pharmacy and the length of time since new medicines "replaced" them. In a sense, they never replaced them, and, if they did, it was just yesterday. It is quite possible that much of the present diversified pharmacy comes not from breakthroughs of science but from a diversionary tactic of the pharmaceutical industry, first in its collective attempt to establish itself as the prime source of drugs in America and second in the attempts of individual companies to outdo their competitors. Thus far, the drug industry has been a fifty- or sixty-year sidetrack from a multimillion-year tradition of planet pharmacy.

Erwin Ackerknecht writes: "It is amazing what an enormous number of effective drugs is known to the primitives. From twenty-five to fifty per cent of their pharmacopoeia is often found to be objectively active. Our knowledge of opium, hashish, hemp, coca, cinchona, eucalyptus, sarsaparilla, acacia, kousso, copaibo, guaiac, jalap, podophyllin, quassia, and many others is a heritage from the primitive."[1]

In fact, up to the twentieth century there was a very vital medical tradition in America (the so-called Eclectic School) based entirely on the adaptation of the North American Indian pharmacy to general public use. Behind this was the common folk belief that remedies native to a locale are most suitable for the individuals living in that locale. A maxim of Asian herbalism, it has been getting fresh attention now that the original Eclectic School is all but dead. West of the Mississippi, notably in naturopathic schools of Oregon and California, courses are being offered again in American Indian native pharmacy amplified by European and Asian herbalism.

Before the general acceptance of American Indian remedies by the drug industry (not, initially, by orthodox doctors), there was universal scorn for the Eclectic tradition, perhaps best summed up by the following statement from Benjamin Rush, an early and prominent American doctor: "We have no discoveries in the materia medica to hope for from the Indians in North America. It would be a reproach to our schools of physic if modern physicians were not more successful than the Indians, even in the treatment of their own diseases."[2]

Time did not bear him out, and among the North American Indian pharmaceuticals adapted by modern medicine were Mayapple (as a laxative), Yellow Jessamine (for tetanus, gonorrhea, headaches, and fevers), Iris, Blue Cohosh, Yellow Dock, Barberry, Indian Hemp, Wahoo, Black Cohosh, Indian Tobacco, Golden Seal, Wild Indigo, Bloodroot, and Spotted Evergreen.[3]

Although there is now general agreement about the efficacy of native pharmaceuticals, there is far less sympathy for the ethnoscience that accompanies it. The usual explanation for the striking "chemical" knowledge of such "backward" peoples is that, during generations of testing materials, groups gradually uncovered workable medicines and dangerous poisons, some of the latter of which were used for murders and fish kills. That is, even if the primitives had no *other* means of discernment, chance cures were inevitable. As the anthropologist George Harley puts it in his discussion of African medicine: "In spite of [the] possible admixture of the magical element, there is no doubt that most remedies . . . have therapeutic value—a value learned, not in laboratories, but by the process of trial and error, in which the successful remedies have been handed down from father to son, or from the midwife to the daughters of the tribe —and continue in use because they are known to work."[4]

We must be suspicious of Ackerknecht's claim of only "twenty-five to fifty per cent" and understand that this means those substances which tested out in modern laboratories. If a substance does not appear objectively efficacious, there are many possible explanations. Perhaps the transmission of information about it was inaccurate and incomplete, and some aspect of the composition or preparation was left out. Perhaps a stage of the preparation was omitted because it was prejudged superstitious. Pharmacists regularly assumed that mythological language or chemically irrelevant instructions were functionally useless. But pharmacy is not so simple. Even the full chemical effects of medicines cannot be extrapolated from conventional tests and formulas. Cultural context determines the range of assimilation of substances, especially substances that have religious or social ramifications. Once we consider the *possible* vital and paraphysical characteristics of substances, the chants, vibrations, rhythms, and sequences of preparation all have ostensible functional consequences. It is not idealistic to assume that a great amount of practical information is always subsumed in "mythological" reference. At very least, ceremony is the original human computer, and myth is a mnemonic device for storing extremely complex and ambiguous data about nature and the world.

Materials can be collected in a number of ways and under a multitude of sanctions: "only in the morning," "from the shady side," "not the first plant, not the second, but the third," "not the lower bark, only the upper bark," "only the petals in the third week of blooming," "under a full moon," and so on. Magical though all of these sound, any of them can have practical ramifications. Preparations differ: the material can be ground up, soaked, pounded, or handled delicately. It can be mixed with other ingredients in different orders. Administration of the medicine can occur in situations ranging from domestic calm to large, adrenalized public ceremonies. It can be given in partial isolation or in concert with other substances or other activities, such as chanting, dancing, fasting, vomiting, etc.

Because all of these phases involve delicate interrelationships, it is impossible to dissociate medicines from their manner of preparation and ingestion. It is therefore impossible to evaluate the different herbal treatments simply by an external pharmacological standard. Some medicines work only in the context of a long and complicated ceremony. So the ceremony requires the herb as much as the herb requires the ceremony.

Before leaving the topic of herbalism, I will quote several examples from different regions and sources. The first one is typical of a thorough ethnomedicinal account. The latter two are more spotty and skimpy, but more typical:

Hawaii[5]

"The pharmacopoeia is very extensive, including mineral, vegetable, and animal elements.

"Some dozen mineral elements, other than fresh and salt water, are used. Salt (*paakai*), particularly Hawaiian red salt, which is colored with dust from red clay strong in ferrous oxide, is made from sea water and hence is rich in iodine. It enters into enemas, purges, and other remedies taken internally, and serves as well as the base for astringents, prophylactics, and counterirritants applied externally.

"Next in importance is a certain red clay (*lepo alaea*) found in only a few pockets or veins on each of the islands and very highly valued by Hawaiians, who will guard the smallest piece with greatest care. It is strong in ferrous oxide and has a rather chalky taste. This red clay, mixed with water and generally compounded with vegetable juices, is drunk to allay all kinds of internal hemorrhages, from the lungs, bowels, or uterus. . . .

"Animal elements to the number of 29 (as counted to date of writing) enter into Hawaiian prescriptions. A few, like spiders' eggs, may represent borrowings from Chinese practice. But others, like sea urchin, lobster, and marine snail are certainly indigenous. The use of the sea urchin in compounds to be taken as tonic for debility is interesting, for this creature's flesh is strong in vitamines. Ashes of human hair and of tortoise shell are used.

"Up to the time of writing this paper, 317 botanical varieties furnishing constituents in remedies have been counted. These include seaweeds and mosses, lichens and moss, water weeds, ferns, grasses, herbs, vines, bushes, and trees. Roots, bulbs, tubers, corms, barks, leaf buds and flower buds, leaves, flowers, fruits and seeds, saps, gums, and resins are used. . . .

"*Popolo* (*Solanum nodiflorum*) is sometimes referred to as 'the foundation of Hawaiian pharmacy.' The raw juice of leaves and ripe berries of the *popolo* is used alone and in compounds for all disorders of the respiratory tract, for skin eruptions, and, when mixed with salt, as a prophylactic and healing agent for cuts and wounds. . . .

"The leaves of the *noni* (*Morinda citrifolia*) are used for sweating when there is fever; crushed or singed, they are applied to bruises, boils, sores, and wounds. The bark of the stem is said to be good for cuts, and the juice of the roots for skin eruptions. The seeds are also mashed and used on cuts. Tiny *noni* fruits, crushed with *popolo* leaves, form a remedy taken internally for womb trouble. . . .

"The oily nut of the *kukui* (*Aleurites moluccana*) eaten raw has a strong cathartic effect. The juice of the bark is used in compounds for asthma. The blossoms and seedlets are also taken raw as cathartics. . . . The fresh leaves serve for poultices on swellings, deep bruises, or other ailments where local concentration of heat and sweating are desired. The oil from the roasted kernel of the nut has many uses: it softens the skin of the pregnant mother's abdomen and of the infant and serves the masseuse as an external lubricant; it becomes an internal lubricant when taken as a laxative or injected (with salt water) as an enema. . . . The *kukui* with long narrow leaves is one of the 'bodies' of Kamapuaa, the legendary lover of Pele.

"Another of the 'bodies' of the hog god, Kamapuaa, is the grass called *kukae puaa* (hog's excrement; *Syntherisma pruriens*). The leaves chewed and swallowed, or juice extracted and compounded with other ingredients, are recommended for stomach and intestinal disorders. Tender shoots are used in a remedy for cataract of the eye. . . ."

BALI[6]

"The violent rainy seasons bring epidemics of tropical fevers, and malaria takes many lives, especially of children. The Balinese attempt to cure the fevers with concoctions of *dadap* leaves, onions, anise, salt, and coal from the hearth, which, after straining, is given to the patient to drink, and he is put to sleep. It is also effective to rub the sides with a paste of mashed *dadap* leaves, onions, anise, and *tinké*, a sort of nutmeg, and to rub the back with coconut oil with scrapings of *dadap* bark. . . . The Balinese love a clear skin and they are disturbed by the prevalent skin disease, from the ugly but harmless *kurab*, a skin discolouration produced by a parasitic fungus, to itches, framboesia, and tenacious tropical ulcers. The *kurab* (called *bulenan* when in small patches) appears as whitish spots on the brown skin and spreads all over if not checked. It is cured by rubbing the affected areas with *lalang* grass, but it has been discovered that it disappears quickly with salicylic alcohol from the Chinese druggists. Itches are cured with lemon juice, coconut oil, and frequent baths in hot water in which *legundi* and *ketawali* leaves are macerated. . . .

"Headaches are cured by massage, but it helps to spray the forehead with a mixture of crushed ginger and mashed bedbugs. For stomach-ache they drink the red infusion of *medarah* bark from Java. A cough is relieved by drinking an infusion of *blimbing buluh* flowers mixed with parched, grated coconut, also sprayed externally on the throat. . . ."

DUTCH GUIANA[7]

"The Bush Negroes possess an extensive system of primitive medicine. Various roots, herbs, and nuts are gathered in the jungle, and their use is mingled with various superstitions. The witch doctor or medicine man who prepares infusions from these herbs holds no exalted position in the esteem of the villagers; he is simply following a particular profession to which no special prestige is attached. . . .

"He prepares several kinds of medicine, among them the *snakee-kutti*, or snake-bite cure. It cures the bites of all reptiles and makes the person immune from future attack. *Snakee-kutti* is made in this way: a venomous snake is killed and the head and the tail-end are cut from the body; the tail is placed in the mouth of the snake and the whole is roasted over a slow fire, along with certain herbs. Incantations accompany the business. After the materials are thoroughly charred they are reduced to a homogeneous powder, which is administered in two ways: first, internally, and second, by making a small incision in the arm and rubbing some of the powder into the wound. . . .

"Minor cuts and wounds may be treated with the bark of the *aproconyo* tree. This is ground up and mixed with the brew prepared from the leaves known as *pekein fol caca* (little rooster)."

The second category of functional ethnomedicine, which I have called mechanical, includes a great variety of techniques. Some of them, such as trephining, scarification, and cupping are extraordinarily ancient and of uncertain usefulness. Processes which apparently arose from some of these, such as acupuncture, bloodletting, and refined forms of massage, are also ancient and current at the same time and represent an evolution of the knowledge of the body.

Surgery is likely the oldest and most typical mechanical technique. Crude surgical methods arise from basic physiology, in crisis situations, or whenever gross physical distress or changes suggest them. Injuries and fractures lead to bandages and splints. Boils and swollen wounds cry out for lancing. Rashes and skin ailments invent their own poultices. Midwifery is perhaps the first surgery; its form is suggested by natural events; from the mechanics of helping a baby out of its mother's body may have come a general science of incision, massage, and exercise.

Surgery was probably born of necessity, but, since then, it has become a tool of the inquiry of modern medicine into the cause of disease and the body's general processes. It now tends to create its own opportunities rather than just respond on an emergency basis.

The most important initial distinction in mechanical ethnomedicine is between surgery and stimulation. Surgery is primarily an emergency manipulation with an emphasis on physical results regardless of how the contact *feels* to the patient. Eventually, with anesthesia, the goal is for the patient not to feel at all. Stimulation, on the other hand, is intended to generate feeling, or feelinglike waves, in the nervous system. Even where there is a physiological goal, as there is in many forms of massage and manipulation, the feeling of the treatment is essential because the patient is responding to his or her system's sensitivity as much as to any gross physical changes.

Manipulation and stimulation mark the poles of mechanical healing. It is at least worth considering whether there is a continuum between them, such that even the most obvious surgery has a stimulating (or deadening) effect on the nervous system (and thus the health), and even the most gentle stimulation has a structural effect on the body. For the latter to be true, in such things as acupuncture and massage, it is necessary to posit some sort of electrical or neural field physically related to the organism and unknown to science. For instance, it is generally believed, among traditional acupuncturists, that subtle changes caused in this field by needles ultimately move the organs of the body and that the field is so sensitive that a skillful physician can alter the internal relationships of the organs in profound ways without even touching the body. We will return to these discussions later, but for now it is necessary to consider mechanical healing, like herbalism, in the context of a possible unknown science.

Paul Pitchford, an American trained in native Chinese medicine, has discussed this in lectures in Berkeley, California. The following is a rough reconstruction of what he says:

"All medicine is making changes in the body. We try to make small changes now so that big changes later will not be necessary. The longer we wait, the bigger the change we have to make. American medicine is involved mainly in big changes, so it waits a long time until drastic action is necessary. The doctor doesn't realize the need for change until it is almost too late. We are going to have to become sensitive to the body to give ourselves time to make small changes. We are going to have to listen to things we have never heard.

"Acupuncture makes very tiny holes in the body. Sometimes acupuncture isn't necessary—pressure is enough. Sometimes even a massage without touching will make profound changes. Surgeons make big holes. They must move the organs like stones. But we mustn't think that is any different than acupuncture. We make small holes and move the organs slight distances without disturbing their rhythm. Surgeons make large holes and move the organs a great distance, but then they wait a long time to act at all."[8]

Aside from explicit reconstructive goals of surgery, the great majority of mechanical healing methods are directed toward either stimulation, relaxation (of an overactive organ), or pulsation (altering the basic rhythm of the muscular and/or nervous systems). Each group has its own variety and range of techniques, but the longest list of different techniques and devices I found is Harley's survey for just one African group (the Mano of West Africa): enema with a long-necked gourd, powder blown up the nose, infusions into the urethra with a long reed, mild juices in the eyes, mud baths, sweat baths, hot medicated baths, splints, fumes, tourniquets, leaves as bandages, incisions over wounds, lying on hot leaves, bloodletting, poultices, chewing without swallowing, and licking small amounts of medicine daily from the finger, plus a basic herbal including effective worming medicines, treatment for skin disease, relief of cough, gas, and constipation, a preventive pharmacy based on swallowing small amounts of poison, and a rudimentary system of vaccination learned from neighbors under Moslem influence.[9]

I will list a number of the more common mechanical techniques, beginning with the mild and moving toward the more roughly manipulative. The scale itself is meant to be suggestive only. In fact, these methods do not lie on a linear axis; some are mild and subtle in different ways from others (for instance, acupuncture is mild with only a minute point of physical contact, but it is also deep and organ-penetrating on the level of the meridians).

BATHING. Bathing as medicine is common in all areas of the world, especially salt-water bathing in the ocean; hot-springs bathing among, for instance, the Pueblo Indians;[10] and stimulation by life-giving stream water.

SWEAT-BATHING. The usual method is to make a special hut beneath which steam or smoke is generated. The patient is bathed in a vapor, sometimes mixed with medicine.

Crow Indian—"He prepared a sweat-bath and . . . then he purified his body again in the smoke of pine needles."[11]

Delaware Indian—"After the fire has burned down sufficiently to form a bed of coals, more logs are added and the rocks, usually limestone, brought in. Twelve stones of medium size are placed in the fire. For handling them, a branch of hickory or any hard wood, about five feet long, is split at one end for use as a fork. After the rocks have been thoroughly heated, water is poured over them to produce steam."[12]

Hawaiian—". . . a little hut made with *hau* branches arched over at the top, presumably erected over a long oven of heated stones. . . . A common practice in treating piles and sometimes in treating a woman who has suffered perineal injury in delivery is to have the patient sit over a vessel containing a steaming decoction of prescribed herbs."[13]

SWEATING. Usually a patient with a fever is wrapped in leaves.[14]

SHAMPOOING. This is part of the treatment of disease in areas as disparate as Southeast Asia,[15] Africa, and the American Southwest[16] where the suds are made from yucca (soap plant) root. Shampooing is used for many different types of diseases and in conjunction with other medicines.

MASSAGE. This treatment is universally favored and, because of its diverse forms, requires a word or two of explanation. Therapeutic massage is more often painful than pleasurable, though the distinction between these two fluctuates; often profound change is initially painful and later more deeply pleasurable. In some cases, the patient cooperates with the doctor, breathing in prescribed ways to relieve congestions and moving muscles by will against pressure.

It is a mistake to think of massage as a muscle treatment: it is a treatment of the internal organs of the body by neuromuscular stimulation. Medicines such as *shiatsu* and chiropractic which claim great range of cure from seeming surface manipulations have a long history of forerunners. Man has always believed in a subtle relationship between muscles, nerves, skeleton, and critical organs.

It is not entirely happenstance that the term "massage" has become a euphemism in our own culture not only for a luxurious treatment, but for prostitution itself; so-called massage parlors are places where sexual pleasure is given under the titillating guise of a massage, or, in some cases, not even under the guise of massage at all, except as a cover. This has two implications: that pleasure is more sought than healing and that pleasure and healing are unconsciously confused with each other.

The latter makes total sense. After all, any contact between humans is potentially therapeutic, a detail which is not overlooked in the subtler systems. Healing by touch is famous, and even the less charismatic doctor imparts warmth and feeling. In our own American vernacular, we speak of physical love as a "medicine"; popular music is filled with such references: "You heal me," "I was sick until you came along," "I'll die without you," and so on. Even *Witch Doctor* and *The Voodoo Man* are love songs. This can be taken either sentimentally or fundamentally. Wilhelm Reich saw through the sentiment and was insistent on the medical importance of sexual intercourse, prescribing it for a variety of diseases, few of them explicitly emotional. It is no mistake to think that the men visiting massage parlors are going to the doctor, and, though few of the women may be involved in conscious healing, the unconscious role is unavoidable. They are unskilled physicians practicing a medicine the body recognizes without the mind. Skilled massage, as well as skilled erotic healing, have extraordinary medicinal effect.

Burmese—"A professional has a most wonderful knowledge of all the tendons and muscles in the human body, and follows them up with a light pressure of the fingers that affords a relief . . ."[17]

Hawaiian—"The exact procedure in Hawaiian massage should probably not be defined more definitely than by saying it consists in both gentle and hard rubbing and stroking, in gentle and vigorous kneading, and in such heroic measures when occasion demands as treading on the backbone of the prone patient with one or both feet."[18]

Called *Lomi,* after the Hawaiian word for "knead," the massage was often done with *lomilomi* sticks—"curved implements of wood with long straight handles and lower ends crooked at an angle of about 45 degrees and flattened. The handle is held with both hands in front over the chest so that the implement curves over one shoulder and the flattened lower end may be pressed and drawn up and down on the upper muscles of the back; or the lower back muscles are massaged by holding the stick so that its crook curves around one or the other side of the body."[19]

The name *"Lomi"* is appropriately preserved in a California school of bodywork and spiritual exercise (the Lomi School) that uses deep tissue massage as a major method. It is literally the school of "kneading."

CUPPING. Very hot cups are applied to the body to bring blood to the surface.[20]

EMETICS. Vomiting is forced, usually by a poison. During the Creek "busk ceremony," the Indians drink a strong hot tea called *assee* (made from cassina leaves) out of a conch shell. There is a special round of drinking for the warriors toward the end of the ceremony, with each participant grunting aloud in a different key after swallowing his portion. This stirs up a very deep regurgitation and simultaneously clears the head and the stomach.[21]

BURNING. Hot irons are used to burn diseases out, and in Bali, fire walking itself is a prescribed healing exercise. The fire is said not to burn when its teeth are taken away by a mantra or prayer.[22]

INCISION. This is one of the most common native practices, with many regional variants. The incision may be a very thin scratch or a deep, painful groove. It may also mean permanent scarification of the body. In some systems, the absolute position of the line on the body is crucial, as, for instance, in Vietnamese medicine, where there are over a thousand vital points, each one related to months, days, and hours by the lunar calendar.[23] A system like this may be ancestral to the even more precise Chinese acupuncture in which needles are inserted without pain or cutting,[24] suggesting that the system may have evolved from an earlier system of incision or trephining joined to a set of astronomical and seasonal correspondences and perhaps an internal geomancy in which power spots on the body are located internally by meditation.

Creek Indian—The Creeks make four deep scratches before drinking herbal medicine during the busk.[25]

Fijian—A short, four-thorned reed is used in the Fiji Islands to cure muscle aches.[26]

Africa—"Throughout the African territories medicine men are well versed in the art of scarification. Fine linear incisions about half an inch long are made in the skin, usually in pairs on the site of pain. Neither medicine man nor patient realizes that, with this treatment and that of cupping, the blood supply to the affected part is increased and so in some instances the remedy is efficacious. Certainly with the incisions into which powdered roots are rubbed the benefit derived is ascribed to the medicines."[27]

Australia—"In south-western New South Wales, other medicine-men, or a cult-hero, performed the central rite in the 'making.' An incision was not made in the postulant's body, but in spite of that, an assistant totem (or familiar) and magical substances such as quartz crystals and mysterious cord, were pressed or rubbed and 'sung' into him. . . .

". . . in Eastern Australia, magical substances and 'agents' were inserted into the postulant either through an abdominal incision, or were rubbed or pressed, and 'sung' into his body and limbs; or the quartz might be inserted in a hole made through his head."[28]

The Australian case brings to mind a point we have made in this book: the magical elements of cures do not prevent the same activities from having a related and simultaneous physiological effect.

BLOODLETTING. What is most enigmatic about this treatment is the assumption that letting blood out of the body releases more of the bad blood and the pressure caused by the disease than it does of the good blood and necessary tension. An ancient Tibetan medical document gives a possible explanation, in an herbal adjunct to the treatment:

"Bloodletting should not be performed before separating the pure from the impure blood; this is done by giving the patient the medicine called *Hbras-bu-gsum-than* which separates good from bad blood, and then bloodletting can be performed."[29]

TREPHINING. This seems most extreme and brutal, but may actually have an ancestral relationship to acupuncture. It involves using a saw to cut disks of bone out of skull or, sometimes, other parts of the skeletal system.

We might consider that just as the modern surgeon is, in spirit, the prehistoric surgeon, the current practitioners of acupuncture, polarity and/or massage are continuing an ancient tradition of manipulation, stimulation, and internal imaging of bodily processes under the direction of a physician.

The third school of practical ethnomedicine exists barely on the functional side of the false functional/spiritual continuum and that primarily because it is the forerunner of psychoanalysis and psychosomatic medicine. My preference here is to call it "psychophysiological healing." What I am describing is basically a healing method in which a shaman combines narrative recapitulation of the disease with the sucking out of the supposed disease entity, usually a feather, piece of down, or like substance. Whether or not the patient suspects the trickery (and clearly he does in many cases), he is drawn into the drama of extracting the externalized, concrete symbol. This is a popular, effective, and almost universal method.

A. P. Elkin explains this in Australian Aborigine terms: "A number of writers refer to the native doctor as an 'imposter,' 'the greatest scamp of the tribe,' or 'as a rule the most cunning man in the tribe and a great humbug.' These opinions are, however, based on superficial observation. When a native doctor sucks a magical bone out of a sick person's abdomen, and shows it to those around and to the patient, he is not a mere charlatan, bluffing his fellows because he introduced and produced the bone at the psychological moment by sleight of hand. Nor is he just play-acting for effect when, having rubbed the affected part of his patient in the 'correct' manner, he gathers an invisible something in his hands, and solemnly walking a few steps away, casts 'it' into the air with a very decided jerk of the arms and opening of the hands. These are two of a number of traditional methods which he has learnt, and in which he and all believe —methods for extracting the ill from the patient, and so giving the latter assurance (often visible) of his cure. . . .

"We should remember that if a medicine-man himself becomes ill, he, too, calls a fellow practitioner to treat him in one of the accepted ways, although he knows all the professional methods (which we might call tricks). But *he* also desires earnestly, like all other sick persons, assurance that the cause of his pain or illness has been extracted and cast away, or that his wandering soul (if that be the diagnosis) has been caught and restored. The actions and chantings and production of 'bones' and 'stones' are but the outward expression and means of the doctor's personal victory over one or both of two factors: first, the malevolent activities of some person practising sorcery on the sick man or woman; and second, the patient's willingness to remain ill or even die."[30]

As with Castaneda's Don Juan, who was a trickster as well as a comedian, something else is happening, something more radical and penetrating than the mechanics of the rite: "He gazes at him silently, after drawing attention to his presence by showing him the feathers—a sign of magical power. He speaks to the spirits and so creates atmosphere, and then gets the patient to gaze through the feathers at his, the doctor's, body, and to see only the latter's 'spirit-man.' "³¹

In the classical version of this kind of healing, the doctor gathers the friends and relatives of the sick person, and, together, they work at healing. He calls up traumatic moments from the past and everyone acknowledges them—violations of taboos, life's griefs. Using a combination of astute intuitions, guesses, striking personifications of questionable data, and actual events he has cleverly researched, he draws the patient into his picture of the illness.

The power of these sessions is not false, certainly not psychologically false, and many scientists have tried to explain the mechanism behind them. Walter B. Cannon's article " 'Voodoo' Death" in 1942 served as a beginning point for inquiry into psychotransference, and many later writers have gone back to it.³²

Cannon points out that death from sorcery is common in an area stretching from Africa to South America and the islands of the Pacific. A variety of especially remarkable cases has been reported throughout Australia. In documented instances, the victim entered the hospital in good health, showing no pathological signs upon examination. The only complaint was that the shaman's bone had been pointed at him. "A spell has been put on me," the Aborigine would say. "I have come here only to die in peace. There is nothing you people, with your medicine, can do to save me." In the ensuing days, he would grow weaker and weaker, but without physical cause. Finally, after death, an autopsy would be performed, without yielding elucidation.

Cannon accepts these reports at face value and so commits himself to figuring out how, in fact, an attack by voodoo could be fatal. For instance, the shock from the awareness of the attack, combined with the terror of social condemnation and alienation, especially in small groups outside whose borders survival was not possible, could cause a drastic response in the victim, much like shock from grief or violence. Profound changes would then take place in the sympathicoadrenal system, with a drop in blood pressure leading to a cutting off of oxygen from the key organs. "In these circumstances," writes Cannon, "they might well die from a true state of shock, in the surgical sense—a shock induced by prolonged and intense emotion."³³

Parapsychologists might ultimately prefer a telepathic delivery of the message, since, in other instances, the victim need not know of the attack in order to be affected by it. But Cannon's article is significant not so much because it offers an ostensible physical explanation for a magical phenomenon, but because it operates on the premise that voodoo *works*. The onus is on *us* to come up with terms that explain it satisfactorily. But the event itself need not be proven. The physical explanation Cannon gives is the only one he can derive: psychosomatic death from social ostracism and fear of a powerful wizard. He thus confers a dignity on a phenomenon that was previously explained as naïve or incomplete observation. "The suggestion which I offer," Cannon affirms at the end, ". . . is that voodoo death may be real, and that it may be explained as due to shocking emotional stress—to obvious or repressed terror."[34] For years afterward, anthropology has gone back to the Cannon hypothesis for new inroads on a puzzling situation.

Lévi-Strauss's 1949 essay, translated into English as "The Sorcerer and His Magic," begins by acknowledging the reality of "voodoo death" and summarizing the Cannon proposition.[35] But Lévi-Strauss is interested in explaining the "psycho-" half of the psychophysical formula: how is belief established in a magical system—belief not only by the victim and community in the power of the magician, but of the magician in his own power.

He retells a heretofore ignored story from Franz Boas' book on the religion of the Kwakiutl Indians of Vancouver Island. We can summarize it more briefly.

An Indian, who is later to take the shaman name Quesalid, does not believe in the medicine men's ability to cure illness. He thinks they are charlatans and intends to expose this. He hangs out with them until they invite him to join their society. Once inside, he learns that they work by a mixture of practical knowledge, acting, and secrets from paid spies. Most notably, he discovers how when the shaman sucks the disease out of the sick one: he conceals a tuft of down in the corner of his mouth which he vomits up, covered with blood from his biting his tongue, at the height of the healing crisis. This hoax is passed off as the extraction of the disease.

Quesalid is now in a position to expose the entire system, but he decides first to learn more. Before he has a chance to make his public statement, he is trapped by circumstance. A sick person, hearing of his apprenticeship, summons him for help. He "succeeds," at least to the satisfaction of this first client and, thereafter, is known as a great healer and hired to cure many other diseases. Although somewhat disturbed by the turn of events, he holds to his original cynicism and passes off his success as the belief of his patients in him.

Numerous successes undermine his cynicism, and he gains a strange confidence and bravado. He transcends methodology and strides around as a healer-at-large. He has no explanation. But he regards the world differently. He sees his power as something authentic, something he has earned.

Eventually, he comes to explore the healing system of the neighboring Koskimo tribe. When he finds out that their doctors do not even produce a bloody down but instead spit into their hands, he is astonished and a bit scandalized. This is even more of a fraud than his own system. And it is a less attractive fraud. Once again, he is trapped by circumstance. Princess Woman-Made-to-Invite of the Koskimo hears of the presence of this great healer. None of her native doctors have been able to cure her, and she wants Quesalid. This situation is handled by his engaging in a contest with the Koskimo shamans before the princess. Quesalid is boastful and superior, anxious to try out his tricks:

"Now I took the water in the cup and rinsed my mouth. After I had rinsed my mouth, I spat the water on the floor near the fire in the middle of the house. Now the four shamans came who had been taking out the sickness of the woman and sat down on each side of me. Also the four praying women came and sat down where they had been sitting before. After I had rinsed my mouth I bent down my head on the back of the sick woman and I did not act roughly when I first sucked, but finally I sucked strongly and I nearly lifted my head. Now I tasted the blood when it came and filled my mouth, coming out of my gums. Now the four women were praying together. Then I lifted my head and I put the blood from my mouth into my hand, among it the down, the pretended sickness. Now I just held the blood in my right hand. . . . When all the blood had come out, I passed it from one hand to the other like a worm with a long round body, the down in my hands being covered with blood. Now this was seen by all the Koskimo and by the sick woman. While it stuck on my hand I was singing my sacred song."[36]

Something is going on here beside fraud, for Woman-Made-to-Invite is cured. She says: "You alone will be my shaman, Quesalid, for you have brought me back to life, although I had already been given up by the shamans of the Koskimo."[37]

The Koskimo shamans, understanding the "falsity" of their own magic, are troubled by this seemingly more authentic system. They argue theory with Quesalid, protesting that the disease is spiritual and can have no physical source, but Quesalid is silent, despite their attempts to lure him into further discussion and even the seductive offers of their daughters. He must next answer the challenge of a doctor in his own tribe of a different clan. Once again he is able to heal the incurable cases of his rival, who begs for the secret, also assuming that Quesalid has found some valid disease object that makes his own stagecraft immoral. Quesalid holds out for an explanation of *his* system, which he gets. It too is rife with sleight of hand and deception. He then refuses to confess his own method, and the poor disgraced doctor goes into exile, returns mad, and dies soon after.

Now Quesalid abandons his career of muckraking and becomes a full-fledged doctor. Not only does he use his knowledge to expose fake shamans, but he comes to believe in the possibility of real ones. He retains a cynical attitude toward the bloody down, defending it as a step in the right direction, but he admits that the killer whale and the toad are the real shaman makers and that the ultimate rectitude rests with them.[38] Surely he understands what this means, even if we do not, for he has been there. The patients know the killer whale and the toad in their own way, and, outside of the objective material equation, these express some truth about curative intelligence and the relation of mind and body, if not about the Linnaean toad and killer whale.

Lévi-Strauss points out the more than superficial similarity between shamanism and psychoanalysis. In both systems, the origin of the disease is relived and, through an emotional participation, the ailment is overcome. In psychoanalysis, the patient retells the event and the psychiatrist listens; in shamanism, the doctor retells the event and the patient listens. However, Lévi-Strauss reminds us, the psychiatrist must undergo, in his training, the same abreaction he requires of the patient in the healing.[39] Shamanism and psychoanalysis share a training: for the shaman it is a dream vision experienced during initiation; for the psychiatrist it is his own psychoanalysis by another doctor. In either case, transmission from the previous generation is more important than explicit understanding of the methodology behind it.

Though neither therapist produces the true disease as a substance in his hand, each locates it in a concrete event, an object or trauma, to which the patient responds immediately. The response itself is crucial and real, even when the method is seemingly a sham. Americans fall for stuff at least as unlikely as the bloody down. The nervous system is what counts, not the mind: the charge can be from a basketball game, a revival meeting, a new car, or a telephone call. The body is pagan and multicultural. At the moment of decision in crisis, it simply responds.

A Kwakiutl patient will react more sensitively and intelligently to a sequence of events within a mythology and sociology with which he is familiar than he will to a supposed Western "biography" of his life, which would omit supernatural and ancestral interconnections and community taboos and obligations. He would rather hear about toad and killer whale than that during childhood his father was aloof and he secretly desired his mother.

"In a certain sense," writes Ackerknecht, "the primitive psychotherapist uses more and stronger weapons than the modern psychotherapist. He works not only with the strength of his own personality. His rite is part of the common faith of the whole community which not seldom assists *in corpore* at his healing act or even participates in singing and dancing. The whole weight of the tribe's religion, myths, history, and community spirit enters into the treatment. Inside and outside the patient he can mobilize strong psychic energies no longer available in modern society."[40]

In other words, shamanism is psychoanalysis, or, since humankind does not lose things altogether but recovers them partially, psychoanalysis is shamanism rediscovered, or those parts of it that continue to refer to our present system.

Let us look at one other different sort of case of psychosomatic "healing," which also enlarges our sense of emetic uses. The African poison ritual, while not literally a medicine, is one of the most famous emetic rites in the world. A man or woman accused of voodoo murder is tried by poison. The defense and the prosecution both have lawyers; the accused's lawyer addresses the poison, asking it to declare the innocence of his client; the prosecution demands of the poison that it do justice and kill the murderer. The prisoner drinks the poison, after which the lawyers continue to argue and the members of the community press around the defendant for the verdict. It is now in *his* hands. If he can somehow neutralize the poison or vomit it up, he is innocent; he is also alive. On the surface, this appears a very unfair trial, at least from a Western judicial standpoint, but, as in all such affairs, we must look twice.

There are various versions of the poison trial in Africa. Harley describes the sasswood ordeal among the Mano. The poison is a dark orange broth made from the bark of the sasswood tree, and the trial is held on a scaffold built beneath the same tree. Harley quotes the head man, who addresses the tree while collecting the poison:

"We are here. We came to call you to settle a dispute. You are a tree that never lies, a tree full of power. You give justice to all alike."[41]

There are countless points at which a bribe can fix the strength of the poison, and even if a direct bribe did not fix it, the unconscious flow of public opinion could direct the brewers. Furthermore, an unsympathetic audience in the court could make the defendant tense enough that he or she would be unable to vomit up the poison.

All of this, however, also suggests that the trial is not fixed. Deep psychophysiological currents underlie the seeming divination. Vomiting the poison is a skill. It may well be, as with a lie detector, that it is difficult to fake innocence, or, in other words, to lie. The physiology of lying works against the physiology of vomiting if they involve different vascular rhythms. Then vomiting becomes truth telling. It is also true that handling poison internally requires medical and martial training.

A trial by poison is extreme, but it suggests a universal attitude: all illnesses are such trials, and the doctor is there as lawyer, to help the sick person marshal his forces against the illness. A sick person is not a murderer, but, in most cultures, even ours, something is transgressed in the act of being sick.

Harley mentions a notable Mano case. "An old woman anxious to show her innocence once drank all twelve cupfuls at one time and vomited it immediately on climbing the scaffold."[42] What a personal triumph!

But now we must put the book in the hands of other more hidden forces.

VII

Spiritual Ethnomedicine: The Works of the Shaman

The primitive world is permeated with spirits of various sorts, and its people live as much among them as among the trees and clouds. Anthropology has used different words to describe this phenomenon: animism, pantheism, and, where it merges with systems of classification, totemism. Spirits have dominion over ceremonies, marriage patterns, crops, hunting, warfare, life, death, healing, science, etc. These animate and sentient manifestations can be ourselves in other forms (i.e., ancestral or unreincarnated); they can be intelligences of another order, interacting with us only incidentally in their business (the stars and planets are sometimes seen as their visible manifestations); or they can be tied to us in a cycle of checks and balances which requires our active participation in maintaining a favorable alliance with them (for instance, in most American Indian societies, plants, animals, rivers, and storms are considered demanding but generous beings in a contingent world). Primitive peoples do not question the irregularity of relations with beings on another plane; they accept such irregularity and develop ritual procedures for maintaining diplomatic relations and initiating younger members of their own society into the discourse.

The distinction between psychophysiological medicine and spiritual medicine blurs, especially for us who lack the latter in our general science. The only Western pragmatic system that has a stake in spiritual medicine is parapsychology. And even parapsychologists work in the relative simplicity of laboratory situations. In the chaos of tribal life nothing can be isolated or proven. Social dynamics cannot be distinguished from supernatural visitations if such should occur.

Spiritual medicine assumes the priority of the spiritual origin of diseases and so attempts to cure them on a spiritual plane. Native doctors do autopsies, study pathology, and know a surprising amount of physiology. But they regard the physicalization of pathology as a late by-product of the real supernatural "infection." African doctors may even locate the seat of a tumor in a corpse and remove it, perhaps to be buried separately, but only because it can corrupt the soul or inflict further curses on the village.[1] It is a spiritual danger, though a physical malignancy. Even this is misleading. To the African doctor, the spiritual and physical worlds work in such complicity that even their twinship is not recognized. Theirs is a unity from start to finish. The physical is simply the spiritual manifested bodily and in matter, sometimes as real entities, sometimes as ghosts and mirages. Any shaman can see this. He does not think: "Here spirit enters into matter." He assumes spirit is always in matter, *is* matter— not only during the disease but from the moment of embodiment and the onset of creation itself.

Earlier we focused on the psychological aspects of shamanism, but here we must consider the parapsychological aspects also. When the shaman removes the disease entity, there is a curative shock on the psychosomatic plane, even if the object produced is a "fake." But the shaman is also trained to observe another plane which we cannot see. If such a plane exists, then we are like blind people trying to explain vision as hallucinations of sound and touch. The following Jívaro example is quite graphic:

"When a curing shaman is called in to treat a patient, his first task is to see if the illness is due to witchcraft. The usual diagnosis and treatment begin with the curing shaman drinking *natemä*, tobacco water, and *pirípiri* in the later afternoon and early evening. These drugs permit him to see into the body of the patient as though it were glass. If the illness is due to sorcery, the curing shaman will see the intruding object within the patient's body clearly enough to determine whether or not he can cure the sickness.

"A shaman sucks magical darts from a patient's body only at night, and in a dark area of the house, for it is only in the dark that he can perceive the drug-induced visions that are the supernatural reality. . . .

"When he is ready to suck, the shaman regurgitates two *tsentsak* into the sides of his throat and mouth. These must be identical to the ones he has seen in the patient's body. He holds one of these in front of the mouth and the other in the rear. They are expected to catch the supernatural aspect of the magical dart that the shaman sucks out of the patient's body. . . . He then 'vomits' out this object and displays it to the patient and his family, saying, 'Now I have sucked it out. Here it is.'

"The non-shamans think that the material object itself is what has been sucked out, and the shaman does not disillusion them. At the same time, he is not lying, because he knows that the only important thing about a *tsentsak* is its supernatural aspect, or essence, which he sincerely believes he has removed from the patient's body."[2]

On one level of perception, diseases are like wild animals and sorcerers who entrap and capture people. They are especially dangerous because they have a spiritual embodiment. They arise spontaneously; they have their own qualities, their own hungers, and when a person has been caught by one of them, these qualities and hungers show through the sick person's personality.

In Vietnam diseases travel as ghosts, dogs, pigs, cats, oxen, and buffalo: "Villagers believe they swarm over the fields after sunset, often getting tangled in the legs of those who tarry too long on the paths."[3]

In Bali diseases have another fleeing visibility:

"Most frequently *leyaks* appear as dancing flames flitting from grave to grave in cemeteries, feeding on newly buried corpses, or as balls of fire and living shadowlike white cloths, but also in the shapes of weird animals: pigs, dogs, monkeys, or tigers. Witches often assume the form of beautiful mute girls who make obscene advances to young men on lonely roads at night. *Leyaks* are, however, progressive and now they are said to prefer more modern shapes for their transformations; motor-cars and bicycles that run in and out of temples without drivers and whose tires pulsate as if breathing. There are even *leyak* airplanes sweeping over the roof-tops after midnight. Children cry during the night because they see *leyaks* that become invisible on approaching to gnaw at their entrails. . . .

"The ever unwilling patients of the modern hospital in Den Pasar claim to have seen strange shadows under doors and flocks of monkeys that grimace at them through the windows; the congregation of sick, magically weakened people naturally attracts legions of *leyaks* and for this reason they fear having to go to the hospital."[4]

In the Fiji Islands, a man described to Dorothy Spencer how his disease approached as a young girl sitting on a fallen log, smoking. She let her *sulu* drop, showing him her genitals. "While they were smoking, he looked at her closely; he saw that she was not a human girl, because her eyes were not quite like those of mortals, her speech was very rapid, and she used archaic words and expressions in talking."[5]

Don Juan warned Carlos about just such people. Only a trained magician can tell spirits from mortals. This Fijian female "disease" seduced her victim, and, after making love to her, he took ill and almost died.

Man's coming into life is a bargain with spirits all the way—spirits who let go of his soul, spirits who give him breath, spirits who battle him and make him sick, spirits who kill him and feed off his remains. The Norwegian anthropologist Knud Rasmussen is given the following lesson by his Eskimo friend Ivaluardjuk:

"All the creatures that we have to kill and eat, all those that we have to strike down and destroy to make clothes for ourselves, have souls, like we have, souls that do not perish with the body, and which must therefore be propitiated lest they should revenge themselves on us for taking away their bodies."[6]

Disease is the primary weapon of the spiritual world, so man's first power is neither fire nor stone, which work in the physical world primarily, but medicine, whose spiritual component sustains its physical being as air in the lungs. Aboriginal man read the world in this context and so became medicine man. From the medicine of spirit power came all other medicines. The code George Harley cites for Africa is confirmed throughout the planet:

"*Nye* is man controlling nature. . . ."[7]

"To the Mano man the medical and religious elements of *nye* are never completely separated, and a certain degree of magic runs through it all. . . ."[8]

"Man bolsters and protects himself from evil human spirits by using *nye*, which is usually the substance and spirit of trees, etc. If a man's soul were so very different from other spirits, the spirit of a tree would have no power over it. Nor would a man seek to strengthen himself by contact with a strong tree such as *wai ba yidi*

which is considered invulnerable because its smooth branny bark
cannot be climbed by monkeys, and because lightning has never
been observed to strike it.

"*Nye* [is] spirit substance, or power under control. . . .⁹

"*Nye* actually does more than fight disease in the interest of the
individual; it also fights tribal calamity in the interest of the community as a whole. Just as *nye*, consisting of the substance and power of
plants and other things, is used in the control of disease and defense
against *wi*, or witchcraft, so *nye*, consisting of human substance and
power, is used in control and aversion of tribal misfortune and the
placation of the spirits of the ancestors."¹⁰

In Fiji the diseases are the manifestation of *vu*; the power that
cures them is *vuniwai*. "Terminologically, magic and medicine are
synonomous."¹¹

In this kind of world, all medicine is either spiritual medicine or
potentially spiritual medicine. All native activity is either spiritual or
potentially spiritual: we are claiming nothing for medicine we would
not claim for boatbuilding. However, in medicine, the spiritual exercise absolutely dominates the technology in a way it cannot in boatbuilding or hunting. The herb doctor, the massagist, and the surgeon
take a back seat to the shaman, the witch doctor, and the master of
voodoo. At least the boatbuilder and hunter construct the basic physical boats and weapons and track down and kill the carapace of their
game. They may require the blessings and protection of the shaman,
but they run their own show. The shaman can absolutely replace the
surgeon and herb doctor, but he cannot send the people off sailing
without a boat.

The spirits can ruin the harvest or give bounteous crops; they can
stir up thunder and lightning or bring soft warm rain; they can wreck
marriages or bless families; they can come from the north or the east
(as the white man did) and totally devastate the land and the people. Shamanistic training is essentially training in how to conduct a
dialogue with the spirits, how to interest them in using their powers
benevolently and sharing them with man.

If we remember that Herman Melville's experiences among native
peoples of the Pacific preceded his writing of *Moby Dick, The
Whale* itself can be understood as an account of supernatural events.
A powerful, perhaps malevolent being hides behind the physical
mask of the white whale. Western man can intuit this, but, without

a dialogue with the supernatural, he is unable to carry on diplomacy. He is, spiritually, a petulant child.[12]

". . . I see in him outrageous strength, with an inscrutable malice sinewing it," says Ahab, says Melville.[13] But for the native, all of nature is so inhabited, and if it is malice, it is also opportunity. It is neither wicked nor incorrigible. It is intelligence of another order going about its own business contiguous with the human world. "Man," writes Melville elsewhere, "seems to have had as little to do with it as nature."[14]

Melville, though he is rarely acknowledged as such, was one of the first American anthropologists to return from the "bush" a believer. Through Ahab, he seems to berate and blaspheme the Church. But he is also the Church's agent returned, to warn "atheistic" civilization about the extent of our spiritual isolation, on which its ministers preach so confidently and vulnerably, given that they are essentially unprepared and unarmed, science equally so.

What's missing in the West is an understanding of the full consequences of an individual human life, to say nothing of entire communities and societies or of the species and life itself. Native medicine stakes its reputation on curing people who must return to spiritual battle, and this means all people, not just priests. Western medicine is based on healing people to go back to jobs and niches. The decay of the cities and the alienation of modern man, the ubiquity of crime and the mass production of meaningless junk: all of these, to the medicine man, are disease, a vast unchecked plague.*

* I say "to the medicine man," meaning from the perspective of another morality. But this contemporary condition is also the fulfillment of many of the medicine man's dreams, especially of power—and literally, insofar as we are our ancestors' realization, physically and magically. The continuum of DNA and culture insures that. The "medicine man" is real, but he is also a fictional character, created by the West to offer its most fundamental self-criticism. Decadent and destructive modern civilization is a myth too. It has a truth to it, and one that is important to this book. In our obsession with the externalization of power, we have suffered a loss in ability to internalize power. On the other hand, any culture gives up some things to gain others. Any culture operates within limitations, unexamined imperatives, cruelnesses, and alienation from something. Just as the African and American Indian were no more backward than nineteenth-century Europe in any absolute sense, so they are no more enlightened than the inhabitants of twentieth-century America in any absolute sense. Both are part of a planetary process that seems, if not inevitable, at least beyond our power to judge or reverse.

This book assumes that the West has lost the key to something. But all peo-

We take it for granted that these are physical, mechanical problems and can be solved by a refinement of industrial and other Enlightenment techniques. We continue to create environmental protection agencies and energy departments and SALT agreements and welfare programs and sedatives. The "natives" continue, out somewhere in the eternal past-present of planet, to wage the spiritual battle. To this day, the Hopis are attempting to send messages about the spiritual crisis in the world to the United Nations, meaning the crisis of real "power"—power transcending nuclear bombs and industrial complexes and partly manifesting through them.

The medicine of the shaman is different because the definition of life is different. The medicine man works on the spirit of the patient; the Western doctor works on his physical body. From a native point of view, our civilization rests on a faulty premise, that the world is physical and mechanical, energy and matter only. We do not pay for it in our bridges, but we pay for it in the meaning of our lives.

Melville's confrontation was neither the first nor the last. Castaneda's experience with Don Juan simply mirrors this. When Carlos is told to kill a rabbit that he has caught in his trap, he refuses. He refuses in classical Western fashion, out of reverence and pity for the singular life of the rabbit and the essentially happenstance event of its becoming snared in *his* trap. Don Juan points out that Carlos has killed many animals in his life, but Carlos responds: ". . . not with my bare hands."[15] Don Juan sees through the physical rabbit. He makes light of the pity and restraint seemingly offered in the rabbit's behalf (and not unlike the pity of the Catholic missionary for the Iroquois war captive as recounted in *Jesuit Relations*). The pity for the rabbit's body shows no respect for its soul. To spare it is to scorn it.

---

ples have lost it, in some way or another. I have no intention of taking an absolute position. I would rather state the different parts of the paradox, for it is from them rather than from any ideological certainty that our lives unfold. I take it that we do not have the answer—not that we have it and do not live it. If we had it, we would live it. There would be no other way. All the rest are ideas that balance our dilemma from one eccentricity or another. All of them are necessary as a map of who we are, despite their over-all internal contradiction. Opinions are cheap, and inevitably transitory and misleading. This book suffers from the initial paradox that, while it describes the loss of healing power in the West, it is itself a product of that civilization, the civilization it is attempting to set outside its own meaning. This cannot finally be true. If the book says anything about non-Western healing, it must also be saying it about Western healing on another level.

"He yelled at me that the rabbit had to die. He said that its roaming in that beautiful desert had come to an end. I had no business stalling, because the power or the spirit that guides rabbits had led that particular one into my trap, right at the edge of twilight. . . .

"I felt nauseated. He very patiently talked to me as if he were talking to a child. He said that the powers that guided men or animals had led that particular rabbit to me, in the same way they will lead me to my own death. He said the rabbit's death had been a gift for me in exactly the same way my own death will be a gift for something or someone else."[16]

Would not the medicine man, archetypally, have the same message for the medical doctor? Heal if you can, with respect—but do not tamper wastefully with disease within a person's destiny. The ostensible result of such cures will be living corpses, individuals who no longer have access to spiritual power because they have bought off a serious disease with their souls.

An important truth is contained here, one whose actual meaning is not explicit because, though we are not primitives or warriors, we still have destinies to live out.

In this context, primitive pharmacy must be seen as both an herbal medicine and a spiritual quintessence. A doctor gains full control over pharmacy by making allies of the spirits who control the plants, animals, stones, and springs from which he makes his tonics. In nature these spirits are free and their power is interwoven with the general power. A naïve herbalist can tap some of this, but a trained shaman can awaken their specific virtues and direct these to a meeting with the disease, all within the aura of a person. In what is otherwise an "innocent" ethnobotany of the Hopi Indians, Alfred Whiting reminds us:

"All the animals, birds, insects, and every living creature, including trees and plants, in the forms in which we ordinarily see them, appear only in masquerade, for, as the Hopi say, all these creatures that share the spark of life with us humans, surely have other homes where they live in human form."[17]

Like diseases, medicines develop distinct qualities in the personality, interacting with diseases on the level of inner hunger where they first occur. Anyone can talk to a sick person, but a medicine man alone, through his medicine, can address a disease. Whether he chants or paints in sand, cuts incisions in the flesh or prepares tonics, he works, ultimately, to establish a link with the disease spirit in its own terms. Making medicine is making power: any medicine man, in his native tongue, will say this. Disease is great power gone wrong. This is fundamental. Medicine is a mastery over the prehuman speech of nature. Shamans intercept messages between agencies of another order, messages humans must intercept anyway, in their depths, by the fine materiality and tuning of their bodies.

The training of doctors is, in most primitive societies, a series of initiations beginning at puberty. It is as protracted and difficult as Western medical training but in a different way. In the western desert of South Australia, where the doctor is also a rainmaker, augurer, and voodoo master, a young initiate is taken from his home by the other doctors (at which time his family mourns him as if he had died); he is blindfolded and fed to a monstrous mythological snake, in the seclusion of whose belly he meditates for many days. The body of the snake, Wonambi, is, at this present time of history anyway, the Djabudi water hole. Later on in the ceremony, the doctors take him into the bush and cover him with red ocher. Fires are lit, and he lies full length before them on his back. At this point, he is said to be a dead man. According to A. P. Elkin's description, the head doctor then "breaks" his neck and his wrists and dislocates his joints at the elbows, the upper thighs, the knees and ankles. It seems improbable that they are actually broken. More likely he is wounded by the charmstone, of black australite, used in this ceremony, and a *maban* shell is placed in each wound, plus additional ones in his ears and the angle of his jaw "so that he can respectively hear [understand], and speak to, everything—spirits, strangers, and birds, and animals." Then a shell is placed in his forehead to give him divine and X-ray vision; one is cut into his neck "so that it may be turned in all directions." A number of them are placed in his stomach to protect him from attack. During this *daramara* rite he is limp, but then he is revived by the singing over him of the doctors.[18]

There can also be medical initiation in a single treatment, as the Mano society for the treatment of snakebite. The initiates learn the correct plants to pick and the proper preparation and application of snake medicine. They also learn how to find and catch snakes, i.e., which snakes to catch by the tail, which by the neck, and how to paralyze them by tapping or spitting on them. But the initiate also learns a whole rite not connected in the usual sense with the handling of snakes—for instance how to behave in the cult house, its passwords, the use of quartz crystal in sending messages, and a variety of other things.[19]

Basically, initiation imposes discipline. Once a shaman gains power, there is no retreat. He must use it or be destroyed by it. This power itself is his medicine. Writes Harley:

"Health of body and of mind are so related that although the so-called medicine-man may be deficient in physical science, his function as a soul-doctor has to be treated as on the whole salutary, given the psychological condition of his patients. His sincerity is attested by the strictness of his training, the severest taboos being judged necessary to preserve his power over the forces of evil."[20]

The medicine man is god, warrior, thief, musician, and doctor. He is the stage master of the healing ceremony, in which medicinal power is derived simultaneously from specific treatment and the mythological context the ceremony creates around the sick person.

By "ceremony" here, we do not mean the sucking ritual of the shaman; we mean a gathering of kin, medical craftsmen, and historians for a participatory healing episode lasting many days. The Navaho case is one of the best documented, so we will stick to it in this discussion.

The central element in the Navaho healing ceremony is the sand painting. This painting represents, simultaneously, the spiritual and physical landscape in which the patient and his illness exist, the etiology of the disease, and the mythology that has been chosen for its cure. Stones, plants, and sacred objects are included inside the painting. Mythological relationships are represented in colored sand. The sand figures may be clouds or snakes or whatever is needed to present the path of the disease through collective ritual space. Dangers and diseases have their place in the matrix too.

Gladys Reichard writes: "[Things] predominantly evil, such as snake, lightning, thunder, coyote may even be invoked. If they have been the cause of misfortune or illness, they alone can correct it."[21]

She goes on to summarize the ritual: "A Navaho ceremony, whatever it may be called, is a combination of many elements—ritualistic items such as the medicine bundle with its sacred contents; prayersticks, made of carefully selected wood and feathers, precious stones, tobacco, water collected from sacred places, a tiny piece of cotton string; song, with its lyrical and musical complexities; sandpaintings, with intricate color, directional and impressionistic symbols; prayer, with stress on order and rhythmic unity; plants, with supernatural qualities defined and personified; body and figure painting; sweating and emetic, with purifactory functions; vigil, with emphasis on concentration and summary."[22]

The chanting and vigil bring the other elements together and get to the heart of the matter. The patient suddenly sees the sickness and his life together, joined in the cosmos, with everyone he knows and cares about singing and praying to that end. The myth is written so that recovery is part of its natural development. "The chant is a recapitulation of scenes in the myth drama. . . . Events of the lower world are remembered and certain episodes are acted out or represented in symbols to preserve the timelessness of power."[23]

Mythology is what holds the ceremony together. The native obsession with the origins of things is not just a charming engagement with tall tales and myth cycles. How things came to be and got their names and powers is the first theorem of spiritual science. Without an understanding of origins, the shaman cannot know essence and is powerless to bless boats, call fish, or plant crops, let alone cure disease. He is not benighted and misled. Like all scientists, he accepts the basic difference between the language used to describe phenomena and the actual phenomena. Mythology is the manual of spiritual science and is more involved in what things are than their precise physical qualities. As Rasmussen's storyteller Orulo explains: "We are content not to understand."[24]

There is tremendous community enthusiasm for these ceremonies. Reichard describes how a young Navaho man will ride fifty miles to bring back a single herb that a chanter needs. The event itself, especially the vigil, is long and monotonous, but no one is bored.

The field of power has the sick person in the center, but everyone in his or her unique state is drawn into the rite. "Since power is to the Navaho like a wave in a pool, always effective though becoming weaker the farther it radiates from chanter and patient, each person in attendance derives benefit from what is done in proportion to his proximity to the ritual."[25]

The larger Navaho ceremony is made up of a number of discrete symbolic events that flow one into another. Reichard has described, with extraordinary thoroughness (800 pages), a single such ceremony, and we can excerpt some brief sections from her account:

"*Thunders and Water Monsters* painting: at the center a blue glass bowl was placed; water was poured into it from the four directions and from above; it was covered with chant lotion herbs, black sand, and four rainbows; then it was sunk into the floor, surrounded by white and yellow outlines, and sprinkled with pollen. The double-tiered clouds at the center correspond in color with the major figures. The Maltese cross is composed of black squash, blue tobacco, blue corn, blue bean.

"The figures are: Black Thunder at the east, Blue Thunder at the west, Pink Water Horse at the south, and Yellow Water Monster at the north. The Thunders' black tails have no rain symbols; they are outlined in white-yellow-blue-red-brown; Yellow Water Monster's tail is outlined in white-blue-black-red. The trail from Water Horse's feet to the center is white."[26]

Earlier in the account, the patient was part of the ceremony and acted in its symbolic space:

"The patient, wearing a piece of unbleached muslin over her shoulders and holding as many as possible of her valued possessions, sat within the corn-meal circle in the hogan, waiting until everything was ready. Then the chanter led the procession to the place of the bundle layout; the patient followed him and the audience followed her—all blanketed and carrying the things they valued most: clothes, small grips, even a baby. At the far end of the hoop arrangement the patient pulled the unbleached muslin over her head, and placed her feet on the bear tracks, then bent over and passed through the hoops; the chanter stood beside the hoop farthest from the hogan. As the patient passed through the black hoop, the chanter pulled the muslin off her head; when she went through the blue hoop, he pulled it off as far as her neck; as she came under the yellow hoop, the muslin was pulled below her shoulders; when she passed through the white hoop, it fell to her waist; and, as she went through the thorny hoop, it fell off completely."[27]

One distinguishing but unnamed element of the Navaho ceremony is visualization, which is also a technique used in Western holistic cures and traditional hermetic medicine. A patient is encouraged to develop images of his own healing process (as in the unfortunate case of the woman with the eye melanoma, cited in Chapter I). The Navaho patient must concentrate on the songs and stories to receive their power. Throughout rural Asia, there are healing images, which people hang on the walls of sick people for either passive or active meditation, for instance, peacocks and hares for headaches.[28]

In a current instance of the Western use of visualization, some cancer patients imagine the cancer cells, the way they form and grow, and the relation of that to themselves and their being sick, and, finally, try to initiate a cure from within by visualizing, in whatever personal or biological imagery they can come up with, a redirection of the malignant cells.

The Westerner must improvise what the native is given by aeons of tradition and mythology. In either case, though, the proper imagery depends on a belief in the process and a trusting of the imagination as real. If that can be done, the course of images will deepen and find its own way. Compare, for instance, part of a magical instruction from Aleister Crowley, a European magus of the early twentieth century:

"Two and twenty times shall he figure to himself that he is bitten by a serpent, feeling even in his body the poison thereof. And let each bite be healed by an eagle or hawk, spreading its wings over his head, and dropping thereon a healing dew. But let the last bite be so terrible a pang at the nape of the neck that he seemeth to die, and let the healing dew be of such virtue that he leapeth to his feet."[29]

If the patient complains, to the Navaho shaman as well as to the visualization doctor, that the illness is more real than the imagination, the answer would have to be that the illness exists also, very powerfully, in the imagination. Certainly cancer is as severe a disease as the Western pragmatist could submit to the test of a seemingly immaterial technique. If the disease is real and its cells are real, why would they respond to the imagination, which is "imaginary"? The answer, Navaho and Western, is that the imagination is the mind of the body as well as of the mind and has access to the same level of reality as the disease. The failure of this method in Western society is really prior to any experiment. Americans are almost born dumb. Skepticism, on a deep subliminal level, is a self-fulfilling prophecy, and even when the patient is enthusiastic, he can undermine the process by never really believing in it. Hoping is far weaker than believing, and passively observing images is different from penetrating through inner visions to their center. It is not a lazy way out; it is so difficult it is rarely tried, except in primitive society which lacks other tools.

Crowley instructed his disciples to imagine deities and spirits under his personal assurance that these were only convincing hallucinations. If the pledges were to be magicians, they came to a point where they understood the apparitions were real.[30]

Everything we have learned so far would tell us that magic and medicine share this issue existentially. The disease "argues" its case within the body, and the body accepts it, for whatever reason of development or crisis. If the body prefers the disease to its health, then nothing can intervene. Ceremonial medicine and magic communicate to the body, to the intelligence—not to the mind. They argue their case, and raw intelligence accepts it or not, regardless of what the person "thinks." Not believing in the ceremony is functionally equivalent to accepting the finality of the disease. Magic and medicine are simply different versions of this exercise.

Aboriginal peoples sense both the nearness of the gods and their skill as doctors. They know that these beings cannot be summoned the way one shouts across a field or prays idly to benign forces. The desire to reach them, to have them be present, must be greater than any fear, lack of faith, or laziness. Trained shamans must be present, with their musical and botanical apprentices.

Nothing is more misleading, though, than to think that the gods come from afar like star dwellers or Olympian strangers. The gods are incarnate. That is why they can heal. The ceremony is a collective invitation to the curative forces to manifest themselves in the personalities of human beings. In our culture, we dress doctors and nurses in neutral costumes, and we forbid them to enter the crisis of possession. We painstakingly ignore the demons. The possibility of possession frightens us and threatens the foundation of our social being. In societies that accept curative possession, it is exactly this profound and disorienting power of the gods that inspires people to call them, to give up their individuality to them. Louis Mars graphically describes the state of possession in a Dahomean voodoo ritual preserved in Haiti:

"And how do the gods manifest themselves?

"They become incarnate in the body of their servants. They eat, drink, speak, and dance in the person of their medium. They are gods who become men throughout the day. Nothing is more common than to meet a spirit at one of these gatherings, and a single individual can experience several successive incarnations during the same meeting. The leader of the ceremony can summon the spirits or send them away. The drummer, because of his talent in beating the drum, can invite the gods to come down from Olympus. . . .

"In the middle of all this confusion of possessed ones and normal dancers, the drums maintain the cadence of the steps under the watchful eye of the priest, who keeps watch over the progression of the ceremony, calling on some to calm their ardor, and bolstering the physical strength of the singers when they begin to falter. . . .

"How condescending these gods are to the men in whom they incarnate themselves, for they borrow men's organic foundation, leaving them with beating hearts gnawed by anxiety, and with the oppression of chests panting in fear."[31]

Yet the gods require men to be happy. They must make men healthy if they are to have health themselves. So they cure.

At the point at which the gods become men, religion also becomes medicine.

Divination is a system that is part of medical diagnosis in a number of cultures and contexts. On the surface, chance operations would seem to be entirely useless, for they encourage passivity and arbitrary choice in place of intelligence, but they are useful for directing attention into avenues it would never seek otherwise. Divination is an admission that man's information is not enough and that he must receive it from other sources. He may go to the gods and spirits, or he may petition nature directly, following coincidences and intersections of meaning.

The Delaware Indian doctor places the chosen medicine in a container of hot water. If it floats, the patient is expected to recover. If it sinks, the ailment will be fatal. Plants are inspected for clues. If the roots are rough, the doctor plans for a difficult case. If they are smooth and well formed, the cure should go easily.[32] The Fiji Island doctor gazes into a bowl of water to find the origin of a disease.[33] The Burmese medical diviner "keeps writing down numbers and characters on his parabaik tablets and rubbing them out, chanting to himself all the time. Sometimes he shakes cowries and seeds together, and when they fall out, decides from their position which of the pictures or rhymes [including a wild figure galloping on a horse, a monkey mounted on a goat, a crow breaking a vessel full of money with its beak] is to be consulted. Each of these gives its own answer, but they are not always as definite in their character as is desirable."[34]

The Navaho system, according to Reichard, combines divination with visualization:

"There are three ways of determining an illness—gazing at sun, moon, or star, listening, and trembling. Listening is nearly, if not quite, extinct; 'motion-in-the-hand' indicates trembling induced by proper ritualistic circumstances. The diviner is seized with shaking, beginning usually with gentle tremors of arms or legs and gradually spreading until the whole body shakes violently. While in a trembling state, the seer loses himself. Guided by his power, he sees a symbol of the ceremony purporting to cure the person for whom he is divining. Gazing may be accompanied by trembling; usually the diviner sees the chant symbol as an after-image of the heavenly body on which he is concentrating."[35]

The Hawaiian system of *iliili* is particularly strange:

"The kahuna laid out pebbles so arranged as to represent the human body and the points on the abdomen that the pupil must be able to feel with his fingers in order to detect the symptoms of various illnesses. When the student's touch had become thoroughly familiarized with pathological abnormalities as represented by the pebbles arranged by the kahuna, he was allowed to perfect his technique by practicing on the sick. The manuscript referred to says in part:

"'In learning this method of diagnosing disease, a pupil was trained by working his fingers over 480 pebbles that we laid down in the shape of a man. And on this pebble shape, he practiced how to feel out with his fingers the different diseases found in man. It was said that by this method of diagnosing, 280 diseases could be found. . . .

"'There were three kinds of pebbles used in learning the art of diagnosing by feeling with the fingers, white, red, and black pebbles. These pebbles were kept in a long gourd called an *olo*.'"[36]

The Method of the Egg is practiced in rural Laos:

"The egg must first be rolled lightly and slowly over the body of the patient, insisting particularly over the aching spot. After a few minutes of this treatment, efforts are made in order to stand the egg on a horizontal board. The operation is repeated until the egg stands somewhat unstably on its appropriate end. At this moment, the operator slightly taps on the board; if the egg topples over the operation has to be repeated.

"If it stands up to the test, the shell of the egg is broken on a clean plate, taking care not to spoil the yolk. . . .

"1. If it is free of any foreign matter, the illness is due to a pathological cause and therefore is of the resort of the quack.

"2. If the yolk is abnormally developed, the illness is due to an evil spirit, and the magician has to be called.

"3. If, however, the yolk is found to contain some impurities, no doubt then that the sick person is under the spell of a sorcerer. In this case, the disease can only be cured with the help of a more skilful sorcerer (witch-doctor)."[37]

Divination puts its trust in hidden inner correspondences which man's peculiar intelligence keeps him from recognizing. Since disease is a mystery and divination is also a mystery, the two seek each other out. Divination may well contain elements of knowledge on an unconscious level, as, for instance, in the poison ritual. Disease diagnosis and weather prediction can make use, simultaneously, of a system of learned signs and symptoms and a system of occult associations, so divination is usually arbitrary only on one level.

There is also an interesting analysis of a very ancient form of hunting augury called "scapulimancy" by Omar Khayyam Moore.[38] In this system, prevalent in the Canadian Arctic, the shoulder blade of the caribou is used to locate the actual animal herds. Prealigned by a traditional method with the hunting territory, the bone is held over the fire to make a map, with cracks occurring where the caribou themselves are ostensibly moving just then. The animal cannot lie.

Because of the probable longevity of this custom in areas of the world where survival is a delicate business, one assumes some sort of empirical efficacy. Moore argues that the divination cuts down on confusion about where to hunt and brings the group together in a suspenseful lottery and that it also randomizes the forays into the territory so that the hunters will not repeat successful or even unsuccessful strategies to which the caribou may have become unconsciously sensitized.

Moore's guess is just a beginning, but it is helpful because it shows that our hasty assumptions about what constitutes useful and strategically promising behavior are not always sound. Roy Rappaport, following Gregory Bateson, has pointed out that purposeful behavior itself is often counterproductive. In seeking immediate goals (food, energy, wealth), men generate unending secondary consequences in the natural and cosmic system of which they are part, a system which is more complex and subtle than their intentions. It is not so much that any one activity or set of goals is in itself disruptive and self-defeating. "Conscious purpose, which aims toward the achievement of specific goals, does not usually take into account the circular structure of cause and effect which characterizes the universe, and this cognitive failure leads to disruption." Rappaport goes on to show that true wisdom may "reside as much in the non-discursive aesthetic sensibility as it does in knowledge."[39] This would include art and religion, as well as divination, for these forms of belief and behavior put their practitioners in touch with the fact of remote hidden consequences and interrelations of events that conscious derivation cannot even imagine. The augurer may pay the usual price in short-term goals, missing the immediate in aiming for the sublime. However, this may not be too large a price to pay. The societies themselves, by their survival until the recent global sprawl of the West, are testimony to the effectiveness of their own systems.

Divination, totemism, and augury are forms of nondiscursive sensibility and pick up things that simple observation misses. In the web of man and nature, which primitive man understands profoundly, nonsense and meaning are mixed and signs and associations replace causal chains. In the development of Western medicine, this kind of analysis has been very common. We need only examine the herbals of Europe to see that the choice of remedy, as recently as three hundred years ago, was made on the basis of mainly nondiscursive clues. We find in William Coles that walnuts are good for curing head ailments because they "have the perfect Signatures of the Head: The outer husk or green Covering, represent the pericranium, or outward skin of the skull, whereon the hair groweth, and therefore salt made of these husks or barks, are exceeding good for wounds in the head. The inner shell hath the Signature of the Skull, and the yellow skin, or Peel, that covereth the Kernell, of the hard Meninga & Pia Mater, which are the thin scarfes that envelope the brain. The Kernel hath the very figure of the Brain, and therefor it is very profitable for the brain. . . . For if the Kernel be bruised, and moystned with the quintessence of Wine, and laid upon the Crown of the Head, it comforts the brain and head mightily. . . . The little holes whereof the leaves of Saint Johns wort are full, doe resemble all the pores of the skin, and therefore it is profitable for all hurts and wounds that can happen thereunto."[40]

This method of discovering pharmaceutical value, known historically as the "Doctrine of Signatures," has obvious difficulties as a final court of appeal. The meaning assigned to a given characteristic may well not be accurate, especially without a microscope for looking inside the chemistry of form. The "correctness" of the native system must be in its classification, simultaneously, of exact human and exact formal qualities, qualities which also intersect in the system of "thought" in which the disease arises. The implication is that the worlds of social man and psychological man are far more dangerous and implicative than the jungle of bears and suns and germs.

The Crow Indians have a rock "medicine" that is simply found, almost as a child might find a coin or a geologist a rare gem. In our cosmology, the event ends with the possession. For the Crow, that is only the beginning. Their most famous rock changed many lives. It was uncanny in gambling. It "led" successful war parties and kept its possessors alive into their eighties and nineties. It also inspired visions, years early, of the coming of cattle and the bizarre houses of the European. The description of its discovery is a matter of recent Crow history:

"This rock medicine was found by One-Child-Woman, wife of Sees-the-Living-Bull, mother of Medicine Crow, and stepmother of Little Nest. Sees-the-Living-Bull, when still a young man, was married to two women. One of them, One-Child-Woman, he neglected, and she finally became so desperate that she decided to leave him.

"Taking her robe and leading her favorite horse, she left camp and went toward the mountains. When some distance from camp she turned her horse loose, saying to it, 'I am going to die on this prairie, but you may roam wherever you wish.'

"She traveled on foot along what is now called Fishtail Creek. Finally she reached the top of a hill where she rested for a while. Suddenly she noticed a glittering object not far away, and she walked to it. Coming close she noticed that it was a remarkable rock with several faces marked upon it. Yet she knew that no Indian had made it. One of these faces resembled her husband, so she thought. Another face was that of a buffalo, a third the face of an eagle, and the fourth resembled a horse. The human face pointed east and the stone was lying in a small depression, surrounded by small stones.

"One-Child-Woman realized she had found a remarkable rock which was undoubtedly a powerful medicine. She sat down near the rock and cried. Then she picked it up, and upon closer examination found that it carried marks of horse and buffalo tracks. Carrying the rock with her she descended the hill. There she found a buffalo wallow and a quantity of buffalo wool. She picked up the wool, wrapped the stone in it and fastened it under her dress against her chest."[41]

It is curious to compare the emotion accompanying the finding of this stone with the power the moon rocks had for Western man. The differences in stones suggest the differences in cultures and times of history. Both mark historic occasions; both are arbitrary geological formations. Western science gains its power from seeming to transcend previous boundaries, while native science gets its power by filling in the equally limitless space internal to its divinatory categories. The rock medicine had some of the emotional impact that the tomb of Philip of Macedon did for the Greek archaeologist who uncovered it. For both, it was an act of touching the roots of the system of time and history in which they existed and from which their lives had meaning.

VIII

Darwinism, Vitalism, New Alchemy, and Parapsychology

Vitalism is, at once, a science, a religious philosophy, and a doctrine which radically alters all other theories of matter and being. It states that life is unique, that it possesses properties in some manner above and beyond its physics and chemistry. In some versions, even inanimate matter contains a slumbering vital force that can be aroused by a form of hermetic chemistry or pharmacy.

There is perhaps no more succinct way to define vitalism than to say it is everything which modern science is not. In fact, vitalism is a nineteenth-century catechism, archaic in both its language and the mechanism that language struggled to represent—ignored after the 1930s. The universal acceptance of Darwinism is what doomed vitalism and continues to. Nothing *marks* contemporary thought more completely than the Darwinist reduction—not necessarily the theories of the man himself, but the translation of those theories into potential laws of science.

Many schools that have found classical Darwinism too simple to handle the complexities of living systems have complexified the theories instead of abandoning them. It is now generally accepted in many scientific quarters that living systems possess aggregate characteristics, emergent properties, that cannot be ascribed to any of their parts, that such systems continue to coalesce into larger and more intricate systems, called "synergistic" in some traditions, and that these higher order systems generate the kinds of special behavior that seemed (to vitalists) to require a metachemical explanation. These would include mobility, reproduction, sentience, intelligence, and civilization.

Vitalism and systems theory are both metaphors or models for the mysteries of nature. Some biologists and anthropologists even believe they are congruent and that the development of systems theory has eliminated the need for vitalism. It is seen as a more precise, elegant, and cybernetic statement of the same events. Despite the fact that it leaves me open to some gratuitous criticism, I have chosen to stick with vitalism here for a number of reasons. First of all, it has a completely different lineage from the biology of systems; it is born outside of Darwinism and continues to represent the possibility of a major rather than a minor revision of the science of nature. As long as it is noncybernetic, it cannot be completely isomorphic with a cybernetic theory. Secondly (which is the same reason restated), vitalism comes closest to the traditional language of the systems I am describing in this book. Since it is not my wish here to modernize that language and try to enforce the ostensible congruency, I will use the vitalistic model with the implicit awareness that other metaphors are also possible. In that sense, I will try to deal with vitalism as though it were *not* archaic and as though it continues to have a stake in the modern world separate of cybernetics and synergy. If the future comes to bury vitalism altogether, then this text will have to be "translated" in order to survive. I am not sure I believe in a future that will not, at least in some quarters, rebel against such a scientific bureaucracy.

A brief summary of the Darwinian universe might go as follows:

The universe is composed of inanimate matter. It was always composed of inanimate matter. At some point in the history of this matter, it condensed and exploded, giving the universe its present geography. There are two climates: hot and cold. The basic universe has no heat. The stars are hot from the condensation. They are the only source of heat.

The planets are small, globular beads from the stars, hot from their relatively recent inclusion in a sun and continued proximity to its fires, cold by their relative lack of density and separation from their source. On these specific planets, chance combinations of matter arise, exist for the duration of their chemical possibility, and disappear by continuing to merge with other chemicals. Event cannot be distinguished from environment, for event *is* environment. This broth of solar matter changes precisely according to laws of chemistry, which themselves are subject to laws of physics. There are no other laws or contingencies. If, from our perspective, the chemical processes seem patterned, it is because there are patterns in our minds, patterns we project onto matter, patterns we now see in the atmosphere of Jupiter. We might even see intention or direction, but this is not possible. What happens, happens only in place of something else which would happen if it did not.

In Darwinian theory, life is said to originate from such inanimate matter, processed in the star cores of the exploding universe and passed in elemental form onto the cooled planets of individual solar systems. For life to originate in this inimical circumstance is nothing short of incredible. It is so incredible it is an embarrassment to those Darwinian scientists, who, themselves, are a product of just this unlikely event. Man is, ironically, an absurd burden to a theory which could not have "evolved" without him. The excuse is that, in an infinite amount of time, anything will happen, even beings with intelligence to know that what is happening would eventually arise and to make a theory acknowledging that fact.

But has an infinite amount of time passed? There is an unacknowledged agreement among many biologists and mathematicians that it has not and that chance occurrence is not sufficient to explain the configuration of living structures on the Earth today. The universe itself is, unfortunately, young enough to present an obstacle to Darwinian theory. The physicist Werner Heisenberg tells the story of the mathematician John von Neumann's debate with a confirmed neo-Darwinist (Von Neumann is known mainly for the formulating of game theory):

"[Von Neumann] led the biologist to the window of his study and said: 'Can you see the beautiful white villa over there on the hill? It arose by pure chance. It took millions of years for the hill to be formed; trees grew, decayed, grew again, and then the wind covered the top of the hill with sand, stones were probably deposited on it by a volcanic process, and accident decreed that they should come to lie on top of one another. And so it went on. I know, of course, that accidental processes through the aeons generally produce quite different results. But on just this one occasion they led to the appearance of this country house, and people moved in and live there at this very moment.' "[1]

A vitalist might laugh and say: "This is the beautiful white villa, this Earth of ours that the Darwinian mechanists have proposed." And this is true, for as unlikely as it is that the villa would be produced by chance, it is a bare step less unlikely that life would arise fortuitously. The Russian astronomer I. S. Shklovskii, in his landmark book *Intelligent Life in the Universe* (the English version done with American exobiologist Carl Sagan), gives the basic odds:

"Four and one half billion years ago the Earth was lifeless. Nowhere—not in the primitive atmosphere, not in the early oceans, nor in the newly forming crust—could even the simplest, most unassuming microorganism be found. Two billion years later, the Earth was fairly teeming with one-celled organisms of appreciable complexity. . . . How? Was it a vastly improbable event which, to our good fortune, occurred by chance in this small corner of the universe, and not elsewhere? Or, starting from the physics and chemistry of the primitive terrestrial environment, was the origin of life a likely event, given only a billion years of random molecular interactions?

". . . the probability of living systems arising, even over 10^9 years, would be $10^{-12} \times 10^9 = 10^{-3}$, a very small number. In this case, we would conclude that the origin of life was a highly improbable event in the time available in the early history of the Earth, and that life is here at all only through an extraordinary stroke of luck."[2]

That particular stroke of luck, later in the book, is considered to be an accidental development of the ability, in some compounds, to distinguish between left-handed and right-handed rotation inside their boundaries. This would have happened, initially, as a spontaneous photochemical response to the polarized light striking the primitive Earth. These compounds would develop a three-dimensional structure with left or right lock and key relationships maintaining their individual integrities. Later, as they came into contact with the environment, the lock and key arrangement would distinguish them from the rest of the external world and allow them to duplicate themselves. Once they were able to reproduce, they would begin to dominate their immediate locale. One hesitates to talk, at this point, about survival of the fittest. The organism would be something more like a chemical anomaly in the environment; as the only such anomaly, it would develop a special relationship with the environment. If it was not absorbed back, it would eventually draw material out of its surroundings to nourish itself, itself separate of everything else. It would not change into the material, any more than we change into our foods; it would change the material into it. These would be the earliest biochemical chains and enzyme systems.[3] Of course, this is not what happened. It is simply an image for how an accidental process might lead to life.

In Heisenberg's account, he next tells the story of Von Neumann's white villa to Niels Bohr, the Danish physicist. Bohr responds:

"Darwinian theory in its present form makes two independent assertions. On the one hand, it states that, through the process of heredity, nature tests ever new living forms, rejecting the great majority and preserving a few suitable ones. This seems to be empirically correct. But there is also the second assertion: that the new forms originate through purely accidental disturbances of the gene structure. This claim is much more questionable, even though we can hardly conceive of an alternative. Von Neumann's argument was, of course, designed to show that, though almost anything can arise by chance in the long run, the probability of this happening in the time we know nature has taken to produce higher organisms is absurdly small. Physical and astrophysical studies tell us that no more than a few thousand million years have passed since the appearance of the most primitive living beings on earth. Now, whether or not accidental mutations and selection are sufficient to produce the most complicated and highly developed organisms during this interval will depend on the time needed to develop a new biological species."[4]

But Bohr knows, as Shklovskii knows, that the time is too short, and that is what makes the whole question interesting to them. A little later, he adds:

"We can admittedly find nothing in physics or chemistry that has even a remote bearing on consciousness. Yet all of us know that there is such a thing as consciousness, simply because we have it ourselves. Hence consciousness must be part of nature, or, more generally, of reality, which means that, quite apart from the laws of physics and chemistry, as laid down in quantum theory, we must also consider laws of quite a different kind."[5]

At this point, the only alternative to an explanation of variation from mutation is vitalism in one or another of its versions. Vitalism assumes that the forms of the world are imparted by a template existing outside of matter as we know it. This entity, or process, in some unknown way, touches the archetypal force of creation and communicates the secret of life to those creatures who then are born.

This process is, of course, permanently inaccessible to scientific measurement.

But, in present-day science, there are no finally hidden conditions; what is not understood simply requires better tools: computer analysis, electron microscopes, tissue samples. Forces from outside nature are impossible.

This is the harsh legacy of Darwinism. It is not an inhumane legacy, for much of enlightened science has sprung from it. It is not even, at heart, an antivitalist legacy. Darwin did not argue the pure chemical basis of life from any profound atheism. He could not find any other influence. The forces that are in evidence, he said, are sufficient to bring this entire world of phenomena into being. That was Darwin's real contribution—not the law of natural selection, which had been postulated many times before—but the statement that there was nothing *but* natural selection. Darwin said, simply, LIFE IS NO SPECIAL CONDITION.

As long as life had its own secret properties, it was possible to have sciences and medicines based on those properties. To paraphrase Thomas Aquinas, we might not have known what they were, but we knew *that* they were. Such notions do not sit well in today's empirical world. Shklovskii's view is standard:

"In primitive times, when very little was understood about the nature of living systems, the most routine biological activities, such as the germination of a seed or the flower of a plant, were attributed to divine intervention. In the early years of the Industrial Revolution, when advances in celestial mechanics gave something close to a complete understanding of the positions and motions of the heavenly bodies, the concept arose that living systems may be nothing more than a particularly intricate kind of clockwork. But when early investigations failed to unveil the clockwork, a kind of ghostly mainspring was invented—the 'vital force.' The vital force was a rebellion from mechanistic biology, an explanation of all that mechanism could not explain, or for which mechanisms could not be found. It also appealed to those who felt debased by the implication they were 'nothing more' than a collection of atoms, that their urges and supposed free wills arose merely from the interaction of an enormously large number of molecules, in a way which, although too complex to use predictively, was, in principle, determined.

"But today, we find no evidence for a vital force; indeed, the concept is very poorly defined, a kind of universal catch-all for anything we cannot explain. The opposite tack—that all living systems are made of atoms and nothing else—has proved a particularly useful idea. An entire, new science of molecular biology has made startling progress and achieved fundamental insights starting from this assumption. And there is nothing debasing in the thought that we are made of atoms alone. We are thereby related to the rest of the universe; and if we are made of the same stuff, more or less, as everything else, then elsewhere there may be things rather like us. We are a tribute to the subtlety of matter."[6]

Vitalism does not challenge the chemical oneness of the universe; in fact, it tends to take this scientific discovery as partial confirmation of its own beliefs; i.e., science has discovered the unity of all things, which vitalism only intuited. However, vitalism takes that unity, as it were, on two planes. The first is physical: the Earth is part of the Sun, the Sun has the chemistry of original matter, bursts of radiation and debris from the cosmos continue to shower the Earth with elements, and galactic and planetary movements keep worlds in their places and set rhythms upon which life on those worlds is based. The second plane is astral or essential: all things have inner bodies; those inner bodies are joined throughout the creation according to affinities and associations; these relationships have no chemical basis (though they are manifested in chemical terms) and pay no heed to relative size of or distance between bodies; the Sun in its essence is the same size as any other planet or moon or person or plant.

Vitalism is the science of the relationships of essence. There are two types of vitalism: biological and hermetic. Biological vitalism vigorously denies any connection with astral planes or occult beliefs. It holds simply that there is a chemistry of life that did not arise from inorganic chemistry; life *is* a special condition, and it has entered the cosmic debris and claimed it for its own ends: direction, shape, freedom, consciousness, and intelligence. This life force is universal and omnipresent and contains the most powerful healing agents possible. In recent centuries, it has been identified, on the borders of biological science, with electricity, radiation, and general energy fields around organisms; but in earlier times, hermetic vitalists read exactly the same characteristics as aspects of the divine or magical specter in nature. Of course, these *can* be the same thing. Either way, medicine is an elixir derived from primary substance.

Hermetic and biological vitalism overlap in a number of ways, but hermetic vitalism is more specifically the quest for a series of acausal relationships between objects—acausal, that is, by the principles of physics and chemistry. Whereas the biological vitalist believes in the single life force and seeks it as an unknown energy within science, the hermetic vitalist understands an enormous variety of occult associations which he derives by intuition and meditation. More important, he has the records of such associations going back for millennia; he can begin his inquiry with the traditionally ascribed affinities in astrology, alchemy, and the traditionary sciences and magics. A great number, perhaps even a majority, of hermetics become so bogged down by the weight and authority of text that they simply expound, superstitiously, the famous connections, which leads these days to an obsession with gross aspects of sun-sign astrology and ritual amulets. But hermetic vitalism is also the discovery of new associations and new dimensions of traditional ones, especially given changes in the world itself and in man's awareness of phenomena. The alert hermetic watches science carefully and borrows images from astronomy, genetics, biochemistry, geology, and botany, for science is a record of unintentional visualizations of the inside of matter (producing, intentionally, a description of externalities). It is also the form which, by hermetic prophecy, explains the current condition and phase of relationships between man and the inside of matter.

Science has often been co-opted by the occult, leading to confusions and distortions on both sides. Medicine is one of the most fertile areas for hermetic vitalism because disease patterns are changing with society and the medical establishment is actively involved in documentation of those changes, and perhaps even complicity in them.

Hermetic pharmacy raises the age-old paradox of the specific, that is, the medicine that works because of its essential relationship to the sick person and/or the disease. Chemical experimentation becomes a wasteful search for impossible combinations; the only source of information about pharmaceutical activity, from a hermetic vitalist perspective, is actual testing of medicines on sick people and the literature describing such testing (though some hermetic vitalists believe that the essential property also lodges somewhere in the shape or

habits of the substance and can be guessed from careful observation).

Paracelsus was one of the most famous occult chemists, and, in his
writings, he denied that it was through any property of hot or cold,
moist or dry, as was traditionally believed, that materials could cure.
They were specifics; they worked from specific unknown qualities
having to do with their own fundamental place in nature. He says:
"In the specifics there are many rare virtues which do not take their
origin from the fact that they are hot or cold, but have an essence
outside of all of these . . ."[7] Another place he says: "So the oil of
cherries and acetum after their digestion produce a laxative, though
neither of them in its own nature has a laxative property . . . Such
specifics are produced out of their own nature by composion of elements. . . ."[8]

In the work of Paracelsus, one finds reference both to specifics and
to general elixir, which he calls "quintessence":

"The quintessence, then, is a certain matter extracted from all
things which Nature has produced, and from everything which has
life corporeally in itself, a matter most subtly purged of all impurities
and mortality, and separated from all the elements. From this it is
evident that the quintessence is, so to say, a nature, a force, a virtue,
and a medicine, once, indeed, shut up within things, but now free
from any domicile and from all outward incorporation. . . .

"Now the fact that the quintessence cures all diseases does not
arise from temperature, but from an innate property, namely, its
great cleanliness and purity, by which, after a wonderful manner, it
alters the body into its own purity, and entirely changes it."[9]

He adds that "each disease requires its own special quintessence,"
though there are some which can be used for any disease.[10]

Throughout the history of science, also, there has been a tradition
of seeking unknown energies, a tradition which, of course, led to the
discovery of chemical compounds, electricity, gravity, magnetism,
etc. Early science, for which alchemy is a prototype, did not distinguish between simple mechanical changes of chemistry and vital
changes of essence. When mechanical change was recategorized and
given its own set of explanations, alchemy and related sciences were
abandoned (historically by the many, that is) in favor of chemistry
and physics. As insight into nature has increased, mainstream scientists have been less and less willing to admit the existence of un-

known energies. Atomic theory has left us with the illusion that research into the infinitesimal will yield the missing relations of cause and effect.

You might ask: What's missing? And, at first glance, nothing is. Every relationship is accounted for, every link of cause and effect is at least tentatively demonstrated. Those things that await description (telekinesis, telepathy, quasars, antimatter, etc.) do not interfere with the daily record of successful experiment and designation. They are rare cases, and life proceeds seemingly without undue attention to them.

We know many things. We know things the alchemists did not know, but we know them about other things than those their actual experiments described.[11] Whether our quest will lead to a concrete formulation of a missing energy or to a wandering about in circles back and forth through our own prejudices and precedents is difficult to know. Medicine is always on the cutting edge of this problem, for a remedy succeeds when the patient is improved, not when the treatment has demonstrated the cause of the disease, which may never be known. Unorthodox methods will always receive more sympathetic audience from those whom necessity has driven outside of convention than from those who must protect the institutions of their scientific heritage and seek consistent explanations for their results.

Meanwhile, "what's missing?" is a question vitalists, hermeticists, and scientists continue to ask. Before psychology and statistics gave birth to parapsychology, some of the most important thinkers in the West were engaged in what we might call "paraphysics." The Rosicrucian scientists of the seventeenth century proposed a kind of solar power that was also an angelic source of light in matter. There was an older Qabbalistic and numerological element to this formulation, but there was also a concerted attempt to understand it in new ways, with respect to the emerging astronomy and physics of the time. Scientists like John Dee, Elias Ashmole, Robert Fludd, Johannes Kepler, and later even Isaac Newton were involved in this tradition. Galileo had marked the first firm step on purely secular ground. These scientists tried to bring characteristics into the world by invoking aspects of their primary nature, such as color, rhythm, shape, affiliation, even as Uriel, Gabriel, and Saturn were invoked in magical and alchemical experiment. The characteristics they hoped to manifest were the same utilitarian ones later revealed by physics: light, motion, transformation, hierarchy, increase, unity. Squares, circles, pyramids, cones, etc., were thought to have intrinsic power, as were combinations of numbers and names, plants and stars. These properties could be released only by an appropriate symbolic arrangement of the constituent elements. If a city was built properly, it would light automatically, have perpetual fountains and inexhaustible wealth, and be impregnable.[12]

Kepler, Newton, and later the physicist Robert Boyle prove the twin meaning of the science of this time. It was angelic and numerological, but it also was objective and mathematical. When we, today, accept the laws of physics and chemistry as they come to us from then, we forget that we have streamlined them and burned off the magical half.

Newton and Boyle were inextricably joined with Philip Sidney and Giordano Bruno in the same professional tradition. It is our choice, not theirs, to make a distinction between Newtonian thought and the thought of Newton, and we might at least consider whether the thought of Newton touches on other problems neither he nor we have yet resolved. One science and philosophy those people made was exploited and confirmed by the future; the other was discarded. For them, though, there was only one science, and when Newton and Kepler discovered the geometric and mathematical laws of nature, they saw them in a full series of which those particular spatial and relational elements were one set, one level of order. From a hermetic point of view, we have found *one* way to light a city and set vehicles in motion, but there are others.

It is pointless to dwell on whether Newton and Kepler really believed these things or whether they were the unknowing victims of religious superstitions which their culture imposed on them. The history of science sees their best work as having transcended the magic they inherited, but it is exactly the longtime association of that magic with science that suggests a possibility we now mainly look back to nostalgically.

The "lost science" occurs in our civilization in a number of ways. People attribute it to the Atlanteans, visitors from outer space, and even the ancient Egyptians and Easter Islanders. In various versions, these magi are said to be able to lift massive weights using intrinsic energy of the Earth and certain shapes (like pyramids) by a system we no longer have. Doctors in this tradition now supposedly dissolve tumors like sugar in water and gardeners grow tomatoes as big as watermelons, both of them tapping power lines of the cosmos that pass through the Earth's field. These lines deliver energy that could not be corrupted in the way we have corrupted and wasted our material fuels and sources of power. This tradition is a myth, neither true nor false but carrying information of another order. Infallibly it says more about us than "them," for if such powers existed, we have certainly lost them, as well as our own sense of our place in time and history; we could not possibly understand the terms for such an event. If the powers did not exist, something else did, or might still, and we are equally cut off from that.

The myth has other versions, less fantastic. For instance, parapsychology, in its many branches, has explored energies which, if they exist, are intermittent and do not follow many of the basic laws of science. They are not "universal"; they are not duplicatable; and they violate fundamental properties of time and space. That is, they are not laws of the science we have. If plants communicate with each other and people dream of the future and lift objects by mental power, we are forced to acknowledge that the twentieth century has two sciences, one revealed and one hidden—even if universal science might ultimately join them into the single universe our senses tell us is here.

The present popularity of books about "psychic discoveries behind the Iron Curtain," "the secret life of plants," "the Kirlian aura," "biological transmutation," etc., is not even as telling as the frequency with which these are referred to in scientific texts, by neurosurgeons, engineers, physicists, and biologists. They are not yet defined enough to be scientific doctrine; yet the attention given them means that scientific problems have also arisen that, at present, have no solution, hence are treated by metaphor with topics in parapsychology and the like. When scientists talk about photography of the aura, fields of energy around plants and crystals, and the geological intuitions of the dowser, it seems that alchemy, as the prototype science for ancient unsolved riddles of nature and matter, still has the greater claim on our future than chemistry.

Whether or not we are headed in such a direction, innovators often reference the past as an omen of the future. For instance, the New Alchemy Institute, which studies wind and solar energy, plant genetics, and fishpond ecosystems, among other things, is named that in express recognition of the Rosicrucians.[13] The members of the institute are committed enough scientists to doubt that the seventeenth-century city could have been lit by squares and circles or that plants have characteristics beyond their biochemical properties. But they do pay homage to the possibility of a miracle within science, a miracle which could change our presently insoluble dilemma of life and resources. They also, perhaps only unconsciously, are acknowledging that a miracle will not be new, and if something like biological transmutation and the making of new elements within living systems is found to be true, it will have also been true then—in the seventeenth century and, in fact, a million or two million years ago— and this may have been intuited by shamans and alchemists.

Psychic healing, homoeopathy, acupuncture, orgone therapy, and various shamanisms and voodoos all suggest there must be an energy outside of contemporary definition. The last two centuries in particular have spawned an international treasure hunt for this energy, a hunt so vast and contradictory in its rules and its goals that it might seem to be a quest for meaning itself in the guise of a palpable and concrete energy source. Certainly the many parallel possibilities of energy, posed in historical sequence, cry out for a single explanation. Wilhelm Reich's later discovery of orgone recalls Luigi Galvani's life force, the mesmerism of Franz Mesmer, the odic force of Karl von Reichenbach, Prosper Blondlot's N rays, Émile Boirac's nerve radioactivity, and innumerable other semielectric, semimagnetic vital energies. Current fashion among parapsychologists is to try to link these by a field theory. Bioplasmic, astral, and spiritual bodies have become, in themselves, a genre of pop literature. Regularly, new models are proposed, showing how these "auras" or "ethers" join and interact with the physical body. Although they are still essentially unknown territory, we "know" them as "electrical" and "magnetic" fields joined by sheaths of energy, wrapped together to form the cosmic body of man.

Healing itself takes place, seemingly, in an astral or plasma body, which transmits it to the physical body in the form of new cells—the same cells which, science tells us, die and are replaced at the rate of five or six million a second, giving the unknown intelligence of our larger body a mode in which to replace pathology with cure. We also know that our bodies are mostly water, the same sensitive and occult water that responds to the moon and the lines of gravitation through the solar system, that shifts its hydrogen and oxygen bonds in curious ways. In the Rosicrucian image, our bodies are universes in themselves placed within the exterior heavens of planets, galaxies, and suns. Within us, there is more empty space than matter. *We* contain solar systems and suns in the minute; we are energy, not substance. We are attunement and phase, not bulk. Unquestionably we are responsive, as flesh, as energy, to subtle forces of nature.

All of this is no doubt correct in a certain sense. It combines the various visions of Hinduism, Buddhism, and the Western occult with modern quantum and relativistic physics and the psychic sciences and includes the languages of the philosophy of reality, science fiction, and avant-garde art. However, it is not where we want to stake our claims which is fortunate, because the territory is already very crowded.

At the same time as we approach a great truth, we get more and more bogged down in our literalisms, our attempts to give one-to-one explanations of things. The ancient astronauts, the conspiracy theories of history (including assassinations), the promotion of LSD as an evolutionary agent, etc., are further examples of attempts to make images for the unknown. It finally does not matter so much whether they are true or false because the elements they contain have not been fully manifested in the processes of nature. Yet peoples' involvement with such theories inevitably traps them in the smokescreen more than in the ongoing world. Intuitions and literalisms contain truths, but they may be different truths from the ones their images seem to betray. There may well be another mystery of which they are passing incomplete visions. Unknown agency, after all, need not be mechanical conspiracy, conscious scheme (of god or space being), or undiscovered energy. The ignorant working out of our own conditions and lives may always be enough to generate complexities and wonders of a profound order.[14] Impossible as it now seems, everything may change in time. We could become the thing we are not, and that alone might resemble, in another way, a thing we were.

In summary, we can say that field theories, so far, have been disappointing. Dozens of books in the last fifteen years alone have explored the similarity of these various systems—vitalist, Eastern and Western occult, homoeopathic, Reichian, parapsychological, etc.—in some combination or other and have offered images of a single energy. Yet they remain only images, blind grasping toward meaning and plot. We are left with a vast world of undiscovered agencies, each of them different, each of them defined by peculiar historical and cultural circumstances. Voodoo (Africa), *chi* (China), *prana* (India), orgone (Reich), *wakonda* (Dakota Sioux), the *astrum*

(Gnostic Europe) need not, finally, be the same things. The unknown science, even if it is single, may be distinguished by the
localism of its effects, its capacity to provide people with forces for
their own systems. *Chi* may always be Chinese, while other healing
energies may have vanished from the Earth forever with the tribes
that practiced them. Despite their tantalizing similarities, these
forces have different heredity and cannot be translated into one another, either in theory or in fact.

In an interview with the parapsychologist Jule Eisenbud, we explored matters of telepathy, voodoo death, and precognition. I asked
him why, if man had these powers, they were not more evident or
accessible: "Did we lose them or have we never really had them
collectively?"

"I have no idea," he replied. "It's beyond me. But you see my own
feeling is that we have a lot of false development, in some way, to
backtrack on, in much the way . . . most people have a lot of backtracking to do to get over hang-ups, bad development in childhood,
the accidents of the way they happened to develop, and I think that
mankind has a lot of backtracking to do too, to get rid of its ways of
looking at things, its ways of feeling and *not feeling* things, its peculiar denial of complicity in each other's lives."[15] Here Eisenbud approached the voodoo issue thirty years later than Cannon (see Chapter VI). A lot had happened in those thirty years for a scientist and
doctor like Eisenbud to go on to say:

". . . thoughts alone can kill; bare, naked thoughts; isn't all this
armor of war, this machinery, these bombs, aren't they all grotesque
exaggerations? We don't even need them . . .

"To put it schematically, and simplistically, and almost absurdly,
because we don't wish to realize that we can just kill with our minds,
we go through this whole enormous play of killing with such, of
overkilling with such overimplementation; it gets greater and greater
and greater as if . . . it's a caricature of saying: how can I do it with
my mind; I need tanks; I need B-52 bombers; I need napalm, and so
on, and so on. . . . I have examples of people who died this way.
Not that I could see them do it, but if I put together the jigsaw, it
looks as though this one was responsible for that event."[16]

At this point I mentioned Cannon's article " 'Voodoo' Death,"
but Eisenbud was markedly impatient with that:

"Yes, of course, of course. But the whole point is that there a man deliberately said, 'I'm going to kill you.' We mask it. It goes on unobtrusively. Which doesn't make a damn bit of difference. What's the difference whether I do it or streptococci do it. We have cover stories, you see. All science has produced cover stories for the deaths we create; it's streptococci; it's accidents, and so on. But, what I'm trying to say is, there must be, I feel, a relationship between this truth, which we will not see, and this absurd burlesque of aggression that goes on all around us, as if we're trying to deny that the other is possible."[17]

The implication could not be more serious: All science has produced cover stories for the deaths we create.

But what can kill can also cure, and these weapons may also be the weapons of healing under other circumstances.

IX

Elements and Humors

Elements are primary units of nature. They give matter all its qualities, ranging from the striations of stone and the color and taste of a beet to the flight of a bird and the lilt in someone's laugh. They are underlying predispositions to form that nature realizes at all its levels of being.

The easiest misunderstanding that one can have about the four original elements of Greek science is that they represent crude but absolute versions of earth, air, fire, and water—i.e., raw soil, gases and volatile things, fire and light, and wetness. In truth, they are unknown as absolutes. Manifested in substance, they take on idiosyncratic local aspects. They are always mixed with each other, and there is no substance that does not contain all four. What we know as air is the aery part of the atmosphere. Lightning is a warm and dry manifestation of fire, but snow also has fire in it, cold and dry fire. The earthen soil gives rise to plants, some of them fiery, some of them cold and moist, some of them dense and clayey, and some of them airlike and ethereal. Earth, air, fire, and water are each expressed in the roots, the branches, the flowers, the fruits, the tropisms, and then again in the over-all coherence of the plant and the properties of medicines made from it.

The elements are in constant motion and flux throughout nature, and nothing that is made of them can remain fixed, as Heraclitus describes: "Fire lives in the death of earth, air in the death of fire, water in the death of air, and earth in the death of water."[1]

Superficially, elementalism seems identical to Vitalism, but, in fact, the elements may express either vital qualities, as in all the ancient systems of Europe and Asia, or simply the structural-mechanical basis of matter, as in the periodic table of modern chemistry. The priority in elementalism is the origin of the basic properties of substance: What is matter? How does it come to have structure at all? How do qualities become mixed and dynamic in nature? How does human life occur from raw material? How is it sustained? And of what is mind made?

There are Vitalist answers to these, and there are also physical explanations. As chemistry in the West became more sophisticated, many "vital" properties were reassigned to compounds, and later molecules. The dilemma of how these properties first came into being remains a Vitalist stronghold, but it is ignored by science as long as most of their interactions can be explained by their inherent material characteristics.

Traditionally, the elements express themselves in human beings through the humors, which are the complex elements of life. The humors respond to environment, diet, habits, and emotional states. They transmit the temperaments and psychic "meaning" of the elements. Man observes the elements, as lightning in the stormy sky followed by mushrooms on damp logs after the rain, but he also feels them circulating within him, passing from one state to another. When they get out of balance, he experiences distortion, though he may not know exactly what it is. The following account is from the Hippocratic writings:

"The human body contains blood, phlegm, yellow bile, and black bile: these constitute the nature of the body, and through them a man suffers pain or enjoys health. A man enjoys the most perfect health when these elements are duly proportioned to one another in power, bulk, and manner of compounding, so that they are mingled as excellently as possible. Pain is felt when one of these elements is either deficient or excessive, or when it is isolated in the body without being compounded with the others."[2]

It is an oversimplification to think of the humors as only the premicroscopic forerunners of a real chemistry of the body. They describe features of mental and physical life that no other system describes; they are a statement of the human imagination of the fluidity, layering, and process going on in the thick, wet layers within. They were real then and they remain real today, particularly as expressions of personality traits and peculiar psychosomatic relationships between emotions, such as anger and melancholia, and chronic illnesses, such as ulcers and arthritis. These continue to be perceived as approximate and humoral. In a sense, the humors are like spirits, are phenomenological insights into the condition of being alive.

The Eurasian elemental system is basic to Old World thought, and it has given rise to a variety of different sciences and medicines. For instance, in Tibet, the three humors are Air, Bile, and Phlegm, as roughly translated into English terms with different connotations.[3]

Air originates in the abdomen, but it has five seats in the body. The Air from the abdomen is important, for it transforms food into nutrition. Brain Air aids in breathing and vision. Chest Air is turned into speech and memory. Heart Air subtly enlivens the whole body. Intestinal Air passes into stool, urine, sperm, and menstrual blood, and it is also felt within as sexual desire.

After the Air of the brain blows food down the gullet to the stomach, the Bile there, aroused by abdomen Air, separates the food into sediment for the intestines and nourishment for the body. Abdominal Phlegm and liver Bile turn the nutrition into blood, some of which remains in the liver and some of which is passed to the different parts of the body as flesh. This begins to answer the question, How is man made of elements?

Refined flesh forms fat and bones, and unrefined flesh is secreted by the body. Refined fat crystallizes along the skeleton, the unrefined part of which becomes the precious oils of the body, some of which are perspired away. The refined part becomes marrow. Refined marrow becomes sperm and egg. Refined sperm passes into the deep center of the heart, where it is life itself, and longevity. Unrefined bone and skeleton become teeth, nails, and hair. Unrefined marrow forms the flesh around the anus, and unrefined sperm is charged by intestinal Air with desire and discharged during intercourse, along with unrefined ovary.

Bile from the heart is translated by the organism into self-awareness and wisdom. Bile in the eyes sees. Bile in the skin is color.

Phlegm originates in the chest, preventing thirst. Tongue Phlegm is the flavor of food. Head Phlegm emerges in the orifices as the sense organs, the eyes, the nostrils, the ear sockets, the tongue, and the skin. Joint Phlegm makes movement at the junctures possible.

There is accurate physiological information in this material, but there is also being and vitality, which merges with the mechanical and chemical operations of the body. Air is not only the respiration of the lungs; it is the will to life, the spark of thought, and the coordination of nerves. Air can also be desire. Bile is the chemistry of digestion, but it is also the sharpness and focus of sight; it is ego and self-perception, it is vibrancy of the blood and brightness of the skin. Phlegm is a liquid and a flavor, and it is also the variety and relationship of the senses; it is movement at the critical points that hold movement together.

Life itself is a function of the continuous transformation of elements and humors into each other. If the organism is in harmony with the transformation, it is healthy. Any excesses in life-style or diet will distort the transformation and cause an excess of fluid or flesh somewhere in the organism. Since the humors are psychological and cognitive as well as physical, the system does not recognize a functional difference between the planned intention of the organism and the unconscious expression of the organism in flesh. The age-old question of which comes first—the pathology or the pathological behavior—is either unanswered or answered by the fact that they are identical humoral distortions. Disease is first an elemental imbalance, afterward a pathology.

Chinese "science" shares in Eurasian elementalism, but integrates it with what-may-be an even older native East Asian cosmology of Yin and Yang:[4]

"The principle of Yin and Yang is the basic principle of the entire universe. It is the principle of everything in creation. It brings about the transformation to parenthood; it is the root and source of life and death; and it is also found within the temples of the gods.

"In order to treat and cure diseases one must search into their origin.

"Heaven was created by an accumulation of Yang, the element of light; Earth was created by an accumulation of Yin, the element of darkness."[5]

Yin and Yang are simple to understand on one level, extremely difficult on another. Where the contrasts are sharp, we can see them; but in most of creation, Yin and Yang are integrated and indistinguishable.

If Yang is the bright day, Yin is the night that must end it. Yang is clearness; Yin is cloudiness. Yang is spring and summer; autumn and winter are Yin. Fire, of course, is Yang, very Yang: light, Yang; sun, Yang. Water, dark, and moon are Yin.

Yang is the body surface, Yin its interior. Yang rises to the upper levels; Yin sinks. Male is slightly more Yang; female is a predominance of Yin. Yang accumulates, compresses, solidifies, holds, thickens, integrates, fattens—on any level of creation. The gravity that drives the hydrogen fire in the center of a star is the same Yang as the coherence of thought. Yin, on the other hand, distributes the light of the star and connects thought to nature and form. It blows out, puffs, softens, disperses. Because Yang is all the time hardening and materializing, Yin *must* disintegrate, lighten, loosen. There is finally only one force, with two poles of expression. As soon as one polar opposite manifests, its counter must come into simultaneous and equivalent being.

There is no good substance or bad substance. Anything in excess is dangerous. Sickness occurs when the underlying forces are not balanced. But sickness is not itself the imbalance; it is the resistance that basic energy must dissipate in restoring its own equilibrium. The ruthlessness of pathology is real enough on one level, but on another level is an illusion. After all, Yin and Yang are responsible for maintaining the universe, not for making life easier for people on the Earth. It has no charitable dispensations. If the organism resists, the flow cannot waste a second before it begins to restore the balance. Otherwise, at any moment, in any galaxy, an imbalance might develop and spread to the rest of creation.

"Yin stores up essence and prepares it to be used; Yang serves as protector against external danger and must therefore be strong. If Yin is not equal to Yang, then the pulse becomes weak and sickly and causes madness. If Yang is not equal to Yin, then the breaths which are contained in the five viscera will conflict with each other and the circulation ceases within the nine orifices. For this reason the sages caused Yin and Yang to be in harmony."[6]

The traditional healing methods of the Far East (China, Tibet, Japan, etc.) directly apply elemental theory, either by external techniques to modify energy flow (acupuncture, moxibustion, cupping, *shiatsu*; see below) or internal remedies (mostly herbs). Even the martial system of *t'ai chi* is based on restoring health (and with it, fighting ability) through an understanding and embodiment of Yin/Yang principles.

The meridians of the body are more important than the organs themselves, for it is through them that elemental energy passes. The restoration of balance is a result of the modification of flow rather than the initiation of a concrete change in an organ. The treatments appear physical because physical tools and techniques are used, but the intention is to adjust the flow of *chi*, or vital force.

Individual organs are joined along meridians, and then meridians are paired and assigned to Yin or Yang at different levels. For instance, under Sunlight Yang, the stomach meridian runs along the leg and joins the large-intestine meridian on the arm. Under Absolute Yin, the liver meridian runs from the leg into the pericardium meridian on the arm. Then each of the five elements is assigned to one Yin and one Yang meridian, such as fire to the heart (Yin) and the small intestine (Yang).

The qualities of Yin and Yang are the basis of the organs. We think we perceive the solid parts and cavities of our interior, but what we experience is the tide and pulse of humors passing along meridians. If the liver is inflamed, wood is literally on fire, and an acupuncture point must be chosen to douse that fire (i.e., to sedate flow). Disease of the liver can also come from the lungs, which are metal, for decayed metal (air) stirs up the wood. Stimulation of earth (stomach and spleen) creates fresh metal.

The system of correspondences goes well beyond this, to include colors, musical notes, associated planets, animals, odors, emotions, etc. Then the body is divided into four seas of energy which flow into the *chi*, and the *chi* itself circulates through the meridians as the hours pass, from the lungs to the large intestine at 5 A.M., then to the stomach at 7 A.M., then to the spleen, the heart at 11 A.M., and so on. Diseases can arise from intense weather—excessive heat or dampness, cold entering the pores of the body through the skin and getting directly into the meridians. The physical wind dilates the pores and brings on the element wind, Yang-Penetrating Wind, which breeds headaches and slows the pulse. Dryness in autumn conceals its own deeper dryness, which parches, cracks, and convulses.

Emotions affect elemental circulation. "Joy injures the heart, anger injures the liver, over-concentration injures the spleen, anxiety injures the lungs, fear injures the kidneys."[7] We do not have to take these rigidly or literally to know what they mean.

The relation between elements and meridians might seem totally mythological without the Asian embryological cosmology. When the fetus is still shaped like a fish, the vein of life begins to sprout between its chest and navel. Branching slowly through the curd of semen and menstrual blood upward along the middle artery of the body, it forms the vertebrae and trails a plexus of tender veins at the right of the sixteenth vertebra of the back and, later, the first vertebra of the neck. From there it rises like smoke, like a snake, to the crown of the head, leaving a plexus and the faint beginnings of sight. Another plexus forms at the heart, one at the navel, and one at the sexual organs.

During the second and third month, the arms and hips and orifices form. The organs become outlined: heart, lungs, liver, spleen, and kidneys; after these, gall bladder, stomach, intestines, urinary bladder, and uterus or spermatic vessels. In the fourth month, the arms are threaded out, and the legs and palms emerge. Ten fingers and ten toes begin growing. Fat, flesh, glands, and sinews differentiate from the remaining curd.

During the twenty-first week, the system of internal air is sealed and a fine film forms on the top of the body, which becomes the skin. In the sixth month the sense organs are completed, so that feelings and emotions begin to gather. The mind becomes extraordinarily clear, and the previous life is visible. It sees that it was "under the illusion there was rain and cold and thunderstorms" and that "people drove it [here]" to "seek shelter in the mother's womb as if it was entering a leafy hut or an earth hole or a cave or a clearing in the jungle."[8] The actual birth will remove this clarity.

Embryology lays the basis for life; and post-embryology is simply the life of the embryo continued in the world. Healing thus maintains a prenatal perspective.

The raw tissue is relatively undifferentiated in the womb. There are rough versions of heart, spinal cord, and gut; and these are imprinted and then carved out by the movement of vital humors along the veins and nerve paths that sprout as they form. Vital connections, such as that between the kidney and the uterus and testicles, or between the throat, esophagus, and stomach, remain from this stage. More subtly, as the body unwraps from its central core, the streams that unwrap it remain active, continuing to hold arms and legs to heart and lungs, brains to stomach and spleen, eyes to hands, etc. The body is the concrescence and fleshing of embryological branchways, and, conversely, the meridian system is the ancient and original connector that maintains the hidden affinities. The contemporary material is the organism, and the meridians are its archaeo-dynamic rivers, currents, and channels. They maintain the functional prenatal intimacy of the organs in terms of the structural anatomy and unity of the body.

The fine needles of acupuncture are not so much physical inter-cessions, or even exciters or sedaters, as they are telegraph keys by means of which messages are sent through the embryological chan-nels from stations called "points." They are of different lengths, di-ameters, shapes, and materials; they can be inserted quickly and removed or left in and twisted and vibrated, the latter by rapid lift-ing and lowering. After application, the virtually invisible hole is "closed" by slight pressure and massage. In certain diseases a cone of herbs is burnt over the point; ginger and garlic are most often used. This is called "moxibustion." Cupping with small jars is another method of directing flow; a vacuum is produced in a jar by heat, and then it is attached to the skin. In Japanese *shiatsu*, finger and espe-cially thumb pressure is used on acupuncture points; the advantage is that there is direct contact between doctor and patient, and the treatment incorporates massage, with corresponding effects on the nerves and muscles.

A 1975 Chinese government English-language publication de-scribes the points themselves:

"Points are spots on the body surface through which the vital func-tion of the viscera and channels are transferred to the superficial parts of the body. They communicate with the viscera, sense organs and tis-sues through the channels. By applying acupuncture or moxibustion at these points, the channels may perform their function in evoking the intrinsic body resistance by regulating the vital energy of the vis-cera, the circulation of qi (chi) and blood, and so cure disease.

"The points of the Fourteen Channels are known as the Regular Points and include most of the points on the body surface. . . .

"Those points that are not listed in the Fourteen Channels are called the Extraordinary Points."⁹

First, there is a series of meridians which flow from the chest over the abdomen, down the inside of the legs to the toes, and down the inside of the arms to the fingers. This set is Yin and, in the upper half of the torso, includes pericardium, heart, and lungs; in the lower half, spleen, kidney, and liver. The Yang meridians go from the head and face down the surface of the arms and legs to the fingertips and toes; they include the upper meridians of small and large intestines and the so-called triple-warmer meridian which regulates metabolic functions (see below) and the lower meridians of stomach, bladder, and gall bladder.

It is important to remember that these are meridians, not organs; as channels they are each given the name of one of the ports they connect. A stomach ailment may be cured on the lung meridian passing through the arm because the ailment rightly belongs on that channel even though it is perceived as the stomach and even though it may have stomach pathology. As all of these points and lines are connected, they pass into and out of specific organs that have solidified from the active humoral fluid. The formative position of the organ may take precedent over its later anatomy. The distances between single organs, or at least our versions of organs, may be overridden by meridianal association. Likewise, space not absolutely lying in an organ may remain in its over-all sphere. Feeling, with its accompanying description of a disorder, is not always an accurate guide to where the current is blocked. The pain may be felt intestinally, but the crisis, or entry, may be in the toe. The triple warmer, sometimes called the "three-burning spaces," which does not suggest any specific function, presents a more accurate image of what a meridian is than one that *seems* to correspond to a known organ. In some writings it is said not to have a form at all, whereas other writings describe it as fatty tissue. It is variously identified as rhythm, breath, temperature, metabolism, sewage, and a link between man and the universe.

The twelve major meridians can be conceptualized as a series of three connected cycles. The first starts with the lung on the chest and goes down the outside front of the arm to the thumb; there the large intestine picks up at the tip of the index finger and proceeds along the outside back of the arm to the nose. The stomach picks it up just beneath the eye and goes along the edge of the cheek, across the throat, down the chest and outside of the front of the leg, ending at the second toe. The spleen begins at the big toe, which has been twisted from its prenatal outside position to the inside of the foot, goes up the front of the abdomen and chest, ending just inside where the lung part of the cycle begins. In this, and the other two cycles, there are various branches, plus partial meridians that form like creases in the main turbulence, carrying impulses between meridians and distributing them to the most divergent parts of the body; in the end, every point is in the center.

The second cycle of meridians begins with the heart on the anterior surface of the chest; it runs down the inside front of the arm to end at the little finger where the small intestine begins. It proceeds up the other way, on the inside back of the arm, across the shoulder, to the cheek. The bladder line begins at the nose, goes past the eye, up over the forehead, down the center of the back in two main branches, down the back inside of the leg, to end at the inside of the embryo, which has been twisted outward into the little toe. The kidney starts on the sole of the foot and runs up the inside of the front of the leg, the abdomen, and the chest, to end near the heart. We can picture each of these systems as expressing either a prenatal unity or a mythology of a prenatal unity, which might be a physiospiritual unity. Although all meridians have their connecting points and watersheds and far-reaching distributions across the body, the triunity suggests three complicated unfoldments of the body like three layers, three creatures, each continuing to channel a coherent stream through the organs that lie in its course.

The third cycle begins with the pericardium, which is the membranous sac around the heart. It continues through the middle of the front of the arm between the heart and lung lines, draining and beginning again at the middle finger. The triple warmer originates on the fourth fingertip and passes up the middle back of the arm between the large and small intestines, draining at the ear. The gall bladder begins beside the ear and runs down the back between the stomach and bladder to the fourth toetip. The liver begins on the side of the big toe, and its course goes up the middle of the leg, the abdomen, and the chest, between spleen and kidney, and ends near the lung on the chest.

This is the rough external map of the meridian bodies. The internal geography is far more complicated. Each point has a variety of influences, and though it lies on one meridian, it may, of course, be stimulated or dulled to effect points, secondarily, on other meridians. There are also single points of great power, classically kept secret because of their danger. There are points which lie on more than one meridian, and points which work in concert to produce strong effects or to reach more deeply into the interior of the body, as well as anteriorly, into the organism's history. The spleen branches into the heart, and the kidney and bladder circulate together at some points of their routes. When several lines pass through a region, as the back and gums, it takes very subtle judgment to know which channel to ascribe a certain difficulty to.

There are also two additional main meridians; the governing vessel originates between the tip of the coccyx and the anus and runs directly up along the vertebrae and the center of the back to its twentieth point at the tip of the head. It has seven additional points continuing down the forehead to the tip of the nose and ending at the upper gum. The conception vessel, the fourteenth meridian, begins at a point between the anus and the scrotum or labia and continues up through the center of the body, with a point on the navel, a point at the middle of the abdomen where the diaphragm attaches, and a final point in the center of the lower gum.

There are also eight minor channels for regulating the flow of energy and fluid through these major fourteen, including one around the waist, which joins all channels together.

Traditional Chinese medicine has been supplanted only in part by global medicine. It is basically a set of principles, and these can be applied no matter the over-all cultural situation. No wise physician, Chinese or otherwise, would challenge the inevitability of the present, including the dominance of mechanical medicine. Now that it has happened, it is our lot and our opportunity.

It is through a misconception that many Americans learn the meridians and their points as if memorizing a color-chart anatomy of the frog. The feel of the system precedes the geography, and a healer with good feeling but no knowledge of the charts can achieve better traditional results than someone rigorously following a map.

Chinese healers in America try to make very small changes in people's lives, either through needles, diet, or exercise. They believe that, just as distortion spreads, so also does harmony. If a prescription is correct and followed scrupulously, it not only works for the person but has ramifications in the world of society and nature at large.

The ancient Hindu system of Ayurvedic healing of India is also elemental and humoral and no doubt linked to the other Eurasian systems of an even more ancient time. To the Hindu healer, the body is made up of five elements: Earth, including all the fixed and solid aspects, such as bone, which give the organism its support and shape; Fire, which is manifested as both the heat and digestion of the interior, including the secretions of the skin; Air, which is the nervous system, perceiving and animating the being; Water, which is glutinous matter like fat, as well as the special bodily fluids, blood, mucus, semen, lymph, hormones, etc.; and Ether, which holds the various bodily elements together.[10]

The elements, present in each body, combine variously at the level of function to form three basic humoral constitutions: Mucus (*kapha*), Wind (*vata*), and Fire (*pitta*). Material ingested, both food and medicine, must be chosen to supply humoral lacks and balance the relationship of these three. Otherwise, indigestion, weakness, and disease will follow.

The Mucus body type is compact, smooth, oily, with dark hair and pale complexion. Mucus supplies freedom of joints, basic normal build, and courage and calmness.

The Fire type is, as might be expected, yellow and pink in color, with soft hair, often blonde, aggressive and tempery, with a tendency to age quickly. Fire brings joy, heat in the body, vision, hunger and thirst, and digestion.

The Wind type is brownish and small, talkative and fearful, with rough skin and hair. Wind brings breath and circulation to the system.

An increase in Mucus leads to dullness, heaviness, and congestion. An increase in Fire leads to hunger, thirst, wakefulness, burning, and incapacity of the sense organs. An increase in Wind leads to flatulence, uncoordination, and dryness.

Likewise, one can diagnose by the lacks of these humors. A lack of Mucus leads to giddiness and trembling and a feeling of emptiness. A lack of Fire leads to chilliness and failure of digestion. A lack of Wind leads to depression and loss of consciousness.

These relationships are dynamic and complementary, so a decrease in one humor will lead to an increase in the others, though one more so than another.

Remedies must take into account both the humoral type of the person and the humoral excesses and deficiencies causing the particular disease. In general, it is considered easier to correct, by diet and medicine, an excess of a humor which is not the constitutional one. So digestive diseases in Fire types are difficult; respiratory disease becomes deep-lodged in Mucus types; and nervous disease persists most in Wind types.

Among the food remedies are: For excess of Mucus, beans, hot spices, honey, sharp vegetables except radish, and fruits with acid are prescribed. For excess of Fire, sweet milk, wheat, grains, beans, and bitter herbs are prescribed. For excess of Wind, wheat, milk, salty and acidic fruits, warm drinks, and sweet vegetables are prescribed.

We have discussed the elements in an herbal context, but mind/body holism in India is preserved in other ways: for instance, hatha yoga can also be used to correct humoral imbalances. The master prescribes postures, breathing exercises, and related life-style changes that purify the system and provide a focus for humoral harmony.

Like Navaho sand painting in the American Southwest, Ayurvedic and Yin/Yang medicines are not simply mythologies but continue to be practiced in Asia and indeed throughout the world. Elementalism may be protoscience, but it is a principle of creation and a methodology of diagnosis and healing, so it has present as well as historical meaning. It exists in dual form: as an extremely archaic and primitive world-view and as a continuously reborn and redefined ascetic simplicity. As an account of original qualities and virtues, it is also a means of returning to them, of understanding and healing ourselves in embryo. Like aboriginal Earth and Fire themselves, it is a part of the Ice Age that is equally a part of our flesh and our cities.

X

Ancient Medicine: Empiricism and Rationalism

Western medical systems have emerged and reemerged from the same basic fragments and dialectics since the dawn of history. Their beginnings are unknown to us, except by our speculations from contemporary shamanism and our reconstructions of a proto-Eurasian cosmology. The healing systems and anatomical beliefs of the original Occidental civilizations to the south and east were inherited by the Greeks as a series of broken messages which they adapted, transformed, and passed on. The Romans formalized, essentially, one aspect of ancient healing. Biblical and Oriental lands were undergoing revolution and revival then. The north and the west remained Ice Age and tribal.

Later, pagan Europe brought its own shamanism to bear. But pagan Europe was also Indo-Europe and mesolithic Eurasia. It would be Christian Europe, mediaeval Rome. The countries of the West, even as they passed through feudalism, rural theocracy, mercantilism, and the birth of physics and chemistry, maintained the Roman medical and legal orthodoxy. They carried it to Africa, India, and America. From America it spread globally.

But it was not just stock Roman law and Roman medicine. New influences came from every region the West visited. The old sources were brought back to life in so many guises they are uncountable. Not only did Europe never take leave of the old Greek quest for the origin of matter and form; it understood that the Greeks were missionaries of an older, hence more sacred temple. Again and again, Europe tried to recover the first rites, sometimes from the Egyptians, or its imaginings of them, sometimes from its own Druids and shamans in cultural memory and present lineage, and later from the magi of the East as well. Paracelsus stands at the crossroads of ancient and modern. He is bigger, vaster than any of his contemporaries and than most of who came after as well as who came before—simply because he acknowledges and embodies the *whole* condition of Western learning and inquiry and not just its passing fashions.

There are many trails leading from the original wisdom, but the wisdom itself was always one. Ancestries blur. Christian and Celtic, Egyptian and Persian, Chinese and Islamic become the same. Alchemy is the most telling offspring of a single planetary tradition long long before there were photographs, from some other outer space, of a Whole Earth.

There is also one scientific truth, one meaning to the genesis and production of matter from nothing, and of life from matter. This has been the fundamental axiom of the European "church" that gave birth to the Industrial Revolution, and it is still the axiom by which we look at galaxies billions of light-years from us and minute particles within the texture of matter and energy.

Contemporary thought is born out of this cauldron—Eurasian, but also global. From the perspective of Indo-Europe, our modern doctors are educated peasants pretending to be initiated chiefs. And medicine is a late product of the sacred aboriginal mines. Its innards are far more primitive than the gloss of its operating room or the flashing lights of its computers reveal. We have shined the ore and sharpened the tools, but it is still ancient metal and gem. We have not solved the old mysteries. But we also continue to solve them.

The expansion of technology has tended to obscure not only important nontechnological modes of healing, but also the historical basis of medicine in the West. As biophysical knowledge has increased, we have tried to map every imaginable unknown territory by its rules. We have become rootless in the sense that we are dependent on new advances to sustain our sense that we have a core and a meaning. Some scientists assume that our insight into disease and its cure has so deepened that we are on the verge, presently, of uncovering the secrets of life. Even doctors who side strongly against the establishment often accept its data and its definition of our medical goals. That so many of the practitioners of alternative medicine and holistic health think of their work as "new" is itself a symptom of the historical provincialism that makes them into a fad.

Although much that is new has been invented, it has not come solely from a breakthrough into the unexplored or higher spheres of knowledge. Our inventions are the products of a changing culture which has required them. After all, we have changed in more ways than in medical practices. The entire world is made up of the new structures in which we live and travel, new jobs and duties, and, along with them, new ailments and deliriums. We have learned most from the sheer process of human civilization on the Earth, and we have learned this by being born into its continuum. "We don't change," said Charles Olson. "We simply stand more revealed."[1]

In order to understand our medical legacy, we must reexamine an ancient rivalry among doctors. On one side are the lineages and guilds of bonesetters, surgeons, and pharmacists. In prehistoric times, the shamans overshadowed them; in ancient and mediaeval times, they were allied with the barbers and smiths more than the priests and philosophers. As university training became a prerequisite for medical practice, their profession gained credibility. By the twentieth century, they have become the medical profession. But they have achieved their status primarily as a trade union, not in the name of healing or of truth.

Their rivals, friendly or unfriendly, interacting or oblivious, are the shamans and charismatic healers, joined, in historical times, by country doctors who stuck by the empirical tradition.

The tradition of healing has never been disgraced or defeated in open battle. It is simply out of fashion and out of power. The modern bias toward visible demonstration and proof is obsessive. Little else might be expected of people from whom such wonderful secrets were kept so tantalizingly and for so many generations. We inherit the hunger of our ancestors for this one kind of knowledge, and we have built a world in which to enjoy all the fruits of recent disclosure. Though healers remain among us, even in the ranks of professional physicians, they are disenfranchised; until very recently almost everyone assumed that the tide stood against them, barring the collapse of civilization itself, for the duration of man.

In particular, healers have rejected the possibility of learning anything about health and disease from the dissection of corpses. As the

first-century Roman physician Aulus Cornelius Celsus put it: "All
that is possible to come to know in the living, the actual treatment
exhibits."[2]

We have since named this the "Empirical tradition" of medicine.
It is opposed by the so-called Rationalist tradition of medicine,
which is based on the accumulation of anatomical and pharmacological knowledge. The Rationalists were concerned with figuring
out how the body functioned, with an emphasis on visible function,
hence on chemicomechanical properties. Understanding these, they
could prescribe on the basis of universal laws, giving chemical solutions to neutralize toxic states, arouse sluggish organs, and dissolve
specific congestions. Later on, as surgeons, they could excise the diseased tissue itself.

Perhaps nothing distinguishes the Rationalist so fully as his search
for a general theory incorporating all the diverse elements that have
been successful in individual treatments. The ambition for this takes
on a significance beyond any single capacity for insight or cure. The
Empiricist, on the other hand, goes from unique situation to unique
situation, developing his art and trying to cure individuals. He has
no uniform set of disease categories.

Not all Empiricists are Vitalists, however. And even those that are,
do not share interpretations of the vital force. The spirits and voodoo of the shamans are as much foolishness to most acupuncturists
and homoeopaths as they are to surgeons. Faith healers and parapsychologists, on the other hand, accept the existence of a telepathy
or telekinesis without believing in the vital properties of plants and
minerals in many cases, properties essential to the rationales of homoeopathy, anthroposophical medicine, and alchemy.

Strangely enough, not all Vitalists are Empiricists. In the last century especially, we have been entertained by a variety of energies,
rays, and auras, most of which are proposed as having a universal
basis. Their advocates would place them in the textbooks of anatomy
and pharmacy, adding the etheric body to the skeleton and the
nerves and the vital power of silver or tansy to the compendium of
active American drugs. Conversely, as psychiatry has proven, Rationalism can give rise to schools as characterological and intuitive as
any ancient Empiricism.

The rivalry is useful, though not as much as we might have first
supposed. We must use it in order to follow the direct lines of medical thought through the tangled history of Europe. Presently, tech-

nological medicine pretends to create its own historical context, explaining itself as the gradual evolution of correct knowledge. But healing does not really fit the role to which our modern scientific myths assign it. It is transhistorical, taking on particular meanings in the different epochs of history. It is exactly *not* progressive, though people will always try to update and reinterpret it—hence "new" medicines, which are really fresh intuitions into ancient skills.

The earliest Greek medicine we know of is from the texts of Hippocrates, which stand in relation to medicine much as Homer's *Odyssey* and *Iliad* stand in relation to literature: they mark the boundaries outside of which we cannot go, no matter how many single islands we visit and planets we discover that were unknown to the Greeks.[3] They state the basic axioms and dilemmas.

The Hippocratic texts, like the Homeric ones, contained not a single dogma but a summary of knowledge from the ancient world. Between the dawn of civilization and the writings of Greece lies a history which dwarfs the one that has passed since the dissemination of ancient Greek thought. The most primitive aspects of the Hippocratic writings appear to be vitalist and humoral in the tradition of ancient Eurasian cosmology: Disease was a mystery within the larger mystery of creation. The body was capable of self-healing by the same elemental process that shaped it from mind and flesh. The Greek physician was a cryptographer, a semeiologist of disease.

When imbalance in the elements occurred, the vital force was excited into action. When disease followed, the vital force was a direct means of transforming the excess humor and detoxifying the organism. This cycle of health and disease was a concomitant of life. The Hippocratic physician could not interrupt it or introduce it; he could only stimulate and deflect it. He could not respond to the symptoms singly or remedially, for this would have disturbed the healing. Instead, he observed and interpreted the character or image of the pathology and interceded at the moment of crisis and flux with a medicine sympathetic to the disease (i.e., healing) process. He chose its intensity as well as its type: too weak or too early a response might have retarded the accumulating current, and too strong a dose might have snapped the vital force and killed the patient.

This natural process of cure was called "coction" (boiling) or "pepsis" in recognition of its similarity to both cooking heat and peptic excitement. The sick organism was "raw"; crude sediment appeared in its urine, stools, sputum, vomit, perspiration, and menstrual blood, though often in very subtle forms. But, as the disease "cooked," digestion improved, the symptoms gradually ended. The physician's skill was in reading the type of coction and picking a medicine similar to it, i.e., which provoked a symptomology *like* that of the disease. He was a musician in an orchestra, playing his note at exactly the point where it should occur in the melody that was already going on. He was also, from the standpoint of the sick body, the inventor of music, for he played his natural instrument, his remedy, in such a way that the organism heard it as music rather than the din of sensation all around.

Prescribing a remedy whose effects are like those of the disease is known as the "Law of Similars." The doctor must choose the right remedy and moment; otherwise his "cure" will not inspire the coction and will not add to it. He must also distinguish between primary disease, which comes from the healthy reaction of the vital force, and secondary disease, which is really a sign of the capitulation of the patient's healing powers—often from the wrong treatment.

For instance, according to the principles of healing in early Hippocratic medicine, hemorrhages, hemorrhoids, nosebleed, diarrhea, and headaches were all signs that a disease was trying to work its way out. For an enlarged spleen, dysentery was considered progress. Diarrhea was usually interpreted as a ripening of white phlegm. Pain in the joints indicated that a long fever was beginning to disperse. Varicose veins and hemorrhoids in an insane person were consequences of the reentry of the disease into the watery and earthen body where the excess humor could be eliminated from the remote aery sphere where it was incurable.

On the other hand, angina followed by lung disease was a sign not of coction but the reverse: that rawness was taking over the body. Rashes were considered peptic, but not if a rash disappeared abruptly without some other corresponding improvement. Diarrhea, nosebleed, and expectoration had to provoke a crisis, with over-all health following, or the disorder was thought to have settled deeper, with a weakening of the vital force, leaving the system at the mercy of the disease process.

Generally speaking, if the doctor interceded in behalf of the vital force, then he prescribed hot baths for those with fever, laxatives for diarrhea, "cold" herbs for chills—in other words encouraging the event which is trying to happen anyway. The implication was that symptoms have no fixed relationships to actual diseases. A fever did not mean that a disease was hot; it also did not mean that it was *not* hot. It was a mystery and absolutely unknowable. Its cause was a spiritual or cosmic variation, an environmental or constitutional change, or some other like thing. Man, made of humors, was immune to direct disease; what he experienced was the change in elemental relationships in his flesh inspired by disease at his core. The characteristics of the disease were auxiliary phenomena caused by the response of the vital force. It was a divine business, and the earliest sources acknowledged this: "The healing art involves a weaving of a knowledge of the gods into the texture of the physician's mind."[4] There would have been no other way.

This type of medicine encouraged lay practice and self-trained doctors, inspirational healers, and an improvisational street medicine. It was a calling more than a profession. It was never wholly divorced from the scientific tradition, but it had little use for most disease categories and explanations. Each patient was a unique event in creation, and the "same" disease in two people was really a similar manifestation of two different disorders.

Whereas the Empirical interpretations probably represented the ancient core of the Hippocratic Corpus, Rationalism appears to have arisen from a later group of physicians associated historically with the Cnidians. Their treatments should be very familiar to us still. If there is fever, it must be lowered. If there is diarrhea, the physician should end it. If there is pus in the lungs, it is to be drained. These remedies also work on a humoral basis, but without the priority of the vital force. That is, if the system has undue wetness, a drying agent is added. If there is an excess of heat, a cooling remedy is given. A typical Cnidian maxim reads: "When the drug enters the body, it first withdraws that constituent of the body which is most akin to itself, and then it draws and purges the other constituents."[5]

As time went on and Greek medicine developed and then merged with Roman and, later, mediaeval medicine, the Rationalists became more and more mechanical and abstract. They revised the body into a kind of animated corpse which proceeded by physical laws, translating food and air into flesh and movement by the breakdown and rearrangement of materials. Coction was simply taken over as digestion and internal chemistry, which was considered a refinement, not a downgrading, of its original meaning.

The Roman Methodist school of the Greek physicians Themison

and Thessalus proposed the body as a porous pipe through which fluids circulate, too fast if the pipe is overrelaxed, too slow if it is too restricted. Sweating and bloodletting were the standard cures for a restricted flow, whereas darkness, quiet, and a diet of thick porridge and soft-boiled eggs was the remedy for agitated flow.

Western medicine throughout its history has gradually removed the idea of the art of healing and the vital force from the literature and methodology to which they gave rise, replacing them with the doctor's own skills as surgeon or pharmacist. The Romans synthesized "laws" arising from intimations of vital energy in the body with laws arising from observation of chemical and mechanical relationships, identifying change with a material quality or quantity, with sensitivity, excitability, nervous energy, etc. The synthesis inevitably denied vital energy by subsuming it in materiality. A vital force continued to exist as philosophical construct, even as the religion behind medicine, but doctors observed it rhetorically rather than actually. Most doctors still think that they observe it actually (i.e., the body's healing power) because the rhetorical observance has also merged with the language of popular chemistry and physics.

Galen, the second century physician, was an Empiricist by practice but a Rationalist at heart. He believed in the vital force, but he attempted to concretize it. Like so many of his successors, he thought the breach in medicine was surely superficial and temporary, and thus he solved it in a naïve way. He saw no reason why an Empiric doctor should not use all the material he could obtain. The more knowledge about anatomy and pharmacy, the less chance there was of choosing the wrong remedy. No doubt in his own practice he balanced experience and theory, but his written prejudice was to emphasize logos and to elevate the physician above the lay practitioner.

Anatomy, physiology, and logic were Galen's cornerstones of medicine. He expected doctors to work from theory to observation, always adding new details in the context of theory. He was to infer the nature of the disease from what he knew of the body.

Galen's writings succeeded, more by assumption than direct statement, in transferring the power of the vital force to the organs of the body. That is, the vital force did not exist except as it was expressed by the individual organs through the humors. Each organ had its own behavior, its peculiar combination of qualities. But when faced with the difficulty of explaining contradictory actions of some organs, Galen returned to the unity of the vital force. By going full circle, he came out nowhere. Ultimately, he recommended collecting more material, licensing physicians, and, in general, developing medical authority. Even though he did not propose a consistent general theory of medicine, his mere attempt to do so *was* the general theory, and it was assumed ever after. He wrote some thirty volumes of medical lore which, at that point, was the medical literature. He left things in the hands of future researchers and logicians who were to continue to resolve the contradictions.

No healer would necessarily take issue with the content of this work, only with the author's assumption that it conferred the ability to cure sick people. The Empiricists and Vitalists ignored the pretense of coherence and continued to treat patients as they always had. For them, physiology might be a matter of great interest, but it was a luxury, always at the service of spontaneous intuition.

So convincing was Galen's synthesis that it has survived all attacks and given medicine its present identity. Not that doctors today see things exactly as Galen did, but those organs he proposed as the locations and centers of bodily process remain our general images of the places and sites where things happen. It is this image that mainstream medicine has observed in place of the healing force, and in place of the cure, too. Homoeopathy, psychiatry, acupuncture, and holistic health have all chipped away at the central image, but its power is great enough for it to suck them in and convert them, for the most part, to itself. A substantial change has not yet come.

The other history of medicine in the West is the history of its outsiders. The most notable of these was Paracelsus, the Swiss hermetic physician (1493–1541), whose original name was Theophrastus Bombastus von Hohenheim. Since his career was both spectacular and unorthodox, he is often ridiculed, but he was one of those rare individuals who stood between remote worlds and joined them for a moment of time. As a scientist, he developed a number of effective medicines, including ones out of flowers of sulphur, calomel, copper, arsenic, and lead. His alchemical experiments contributed equally to divination and laboratory chemistry. He traveled widely in the Western and Arabic worlds of the sixteenth century, healing the sick and learning new folk cures wherever he went. In his research, he journeyed back to the Hippocratic roots fourteen hundred years after Galen, taking for himself the name of his predecessor Celsus and placing himself squarely outside the Roman synthesis. He considered the Romans and their followers the squanderers and despoilers of the true ancient medicine: "I am Theophrastus, and greater than those to whom you liken me; I am Theophrastus, and in addition I am *monarchia medicorum*, monarch of physicians, and I can prove to you what you cannot prove. . . . Let me tell you this: every little hair on my neck knows more than you and all your scribes, and my shoebuckles are more learned than your Galen and Avicenna, and my beard has more experience than all your high colleges."[6]

Paracelsus gathered so much information from the streets that he considered himself beyond the isolated medical establishment: "I went not only to the doctors, but also to barbers, bathkeepers, learned physicians, women, and magicians who pursue the art of healing; I went to alchemists, to monasteries, to nobles and common folk, to the experts and the simple."[7]

It is not as though the Hippocratic Empiricists stand at the beginning of time. Their writings mark the end of a long and distinguished lineage of healing; Paracelsus not only summarizes the mediaeval hermetic tradition; he taps other esoteric traditions in the outlands of the West, and no doubt by doing that, he gains access to the pre-Hippocratic corpus as it was honored and maintained outside the Greco-Roman orbit. A hundred years after Paracelsus, the Flemish physician Jan Baptista van Helmont practiced medicine and wrote books in this same tradition. Like Paracelsus, he placed great emphasis on folk remedies, "for truly the Arabians, Greeks, or Gentiles, barbarians, wild country people, and Indians have observed their own simples more diligently than all the Europeans."[8]

Paracelsus believed in a fully spiritual universe. The stars may move outside the Earth and outside the body, but that is only in their physical manifestation. The inner harmonic progression that occurs in the planets also occurs among the metals and, in another sense, among the plants of the field. The duty of the physician is to discover the inner virtues of these things and extract from them the vital elixirs of alchemy and occult botany.

Within the same science, he made two different types of medicine, one we might call "conventional herbal," that is, mixtures of vegetable oils, ground plant parts, spices, liquors, etc., given in his writings as precise recipes; and the other, purely astral and alchemical, based on the extraction of unknown qualities of metals like antimony and tin and the long-term coction of them under low-grade heat. The former involved traditional formulas of European pharmacy, of which Paracelsus was obviously a scholar; the latter required the spiritualization of inorganic matter by activating the vital force in minerals.[9]

The hermetic scientist sought to bring out the latent in nature, so that he isolated not just silver, but the silver of silver, the gold of gold, the sulphur of sulphur, all of which were elemental medicines. This kind of alchemical pharmacy has been almost abandoned in recent times, though a form of it reappeared in the anthroposophical medicine of Rudolf Steiner, and there have been a handful of documented twentieth-century instances of the attempt to prepare this elixir of the metals. Paralab, a laboratory in West Jordan, Utah, near Salt Lake City, named for Paracelsus, prepares a variety of remedies in the alchemical tradition.

The remarkable feature of Paracelsus' work is that the Vitalism, so fiercely held to and richly integrated, does not keep him from an involvement in particulars. He gives us enduring images of the colors of burning metals in their flasks, the trees and flowers springing up individually from the original seed, the intricate wetness of water and the fieryness of fire, the feminine and masculine qualities of minerals and solutions, the brilliance of gold, the explosion of blossoms in the spring, the special light of the Sun, and so on. For all his involvement with the single spirit, he was equally concerned with the diversity and beauty of matter. He remarked that it was preferable to know one herb in the meadow absolutely and well, root and flower and seasonal change, than to gaze piously on the whole meadow.

He took medicine back to its folk origins, and at the same time, he took medicine forward into new experimentation. He lived an ancient law that was no longer believed: "The art of medicine is rooted in the heart. If your heart is false, you will also be a false physician; if your heart is just, you will also be a true physician."[10]

Van Helmont was the best-known inheritor of the Paracelsian tradition, though he was more of a conventional protoscientist. Paracelsus was a traveling minstrel, healer, philosopher, and poet. Van Helmont was a healer, too, and a Vitalist, as well as an advocate of folk and ancient medicine, but he was a general theoretician. He explained disease as an idea or form imprinted on the vital force, or *Archeus* (in his terminology), which then "frames erroneous images to himself which should be unto him as it were for a poison. . . . which images or likenesses, indeed, as being the seeds of disease beings, should be thenceforth wholly marriageable unto him in the innermost bride-bed of life."[11]

The medicines work as specifics because of the ideas imprinted on their own *Archeus* which overcome the idea of the disease. Ideas precede human consciousness; hence the rudiments of the various emotions, the seals and characters of the personalities of individual people and plants and animals, are contained archetypally in the raw effluvia of nature.

By his own declaration, Van Helmont was not a mystic. He considered magic a false authority like Galenism, hence an enemy of Empiricism. He dreamed of a spirit handing him a bottle of medicine that he could not experience or perceive, but he would not accept it on occult faith. He had to know the medicine through his senses or refuse the gift.

In the early eighteenth century, one of the strongholds of Vitalistic medicine was the medical school at Montpellier, in France, that followed from the German Georg Ernst Stahl. Because Stahl was a leading chemist as well as a physician, his comments on the role of chemistry in medicine are striking. He rejected chemistry not only on a material basis but a humoral basis, and, in its place, he proposed that an intelligent force called *Anima* regulated the body. The circulation of the blood, demonstrated a century before by the English anatomist William Harvey, was essential to Stahl's theory, for it was by the movement of fluids that the *Anima* kept the organism healthy and removed toxicities.

The *Anima* and *Archeus* are Vitalistic, but the blood is mechanical. It is difficult to know whether Van Helmont and Stahl were more scientific than mystical or vice versa than their predecessors because science and hermeticism have a way of stealing from each other what they think is rightfully theirs. Clearly these men were not street doctors or astral chemists, but rather carried the weight of Paracelsian medicine in their time.

Théophile Bordeu, a student at Montpellier, stood somewhere between Stahl's *Anima* and the surgeons and physiologists who represented the medical establishment. He upheld vital-force dynamics but tried to define them more physically. The *Anima*, he said, regulated the flow of fluids through the body as a *chair coulante*, a circulating flesh, filling the pores and crevices, picking up extracts from the glands and carrying them to the organs. Bordeu thus was one of the fathers of hormonal medicine with its insight into the sympathetic nervous system and the involuntary responses of the body. He wrote that "a knowledge of the composition of the blood is inseparable from a calculation of the effects it produces unceasingly upon the sensitive organs."[12]

Secretion is not a brute mechanical force; the *Anima* guides it intelligently and selectively through the organs.

In line with the Hippocratic and Paracelsian tradition, Bordeu believed in curing by similars rather than contraries, and he accepted the principle of coction. Quelling the symptoms at crisis, he said, insured a history of chronic disease. He believed that mineral springs were powerfully medicinal because they could transform chronic diseases back into acute ones through inciting coction. He even praised the cure-all theriaca, which was made up of all the leftover medicines from an apothecary's shop at the end of a day. He saw it, like mineral waters, as peppy and stimulating, awaking the vital force from its languor or from its dwelling in melancholy and suppressed anger.

The other tradition in the West, preserved from preclassical times by the Hippocratics and practiced by Celsus, Paracelsus, Van Helmont, Stahl, Bordeu, and their countless colleagues, stumbles through the centuries as both a brilliant healer and a mysterious stranger, a familiar to science and a vestigial witch whom science cannot purge. Western medicine put its hopes into visible disease and knowable cure, but it paid a price, both immediate and gradual, for its neglect of mind and spirit. It would have paid a different price had it wrestled with them throughout and it would not have spawned science as we know it. But the ghosts have been inherited all the way: voodoo and vital force, quintessence and X-ray quartz, elements and similars, *Anima* and *Archeus*, folk medicine and faith healing. And they are not merely empty baggage or cast-off placentas. They are something we keep coming back to, forever.

Transitions

XI

Homoeopathy: The Great Riddle

Homoeopathy was developed by a German physician Samuel Hahnemann (1755–1843) in the late eighteenth and early nineteenth centuries and became a dominant medical practice in much of the Western world until the early twentieth century.[1] Its success was greatest in North America; its decline was most swift and thorough there, too. Homoeopathy ran into insurmountable internal contradictions and ultimately lost its identity as a single consistent system. The policies of the American Medical Association and Abraham Flexner's *Report on Medical Education in the United States and Canada* (1910) finally took away its professional sanction, and it was isolated as a *nonscientific* medicine.

From the beginning, homoeopathy has been a mystery. The issues it raises are so complex and on so many different levels that any description is misleading in one fashion or another.

Homoeopathy is first, and perhaps foremost, a continuation of the Vitalist and Empirical tradition of Western medicine. Its science and philosophy arise directly from the treatment of the sick, and historically its claims have been based more on inexplicable results than on a logical and self-evident mode of treatment. By today's definition it is not a science. Despite the arguments of some supporters that it is "another scientific medicine," we more likely could conclude that it is "the medicine of an unknown science."

Homoeopathy is based on the responsiveness of the defense mechanism rather than the intercession of the physician. This defense mechanism is neither visible nor associated with any organ or system. It has the power to respond appropriately to any disease and thus is a direct descendant of the vital force of Greek and mediaeval medicine and a derivative from Paracelsus and Van Helmont.

Homoeopathy also makes its own excursion into "Stone Age medicine." It is holistic and dynamic in the same way that Navaho and Australian Aboriginal medicine are, though not for the same reasons. At a hypothetical "Cosmic Healing Conference," witch doctors and homoeopaths would go at once to opposite sides of the room.

Homoeopathy is neither the first nor the last attempt to develop a scientific Vitalist medicine. Alchemists, gnostics, animists, and other naturalist-magicians worked for millennia toward a cure based on the life force and the primal energy of nature. Goethe, Steiner, Jung, and Reich followed. Homoeopathy is notable, though, for its odd and unlikely combination of elements and its time of birth. There seems no reason why it should have arisen when it did, at the turn of the nineteenth century, when the hermetic and magical sciences were in active decline and the scientific revolution was building toward a crescendo. Surely, if there were such a principle of healing, the ancient Egyptians or Greeks would have known it, and Paracelsus would have incorporated it in his hermetic medicine. Why a new hermetic science at the very end of active occult research? It would seem that if homoeopathy had not been inherited by the Middle Ages, it would at least have been left for the unknown sciences of the remote future. Yet it appears, no doubt for some profoundly right reason, at a hiatus in magical-psychological inquiry, and it persists as a clinical occult discipline through the entire period before the rebirth of paraphysical studies.

Homoeopathy is either ancient medicine, nineteenth-century medicine, or twenty-second-century medicine, but, in our current time, it has no clear resolution or historical meaning, except in its practice.

Homoeopathy, as we know it, is the invention of Samuel Hahnemann. His discoveries define it more thoroughly than even the laws of Newton define physics. Although aspects of homoeopathic thought were in existence before Hahnemann, the system itself arises as suddenly from his mind as Mormonism did from the golden tablets of Joseph Smith. Before Hahnemann, there was no homoeopathy. Since Hahnemann, homoeopathy has changed only to a minor degree, much less than biology and physics during the same time. To his supporters, Hahnemann is the single genius in the history of recorded medicine, if not the history of science. To his detractors, he is a bizarre case in the history of delusion.

It is a mistake to assume that homoeopathy began as an unorthodox or even an alternative system. We tend to forget the very different conditions into which it was born. In Hahnemann's day, medicine was in a totally experimental phase, and few theories or facts were firm. Mainstream medicine relied on procedures and drugs which today would be considered primitive, dangerous, and ineffective. Even a hundred years later, by the acknowledgment of modern doctors and historians, physicians stood an equal chance of harming or helping a patient.

Hahnemann intended only methodological reform. He made a reasonable contribution to the general research of his time. He assumed that he had isolated the laws of medicine that others were also seeking and that mainstream science would vindicate him and do away with the rest, as error and superstition. The initial response was not totally out of keeping with this expectation. This does not mean that he was received with open arms; in fact, he found himself in immediate conflict with the medical profession. But that conflict was part of the fabric of medicine in his time, and there was no higher body, scientific or legal, to decide between interpretations, nor was there any generally agreed upon principle of physics or chemistry that challenged homoeopathy's claim to science. Hahnemann was one more candidate seeking a constituency, and he was allowed to go to the marketplace without interference from a scientific establishment or medical regulatory body. The resistance, at times, might have seemed official, but the rapid growth of homoeopathy as legal medicine shows otherwise. It lost many local battles, but it was not until the twentieth century that it was exposed as an "imposter" in the field of scientific medicine.

Hahnemann was a pariah, but the full import of his discovery was unknown to him. He stumbled through a series of inexplicable experimental successes and left a new set of rules. His discoveries were so radical and their implications so far-reaching that they could never be included in the mainstream of medical thought, not then, and not now. Even today some homoeopaths would like to see homoeopathy accepted as an ally of general medical orthodoxy, but without absolutely revolutionary change at the very roots of medicine and science, this is clearly impossible.

From our perspective, Hahnemann's career reads, in part, like a science fiction story, in part, like a metaphor from quantum physics. Clinical homoeopathy cannot be verified in the laboratory, which means, pessimistically, that standard scientific testing has already disproved *all* homoeopathic claims. Many homoeopaths would deny this, and they have cited various experiments in the chemistry of enzymes, colloids, trace elements, hormones, and drugs. These experiments with microdilutions are interesting and provocative, but they are isolated events, without controlled retesting and general orientation to the rest of science, nor do they test the exact claims of homoeopathy.

If we were to side with orthodox science here, on the basis of the impossibility of homoeopathic pharmacy, we would be left still with two significant events: one, the startling and repeated success of thousands of homoeopathic physicians in all parts of the world for over a century of practice, and, two, a homoeopathic attack on the methods and goals of mainstream medicine that is homoeopathic in perspective but does not require the proof of homoeopathic pharmacy for its own relevance. Furthermore, we seem to require some explanation for the unusually stellar reputation of this one system from among all the Vitalistic sciences attempted in the West.

The next chapter will explore the principles and methods of homoeopathic medicine. But there is a major difficulty to this proposition, and it would be useful to present it here in outline, and then in more detail later. Homoeopathy has been defined in a variety of ways, and, although most homoeopaths will argue that there is a single orthodox definition, nothing has marked the history of this medicine more than the disagreement about what it is and, equally, what it isn't.

The fundamental split is between pure Hahnemannian homoeopathy and either weakened or more pragmatic adaptations of that form to actual medical practice. Few people, especially in the United States, practice pure Hahnemannian homoeopathy today.

Underlying this split, however, is another more basic one between the purists and everyone else. The purists insist on following homoeopathic procedure literally and to the exclusion of all other methods. Hahnemann was a purist insofar as his thought set the very axioms on which purism was based, but, over his lifetime, his interest and pursuits included a large number of things that were not homoeopathic. He was a physician before he was a homoeopath, and he was a general medical philosopher whose innovative theories were rooted in homoeopathic thought. But Hahnemannian medicine, as it was proposed in its time, was not even entirely homoeopathy, let alone Hahnemannian homoeopathy. That definition comes at least a century later from the use of his writings to establish an orthodoxy. There has also been a series of significant disagreements about the relative importance of different aspects of Hahnemann's homoeopathic thought. In general, homoeopathic thought has been free to interpret disease and civilization in complex and profound ways, while homoeopathic practice has been forced to deal with the reality of discrete disease in individual persons. The result has been a substantial difference between the treatments and their supposed meaning. We can deal with these separate splits gradually.

Although Hahnemann invented the unique system we call "homoeopathy," many of its elements were in existence in different forms before Hahnemann. The practice of giving a medicine that initially heightens symptomology (i.e., feeds the symptoms) has existed since prehistoric times and was, as we have seen, an important part of Hippocratic and Paracelsian medicine. But in both these systems, the use of similars as remedies was mixed with the use of contraries, and most doctors treated cases on an individual basis. By basing homoeopathy on the Law of Similars, Hahnemann formalized the distinction between a medicine that respects and encourages symptoms and all other medicines. He called the first, of course, "homoeopathy" (from the Greek for "*like* treatment of disease") and the second "allopathy" (from the Greek for "*other* treatment of disease"). He meant to include in allopathy the medicine based on the supposed Law of Contraries, plus all other treatments that were not based on responding to symptomology with similar-acting medicines. Today, allopathy has become synonymous with the medical establishment, a word used not only pejoratively by homoeopaths but proudly by physicians who have no sympathy for treatment by similars.

Hahnemann regarded his own work as general medicine, and he made many contributions, of which homoeopathy was one. But at the time he presented his ideas and throughout most of the nineteenth century, the full body of Hahnemannian science was considered homoeopathy. After all, that is what Hahnemann named it himself. Much of the material, however, dealt with diet, hygiene, immunization, the preparation of medicines, and even the origin of germs and techniques of surgery (nonhomoeopathic topics).

At the same time, nineteenth-century allopathy bore little resemblance to current allopathy, or mainstream medicine, which is actually a mixture of traditional beliefs, innovations during the nineteenth and twentieth centuries, and the single self-critical thread of scientific experiment that runs through its very fiber. The innovations came partly from American science, but even more from early twentieth-century British medicine; in addition, Hahnemann's nonhomoeopathic philosophy of therapeutics was adopted almost *in toto* by the establishment. Only his homoeopathic principles were "invalidated" and dropped from general practice.

The division into allopathy and homoeopathy is currently based on the elimination of homoeopathic techniques from general medicine. Although, from a homoeopath's point of view, this is the primary event, it is actually only part of an over-all trend. In its struggle for consistency and accountability, medical convention did away with or adapted all alternative methods and questionable techniques. Most people know nothing of either homoeopathy or allopathy: there are just doctors.

Homoeopathy, then, had its heyday before the formal split into allopathy and homoeopathy, i.e., as a different system than it presently is. By the Civil War, it was *the* American medicine and what we know as standard medicine almost became extinct. Homoeopaths were wealthier, more popular, and maintained a network of prestigious medical schools and hospitals. Through their joint efforts with other sectarian medicines, bloodletting and dosing with mercury, which were the mainstays of regular medicine, were successfully criticized and gradually eliminated. Allopathy eventually replaced them with other surgeries and dosing with other drugs, but homoeopathy scored a permanent victory on at least these specific items. Hahnemann's philosophy, though it did not succeed in establishing homoeopathy as universal medicine, led the way to a general revision of the medical profession in the United States. After that, it no longer existed in its traditional form, though it came to exist in its purest form as simply the homoeopathic principles. Only after mainstream medicine adopted general Hahnemannian thought was it equipped to dismiss specific homoeopathic thought.

Although homoeopathy did finally succumb to a no-holds-barred attack by the American Medical Association (AMA) backed by the pharmaceutical companies, its inherent position was untenable, and it would have split from within eventually. Many homoeopathic physicians saw themselves simply as doctors and came not to distinguish between homoeopathy and allopathy, adopting new procedures and drugs as they appeared on the market and generally participating in technological progress. They held the ideal of universal medicine without a corresponding rigorous commitment to homoeopathy as the only candidate, so they strayed without even knowing it and without any certainty as to what was pure homoeopathy and what was violation. Hahnemann's writings were the only referee, and they were not decisive on many issues.

Then, experimental science, without even knowing of the debate, sided strongly and fatally (for homoeopathy) with the allopaths. That is, it sided with the mechanics and chemistry that allopathy had come to use in its diagnosis and treatment and which it continued to refine by experimental technique. As science set the guidelines for accountability in medicine, homoeopathy was considered not accountable, hence unethical. It was, by principle only, unable to cure the sick.

Many homoeopaths accepted this verdict. They did not want to be considered quacks, nor did they want to lose their connection to the cutting edge of science. A decade into the twentieth century, homoeopathy became only marginally legal, and to practice it involved economic sacrifice. It became an almost insurmountable problem for homoeopaths to gain both AMA credentials for practicing medicine (the M.D. license) and the education necessary for practicing homoeopathy. It was not long before being a doctor of homoeopathy had about the same credibility as being an alchemist. Yet a bare moment of history had passed since homoeopathy's widest acceptability.

Today, for the first time, the difference between homoeopathy and allopathy is a pure difference of medicinal principle. No side issue clouds this any longer. If homoeopathy has won all the secondary issues, that is no longer relevant, for the allopathy it now stands against has incorporated these Hahnemannian concerns.

If Hahnemann were to view the present situation, he would find not only that his great discovery had been abandoned and rejected beyond his most paranoid fears, but also that he had strangely succeeded as well. With much of modern medicine he would not be at odds, for it has progressed beyond the stubborn fallacies and errors of his time. It has developed a system of controlled laboratory experiments, and it has come to a clear-mindedness of procedure, but a clarity, from Hahnemann's standpoint, around dangerously false principles. He might even understand that homoeopathy was never actually defeated within the context of the practice of medicine, but by what chemists and biologists chose to agree on and, as the lawmakers of the scientific community, imposed on all systems purporting to be science.

The homoeopathy of today, which has been revived as an alternative medicine, is not the original homoeopathy. It may subscribe to the same rules, procedures, and principles, but it also subscribes to a late twentieth-century thought that is incompatible with some parts of homoeopathy, and it occupies a different place in relation to the rest of the medical profession. Before antibiotics and medical specialization, homoeopathy was proposed as a revolutionary new discovery, and it was heralded or vilified for years as "The New School." Today homoeopathy struggles between datedness and futurism, under one aegis attempting to propose the unknown science that will vindicate it and open new perspectives and under another aegis attempting to reestablish Hahnemann's original orthodoxy.

XII

The Principles and Methodology of Homoeopathic Medicine

Homoeopathy contains elements of vitalism, elementalism, empiricism, hermeticism, and science—all conceived of simultaneously as part of the same dynamic. One must listen to the details and definitions very carefully in order to hear the subtle interwoven echoes of these things through each other. In a certain sense, homoeopathy is the only branch of hermetic science that has succeeded, if temporarily and incompletely, in gaining quasi-professional standing as a secular institution.

Homoeopathy differs from mainstream medicine on the most rudimentary level of disease definition, for it retains the Hippocratic tenet that the core itself is unknowable. According to homoeopathy, the disease categories of standard medicine are classes of pathology representing lines of weakness in the defense mechanisms of individual organisms. They are not the diseases. The diseases are too profound and spiritual for man to locate them. In his *Lectures on Homoeopathic Philosophy*, published at the turn of the century, the American homoeopath James Tyler Kent stated this in vintage homoeopathic language:

"Causes exist in such subtle form that they cannot be seen by eye. There is no disease that exists of which the cause is known to man by the eye or by the microscope. Causes are infinitely too fine to be observed by any instrument of precision. They are so immaterial that they correspond to and operate upon the interior of man, and they are ultimated in the body in the form of tissue changes that are recognized by the eye."[1]

The tissue changes are the visible result of disease on the inner plane. Any actual disease can generate a variety of widely different symptoms and symptom complexes in different individuals, none of which are the disease itself, none of which contain even a morsel of its actual fabric. Instead, they are the body's idiosyncratic response to the presence of disease.

In homoeopathic cybernetics, the organism is presumed always to have the best possible (i.e., least destructive to itself) response to an underlying disturbance. It may develop painful and exotic pathologies, but even they will be the best it can do under the circumstances. Its response is actually a system-wide recognition of the existence of disease within itself and a synchronous attempt to allow the disease (which is contemporary and inevitable) to express and vent itself with the least damage to the vital organs.

If the best possible response is frustrated by medical treatment, then the organism will find the next best possible integration of the disease, i.e., the best possible response under the new contemporary situation. Although the curtailment of symptoms might be considered cure by allopathic definitions, this is not the case in homoeopathy. The difference between the best possible response and the second best (or between any two sequential possibilities on this scale) may be the difference between eventual cure or lifelong illness.

The conflict with allopathy is head-on here. If the visible disease is not the disease and if its alleviation is countertherapeutic, then the whole of medicine is involved in a system of superficial palliation leading to more serious disease. Doctors do not cure; they merely displace symptoms to ever less optimum channels of disease expression, each of which they consider to be a separate event because of its location in a new organ or region of the body. The disease meanwhile is driven deeper and deeper into the constitution because its mode of expression is cut off each time.

As disease becomes more serious, it tends to change in the following manner: exterior organs improve, internal organs are affected in place; symptoms move from the periphery of the body, typically the fingertips and toes, toward the center of the body, notably the heart and nerves; symptoms also move upward toward the head; life-sustaining systems are attacked latest in the disease process; the acute becomes chronic with more severe and new acute phases in its cycle;

temporary alteration of function becomes permanent alteration of structure; pathology moves from the physical level to the emotional level to the mental level, its ultimate expression being insanity and loss of reason.

On a simple physical level, homoeopaths note sequences of worsening disease, for example, like the following: first herpes on the lips, then canker sores in the mouth, then canker sores deeper in the digestive tract, then duodenal ulcer, then colitis; or, first a urinary infection, then a kidney infection, then cystitis, then nephritis, finally destruction of the kidney. These sequences are single diseases, respectively, not different consecutive ailments.

A passage indicating improvement could be, for example, severe heart attack followed by mild pneumonia (as a disease releases its hold on the heart and fans out into the lungs), then painful arthritis as it is dispersed to the joints. Its ultimate stage might be a skin rash. If the original condition was serious, the skin rash itself may remain chronically for the patient's lifetime, a weakness grafted permanently onto the system. But certainly such a rash would be less debilitating than the other expressions.

It should be added that this kind of improvement, in the opinion of virtually all homoeopaths, can occur only from homoeopathic medicines, though some admit the possible effectiveness of other dynamic medicines with which they have not had experience.

The disease, like the organism, vibrates through three planes, which it integrates in its unity: the physical, the emotional, and the mental. In the spontaneous transfer of a disease from one plane to another, the new pathology must occur roughly on the same level as the old one, or a slightly worse level, but, in jumping plane of manifestation, it can never improve. The jump itself is an inflammation only. A skin ailment may appear to vanish without a trace, but the patient is suddenly depressed. A conventional doctor might wonder why. Shouldn't the patient at least be happy that the skin condition has cleared up? The homoeopath knows why: the skin ailment was painful primarily because it expressed a deeper disorder. As the condition deteriorates and the disease itself comes closer to the core of the organism, it jumps to the emotional level and expresses itself as depression. The patient feels worse because he intuitively experiences the disorder closing in on him. The skin improvement is superficial; conversely, the heart patient might well consider a rash to be minor and restorative after having felt the same disease in his heart. The skin ailment *is* the depression, or, more properly, they are both functions of one aberration. A stomach ulcer might, similarly, be transformed into violent irritability and paranoia. It is the environment and defense system of the patient that determine how any condition will change and whether it will go deeper on the same plane or be passed to a more inner one.

Diseases never just "go away." That is too shallow and naïve a prospect for the homoeopath. A new pathology always replaces an old one. The old one may appear to be cured, but only because the organism's defense has retreated by a degree.

Standard medicine, in treating visible pathology, must, by homoeopathic rules, always drive disease deeper, for it deprives the organism of the best defense it has. But standard medicine will not recognize the translation; instead, the doctor will declare a cure or an alleviation. It is not that all physicians are fools; any competent doctor understands the defense mechanism. Fevers, coughs, even ulcers are generally seen as healing responses, preventing more serious disease and useful except when they begin to cause organic damage themselves. Psychiatry regularly recognizes, as a first law passed down from Freud, that the organism arranges the mental disorder that best allows it to continue to function and that without the disorder, the organism would sink into more fully developed insanity and emotional distortion. Where standard medicine fails, by homoeopathic standards, is in choosing a seemingly arbitrary point at which to break off its acknowledgment of defense priority and to begin an interventionist strategy. Allopathy believes that the skill of the physician can reverse certain conditions when the system cannot. Homoeopathy believes that the system alone can reverse pathology and that intervention on a symptomatic level must always not only fail but do deeper damage by disturbing the organism's extraordinarily refined response.

In homoeopathy, the visible disease is understood precisely as the working of the cure. If someone is interested in its nature and the progress of its pathology, the germs and microorganisms it attracts, the way in which it spreads and chemically alters the body—that in itself is an innocuous pursuit, irrelevant to the actual dynamics of cure. If that same physician lets himself believe that he can improve the health of the organism by changing what he sees, reversing its disruptive process in the tissues, he is dangerously misled. Temporary relief is always given the organism only at the expense of an ultimate return to full health. From the point of view of homoeopathic philosophy, the present symptomatic medicine is so widely accepted now in part because people do not know how true health actually feels.

The allopath is confused by the temporary improvement because he does not view the organism as a complete entity with a single expression of disease. He never takes a full enough picture of the symptoms to get beneath the workings of the deplacement and see the consistency of relationship between things he considers separately occurring conditions. If, after allopathic treatment, a person with kidney disease has less albumin in his urine, the assumption is that the kidneys are working better. The patient may feel worse, but the doctor assumes that the feeling is either a side effect of the disease, a matter for the psychiatrist, or an irrelevant concurrent happening. The homoeopath is trained to see nothing as a totally separate event. His experience tells him that suppressed kidney disease may well be followed by deeper discomfort, that the discomfort will not go away by itself, and that its cure demands, on some level, the reexperiencing of the kidney disease. If that should happen, the original physician would consider it an unfortunate relapse. For the homoeopath it is the reversal of suppression. It is a homoeopathic law of cure that old suppressed pathologies return in reverse order when present ailments are correctly cured. This kind of unity of expression is one of the keynotes of original Hahnemannian thought, as it was set down in *Organon* (1810), Hahnemann's basic textbook of homoeopathy:

"All diseases are, in fact, diseases of the whole organism: No external malady . . . can arise, persist, or even grow worse without . . . the cooperation of the whole organism, which must consequently be in a diseased state. It could not make its appearance at all without the consent of the whole of the rest of the health, and without the participation of the rest of the living whole (of the vital force that pervades all other sensitive and irritable parts of the organism); indeed, it is impossible to conceive its production without the instrumentality of the whole (deranged) life, so intimately are all parts of the organism connected together to form an invisible whole in sensations and functions."[2]

It is certainly clear from the above why a rapprochement between standard medicine and homoeopathy is impossible. Just on the principles alone, without even including the exotic and spiritual pharmacy, homoeopathy condemns orthodox medical science to a wild goose chase of symptom classification when the dynamics of symptoms in no way reflect the dynamics of the disease. In treating imaginary categories, physicians were doomed to make their patients worse. Hahnemann wrote in *Organon:*

"Two thousand years were wasted by physicians in endeavoring to discover the invisible internal changes that take place in the organism in diseases, and in searching for their proximate causes and *a priori* nature, because they imagined that they could not cure before they had attained to this *impossible* knowledge."[3]

Modern homoeopathy has developed new language to explain how conventional medical treatment must always make the patient sicker, even if it gives him the delicate illusion of health. It accuses the establishment of transforming the old well-known diseases into a new class of iatrogenic ailments that are difficult to unravel and often impossible to cure. If they prolong life, they do so at a weaker level of vibration, so that the organism does not experience its own being with any richness and never can know real health. George Vithoulkas, a contemporary Greek homoeopath, explains the dynamics of false cure:

"*Since allopathic drugs are never selected according to the Law of Similars, they inevitably superimpose upon the organism a new drug disease which then must be counteracted by the organism.* Furthermore, if the drug has been successful in removing symptoms on a peripheral level, the defense mechanism is then forced to re-establish a new state of equilibrium at a deeper level. In this way, the vibration rate of the organism is disturbed and weakened by two mechanisms: 1) by the influence of the drug itself, and 2) by interference with the best possible response of the defense mechanism. Consequently, if the drug is powerful enough, or if drug therapy is continued long enough, the organism may jump to a deeper level in its susceptibility to disease. The real tragedy of such a consequence is that the defense mechanism of the individual cannot then re-establish the original equilibrium on its own; even with homeopathic treatment of very high quality, it may take many years to return to the original level, much less to make any progress on the original ailment.

"It is a strange but true paradox that people who have been weakened by allopathic drugging become relatively 'protected' from certain infections and epidemics. This, of course, occurs because the center of gravity of susceptibility has moved so deeply into the more vital regions of the organism that there is not enough susceptibility on superficial levels to produce a symptomatic reaction. In such an instance, this is not a sign of improvement in health, but rather a sign of degeneration."[4]

Hahnemann presented the example of suppressed syphilis. First the external chancre is removed palliatively, the physician is satisfied, but the disease is deprived of its least dangerous outlet. It may fester at the same level for several years, but eventually it will lodge more deeply, damaging the nervous system or distorting the brain. It is as though the hole in a steam kettle were blocked, causing it to erupt within.

Take, for instance, the following sequence:

A sick person goes to a regular doctor. His disease is treated and he is considered cured.

The next time he is sick, he goes, perhaps unaware, to a homoeopath. The doctor discovers that the new disease is primarily a result of the suppression of the earlier disease. Good therapeutics demands a return of that disease, which was ostensibly cured and the successful treatment of which was paid for.

By homoeopathic standards, the patient is the victim of poor medical treatment. By allopathic standards, the patient was cured and came down with a new ailment. If he should return to the allopath, he would be told there is no invisible disease and that the two separate physical diseases he has contracted are in fact different diseases. If he should return to the homoeopath again after that, he would find out that they are not different diseases, merely different symptoms from the same underlying disease. Ultimately a choice must be made. The allopathic establishment made that choice, collectively, for the American public, but this does not do away with the problem. From a homoeopathic point of view, the allopathic medical care provided in civilized countries has driven disease inward to such a degree that we see an exponential increase in the most serious pathological expressions—cancer, heart disease, and mental illness.

Seventy years ago Kent said that if we continue to treat skin disease palliatively, the human race will cease to exist. What a gargantuan exaggeration by the usual standards of medical theory! It is, in fact, meaningless as stated. But homoeopathy considers the skin a great drain of bodily poisons and the first line of defense against disease taking deeper root. If the outer layer reacts strongly, it protects the organism; such is its power and sensitivity.

The cumulative charge of poor medical treatment against the doctors of the West is so serious as to be mind-boggling, and, as we have suggested, it places conventional malpractice in a totally new light. It is, finally, *all* malpractice. The difference, seen homoeopathically, is between the sanctioned malpractice that makes up most of modern medicine and the occasional intentional or careless violation of a meaningless code of ethics.

The implications, to the homoeopath, pyramid from here. If the disease is invisible, then all the research is for naught. If medical treatment produces more serious ailments, for which patients must again be treated and charged, then the entire medical profession becomes an extortionist gang. The "sting" would outdo any "con game" on record. The older, sicker people, their diseases assured by earlier treatment, require extraordinarily expensive hospital treatment. By this stage, the disease causes are so deeply internal and refined in nature that a full supporting army of laboratory, pharmaceutical, and surgical aid is required. The result can only be either the death of the patient or the postponement of jackpot until a later, even more serious expensive ailment. Ultimately the patient dies, and the sting is complete, with perfect above-ground legal disposal of the body. What makes the whole thing a mockery (again, we must emphasize, seen homoeopathically) is that the *real* disease cause is invisible anyway. Any quest for an impossible object will become exponentially more expensive at each level of refinement, for, as long as there is no limit to the variety and subtlety of equipment that can be developed to aid in this grand delusion, there is also no limit to the cost. It is not that disease treatment has gotten more expensive with the improvement of techniques and the expansion of health care. It is that the medical profession has launched a Moon-voyage style research expedition, with the public as unknowing guinea pigs. The research has become ultraexpensive, but actual health care has not improved, except to prolong the life of the subjects. Unfortunately, the prolongation merely subjects them to more exotic diseases, even previously unknown diseases, with the result that they must pay more to have their cases thoroughly researched, not cured.

The responsibility all falls on the sick person, the victim. He is a participant in an ongoing lottery. He is even allowed to gamble on the results with health insurance companies. He bets with his money that he will get sick and with his body and life that he will stay healthy. Either way, he wins, but either way, he loses. If disease happens, it is like an unlucky throw of the dice, but he is held responsible financially.

An individual's control over his destiny, under this present medical regime, is limited to diet, exercise, and avoidance of certain obvious health hazards—all very important and early Hahnemannian precepts anyway. But he may follow them to a tee and still get sick. Then he is subjected to medicines which prolong and deepen the illness.

If there is any truth to these homoeopathic views at all, here in our age of technological progress, when people are glad not to have been alive during times of plague, then we are somewhere else entirely, somewhere other than we thought we were. We would not be the first people in history to tread that ground. The age-old fear of doctors that some people have may prove to be prophetic. It was once considered indulgent paranoia to fear the doctor, to believe that he somehow carried the illness and passed it on. Not by homoeopathic standards!

Symptomology is very important in homoeopathy, but it is used diagnostically and according to a very different system of symptom reading. Since the doctor is searching for a similar to the disease among the remedies, he must learn to read the symptoms profoundly, not superficially. They are the sole basis he has on which to select a remedy. The disease *cannot* be assigned to a category and understood by characteristics common to the category. The disease is specific only to the one occasion of its appearance in the single patient, where, in delicate interaction with the defense mechanism, it gives clues to the dynamic of its action, its direction, and hence the direction in which the proposed cure must work. This allows the disease to be cured on the basis of the language of its symptoms, sparing the doctor any involvement in its nature or degree of pathology. In Hahnemann's words:

"'The disease, being but a peculiar condition, cannot speak, cannot tell its own story; the patient suffering from it can alone render an account of his disease by the various signs of his disordered health, the ailments he feels, the symptoms he can complain of, and by the alterations in him that are perceptible to the senses."[5]

The full import of this methodology may not come across in a first reading because we are accustomed to think of actual disease causes and remediation of what has gone awry. Our unconscious prejudice runs deeply enough for us to tend to understand homoeopathic language only by reference to allopathic clichés. Since the disease cause is unknowable, the cure cannot come from knowledge. The worst damage an ailment causes tells no more than a minor symptom, for both are expressions of the unknown. The ravages of pathology seem to require the doctor's attention; and it is no wonder that he seeks to learn not only how such damage could come about in the natural order of life but also how to reverse its mechanism. Hahnemann, however, bypasses the whole matter of the relative importance of symptoms with a master stroke. All symptoms are equally important because all are clues to the nature of the disease. The disease is a property of the constitution itself and lies beneath any concrete manifestation, beneath any separation into mental and physical. Everything potentially reflects it: a wart, a nightmare, a taste in food, a sensitivity to cold, diarrhea, weeping, anger, messiness, fastidiousness, fear, restlessness, loss of memory. Among symptoms recorded in a standard repertory (with the medicines of which they are descriptive) are: time passing too swiftly (*Cocculus*); crawling as of ants over the surface of the head (*Picric Acid*); calls his boots logs of wood (*Stramonium*); moved to tears welling at the sound of bells (*Antimonium Crudum*); symptoms worse at 2 A.M. (*Kali Bichromicum*); wounded pride (*Palladium*); feeling of a mouse running in the lower limbs (*Sepia*); feeling of a living animal in abdomen (*Thuja*); ridiculously solemn acts carried out in improper clothing (*Hyoscyamus Niger*); and a woman's dreaming of a large snake in her bed (*Lac Caninum*).[6]

Odd as some of these may sound, each is a clue to an underlying process. The body wastes no energy. It would not be able to produce these idiosyncrasies unless it meant them (i.e., unless something inward spoke in terms of them). Hahnemann precedes Freud, Lévi-Strauss, and the whole of twentieth-century humanistic and linguistic science in the dictum "Either everything has meaning, or nothing has meaning,"[7] to paraphrase Lévi-Strauss in *Totemism*. Freud used dreams, jokes, and strange compulsions as his clues to the unconscious; Lévi-Strauss later used ceremonies, kinship structure, and myths as the keys to unknowable essence of a culture.

The differences between Hahnemann and Freud or Lévi-Strauss are vast, but they share the perception that mind and body shape their extenuations out of underlying content that either they or the complexity of their situation tries to conceal but in fact betrays.

Alfred North Whitehead, the British mathematician and philosopher, has his own version of this holism:
"Every proposition proposing a fact must, in its complete analysis, propose the general character of the universe required for that fact. There are no self-sustained facts, floating in non-entity. . . ."[8]

Hahnemann's insistence on replacing value scales with infinitesimally precise record keeping is also decidedly modern. He understood implicitly that the evaluation of symptoms was a red herring that predisposed physicians into familiar disease categories. The only reason for emphasizing certain symptoms of a condition was to locate and name that condition in comparison with other conditions sharing those symptoms, then to treat it in a manner already set down as biomechanically effective for that pathology.

Ironically, homoeopathy may give the appearance, to the outsider, of being obsessed with trivial and odd symptoms. A patient having recently suffered a heart attack may find the homoeopathic doctor more interested in hand gestures while speaking or a minor ailment that was treated and cured several years back. If, in truth, homoeopaths collected exotic symptoms because they believed each one needed to be improved, *sui generis*, homoeopathy would be guilty of irrelevance.

This was never Hahnemann's intention. The doctor elicits symptoms only in order to learn the disease. He encourages the patient to talk because the talk, in its intensity and rhythm, must be a manifestation of the disease too. He asks about tastes in food in order to see what the person is seeking or avoiding, or even what he thinks he is seeking, thinks he is avoiding. It takes a brilliant diagnostician to work through such a puzzle, but the good homoeopath must be this. The symptoms are the clues of the mystery, the only visible remnants of an invisible and unperceived attacker. If this intruder happens to track in a few grains of sand that show where he came from, the alert observer will use these and ignore the lamps he has knocked over and the bureau drawers he has pulled out.

Hahnemann knew that, in a system of signs, unusual items carry more information than common ones. He writes: "In this search for a homoeopathic specific remedy . . . the *more striking, singular, uncommon, and peculiar* (characteristic) signs and symptoms of the case of disease are chiefly and most solely to be kept in view."[9]

The patient, especially when badly "trained" by allopathic symptom collection, will often ignore the most deep-seated and diagnostable symptoms and give the ones which are most transitory and least indicative of the disease. But this is, of course, because allopathy does not make the same distinction between symptoms and diseases, and in many cases does not make any distinction at all. When an allopath examines a diseased organ or a corpse, he is looking directly at the active pathology. In homoeopathy, these are only the hit-and-run effects of an assailant that has long since fled.

Esoteric homoeopathy, as we shall see, believes that the disease core is inherited and develops early in infancy. Hence, the homoeopath is interested most in those symptoms which appeared earliest or which have persisted the longest, even if they were once healed allopathically. Acute conditions mark telltale outbreaks of the underlying disease in coordination with the defense response. The homoeopath is interested in discovering the chronic sequence that manifests in an acute susceptibility. But the patient may well have gotten so used to his long-standing problems that he discounts them and despairs of ever having them improve. No doctor has been interested in them before, so he forgets self-protectively and by habit.

The homoeopath tries to draw the patient out with a new set of questions. He asks: "How do you feel before a storm?" "Are you often dizzy?" He wants to know about susceptibility to heat and cold, low points and high-energy times of the day. He asks: "In what position do you like to sleep?" "How do you feel when your collar is buttoned?" "Do you like or dislike a belt around your waist?" "How do you tolerate waiting for a train?" He wants to know about times of anger, sadness; about sources of frustration. He wants to hear fantasies and fears and dreams. He observes the exact location and pattern of itches and pimples. He inquires into the color of urine and stools, the shape and consistency of stools. He observes whether the patient is neat or sloppy. If he is neat, is he normally neat, or fastidious? He may also get at some hidden characteristic by asking: "How do those around you think of you?"

As in psychiatry, the verbal account of the symptoms is used as the patient's conception of the disease; the manner in which he gives the information may itself become the dominant clue. The symptoms then become less useful diagnostically than the incidental office behavior. Even so, subtleties of analysis are involved. Vithoulkas points out that many remedies (i.e., diseases, which mean, homoeopathically, people with those diseases) are hypochondriac, talking about their ailments incessantly. But *Nitric Acid* is basically nihilistic and will produce new more dread symptoms if previous ones are relieved. It is a sterile anxiety with a conviction that no one can help under any condition. *Arsenicum Album* is just as anxious about his health, but he is convinced that the doctor can save him if only he will hear him out and get to the bottom of it. *Phosphorus* babbles about ill health, but not specially to the doctor and not with any sense that either his health or the doctor make a great deal of difference.[10] The interpretation of such subtleties determines the course of the treatment, but there is no value placed on them as such. The doctor does not try to remedy them per se; in many cases, they are neither desirable nor undesirable, but infallibly expressions of the whole.

Hahnemann knew that a heart attack was more serious and worrisome than a wart or a craving for a particular food like broccoli, but as an expression of the constitution they are comparable. In fact, the craving for broccoli may be far more significant if its specificity suggests a medicine that the heart attack does not. The treatment by diagnosis from the broccoli will then improve the heart condition in a way that emphasis on the immediate mechanical causes of the heart attack could not.

The visible effects of pathology that stand out boldly and define the common disease groups of allopathy are often useless, for they define the immediate acute phase rather than the underlying affliction. Standard medicine not only emphasizes these but names its diseases after them and the classes they create: tuberculosis, cancer, influenza, kidney stones, whooping cough, colitis, schizophrenia, acne, etc. But in homoeopathy, diseases do not exist at all apart from their manifestation in individuals. "There are no diseases," wrote Hahnemann, "only sick people."[11] A person has one constitution, and although the weakness in that constitution may be expressed differently at different times in his life, there is a sense in which he has only one disease and can have only one disease. This is why a homoeopath may claim to be able to cure one person's disease whose presenting complaint is a cancer, but after examining another person's skin rash may declare the disease incurable and predict death within twenty years. To an allopath, this is a violation of fundamental reasonableness. But, homoeopathically, names like "cancer" or "eczema" are simply shorthand for stages of totally different diseases that momentarily resemble each other in a stage of pathology, or that may have a transitory susceptibility to the same bacteria.

It is not biased to say that allopaths treat the *symptoms* of homoeopathic disease—because allopaths do not believe there *is* a disease core. They consider the homoeopathic list of illnesses a fantasy of vitalistic science; they are content to know the palpable disease. If homoeopaths want to claim they can cure something more profound, allopaths leave them with the burden of proof that something more profound exists.

Homoeopathic treatment naturally follows from the definition of disease. The patient is given a remedy that would produce symptoms similar to his disease in a healthy person, i.e., a person who does not have the disease (or any other complicating condition) and thus can respond to the pure medicine. A successful cure combines a profound diagnosis with an insight into the matching medicine. If the doctor does not know the medicine from experience, he must painstakingly find it by key in the Homoeopathic Repertory, which is essentially the collected history of individuals' responses to the remedies. From there, he limits his range of selection to the few medicines that are listed for the important symptoms. After that, he must choose the Similimum, the specific remedy, on the basis of his comprehension of the wholeness of the disease and the wholeness of the remedy. Individual symptoms and characteristics are useful in finding one's way through thousands of possible remedies, but, ultimately, the doctor must deal with the fact that the remedies and the diseases to which they correspond are functional wholes and express characteristics and tendencies that go beyond the multiplicity of symptoms. In practice, homoeopathic diagnosis falls somewhere between an on-the-spot encyclopedic research project and an instantaneous comprehension of a unity.

There is no consistent pharmaceutical code linking diseases and remedies. There have been attempts to discover one, ranging from that of Paracelsus and his Doctrine of Signatures to Edward Whitmont's medicinal archetypes, which we will look at later in this chapter. At this stage in the development of homoeopathy, though, the only body of information about remedies comes from their testings and uses. Medicine and disease are matched without insight into the mechanism of the former or the chemistry of the latter. It is Hahnemann's first law of homoeopathic pharmacy "that it is only in virtue of their power to make the healthy human being ill that medicines can cure morbid states, and, indeed, only such morbid states as are composed of symptoms which the drug to be selected for them can itself produce in similarity on the healthy."[12]

Homoeopaths often know as much physiology and pharmacy as their allopathic colleagues. But this knowledge is of little or no use in the treatment of disease, they feel, unless it helps link remedies and diseases or makes the doctor more sensitive to clues. It is difficult enough for the average patient to accept that the doctor may have no understanding of or insight into the mechanism of their discomfort. But to accept that such information—the pride of the medical establishment and twentieth-century enlightenment—is of no help in the treatment of disease is almost impossible. Yet this is what homoeopathy implicitly claims, even though it may not advertise this out on the streets. It is a system based on the acceptance of inevitable and natural law, so it does not require chemicomechanical data at all.

Ideally, the disease itself could be the medicine, but for reasons of constitutional weakness, environmental and social disruption, and, according to some homoeopaths, the psychospiritual condition of mankind, this is not the case. While an organism is able to improve within certain symptomatic limits, it cannot spontaneously throw off an entire illness that matches its own basic susceptibility. For one, the illness exists in layers, without a single shape or manifestation. In theory, each remedy allies with the defense mechanism and jars the system out of the disease configuration, but many additional remedies may be needed after the first one before the full archaeology of the condition is engaged.

Past conditions cannot be treated unless a removal of present symptoms brings them back. Hence, chronic ailments that are in temporary dormancy cannot be diagnosed and dislodged until they actually reoccur.

Each remedy, as it is given, changes the picture. It is the single remedy, but, as soon as the picture changes, there is another single remedy. Ultimately, a series of these "single" remedies will unravel and dispel the entire condition. It is crucial that they be given only one at a time, for no collective cleansing is possible, and each new picture is interpreted only in terms of its present priority and the response of the system to the last remedy that has been given.

By the standard of an eventual, complete cure, the symptomatic alleviation is not as important as the successive pictures, for as long as the picture is clear, a more correct remedy can follow a less correct one. The only incorrect choice is the remedy that clouds the picture and confuses the sequence of prescription.

The levels of disease must be separated, one by one, and the physician must go, etiologically, from one whole picture to the next whole picture. He cannot predict what should appear next, and he cannot be dismayed if a newer condition brings more suffering than a previous one. Homoeopathy is nonpalliative by principle. It often requires suffering. It proposes only an unwinding of the disease by a passage through the elements that make it up in time and space. A promising sequence may have the most painful eruptions, especially if the disease is deep-seated and has been suppressed by things like cortisone. Superficially, things get worse. However, if the flare-ups did not occur, the entire disease would not be removed. The process would stalemate around a particular pathological equilibrium.

One does not know, before the fact, what will happen, for the process reveals its own dynamics, its own history, as it goes. The basic homoeopathic law holds things together at each new level: prescribe by similars; take a total symptom picture and give the remedy that would cause those symptoms; wait while the organism fights for a new equilibrium; and when the result of the treatment is finalized, take a new picture; prescribe again if necessary.

Each prescription assumes that the organism will cybernetically make the best possible use of the dose, even if it is not on exactly the wavelength of the disease, and that, then, the results of the prescription and subsequent reorganization will be the next place from which to continue. The patient is improved only if he is organized around a less inward and profound center of gravity of disease. If he is reorganized around a deeper center of gravity, the medicine has made the condition worse. If the medicine is totally off the wavelength of the disease, then nothing will happen and the doctor will have a new chance. A very errant prescription does not alter the case at all, whereas a near-miss may cause a disruption which, if it is not antidoted, will make either the disease worse, the picture muddier, or both.

Each condition, as it comes into being, is real. The homoeopathic remedy, like the allopathic drug, changes the condition finally. It does no good to say: "That *was* the disease. Let's go back to it." It is no longer *the* disease after the remedy.

By esoteric homoeopathy, the same thing is true of the collective health of humanity. The supposed global improvement betrays on the deepest levels what it conceals by its superficial well-being. We might say that some things are better (smallpox, for instance), while other things are worse (like cancer, mental disease, genocide), but that would violate holism, and, from a homoeopathic standpoint, social and economic problems are the collective result of disease driven inward. The same solution must then be applied to the planet as to any individual: its case must be taken now, and the prescription must be given for present symptoms. Only when they are changed can a new prescription be given. There is no way to return now to the simpler times of simpler diseases and apply homoeopathic remedies on that basis.

In an ostensibly healthy person, the effects of the homoeopathic remedy are manifested as a brief artificial disease called "a proving," because it is the only proof of how the medicine will behave in a sick person. If the homoeopathic aggravation occurs in a sick person, this is, in a sense, the result of the artificial disease and the actual disease combining before the dynamics of that situation provokes a new condition. But the aggravation is not always noticed. Since the condition may already be painful and intense and since the vibration of the medicine may well occur on a deep organic level, its shock may blur with one's general kinesthesia. Contrarily, if the person has been under suppressive allopathic treatment which has been halted for the substitution of homoeopathy, the aggravation may be more painful and symptomatically severe than the disease, for it will activate something that had previously been drugged and to which the organism had been artificially numbed.

If the remedy is right, though, patients always feel they are somehow better. Every obvious manifestation may be worse, but there is a sense that things are under control and will improve.

The initial effect of a homoeopathic remedy is to aggravate the disease, and the initial effect of the allopathic drug is to alleviate the symptoms. However, it is not the initial effect of the medicine that is of concern homoeopathically. The homoeopathic aggravation must be followed by swift and complete cure in the case of the final and correct remedy. The allopathic alleviation is palliative and insubstantial; it drugs the organs without strengthening their response. The only lasting effect of an allopathic pharmaceutical on the system is its side effect, which is chronically and ultimately aggravating.*

* Devout, esoteric homoeopaths say that we have not yet earned the right to have such a swift righteous medicine as allopathy claims to be.

Homoeopathy is, from the beginning, the medicine of side effects and secondary responses. These are the fully integrated and permanent decisions of the organism after it has had its first startled reaction.

The question then is: Why is the homoeopathic remedy so much more noticeable to the organism than everything else in the environment? Homoeopaths give two answers: 1) because it is exactly specific and 2) because it is on the dynamic plane. In order to understand the first, we must review why the disease itself, as an elegant response of the defense mechanism, is not the self-sufficient cure.

Because the disease is the exactly correct response, the organism engages with it in a deep romantic folly, often to the death. The medicine resembles the illness, often to a tee, but it is *not* the illness. The vibration of the correct remedy somehow provides a safe context, somewhere deep in the internal language of the body, in a patterning like gene transmission and cell growth. The sickness is expressed through *its* nonpathology instead of by deteriorative disease.

That is one model. We might also say the medicine supplies what was constitutionally lacking so that the need is not expressed pathologically. Perhaps the medicine shocks the system into action, causing it to cure itself.

Homoeopaths understand that it is ultimately the vital force that initiates the cure, not the medicine. Their respect for disease is almost religious. It is a force of nature, like gravity or procreation. To assume that it could be manipulated by the crude machines and concoctions of physicians is arrogant. One might as well, with Ahab, attack the Sun. The only thing equivalent to the disease is the life of the organism. If that can be sparked into countering the disease, then the disease can be overcome. Any use of crude substance to alter its course must be as much an attack upon the organism as it is upon the disease.

Hahnemann laughed at the idea that a medicine could be instructed to do only good when in the body. One might as well, he wrote, instruct the carbon, nitrogen, and hydrogen in a meal of cabbage, roast beef, and wheatcakes, telling them what part of the body to nourish and what part to stay out of.[13] The only escape from this dilemma was to give nonmedicines for medicines, i.e., substances which affected the system not by digestion or inclusion but by the information they carried to the deepest levels of somatic process. Then the native intelligence of the body and the disease, matched by the insight of the physician, might meet on meaningful ground.

Theodore Enslin, at a seminar in 1977, gave some notable insights into the action of homoeopathic medicines:

"It is a parallel. It is a recognition of the fact that the unwanted manifestations can only be braked by producing other unwanted manifestations which are similar. And there's a great difference between similar and the same. There's a popular conception: if the guy gets gas from eating cabbage, you give him a high dilution of cabbage, and that's going to cure him. That's not what's done at all. Actually, the medicines are not medicines at all. The process is an outrage of the system itself. A diseased system is an apathetic one: it just doesn't give a damn. But in many—most cases, unless the thing has gone too far—that apathy can be overcome by introducing a parallel. When that parallel becomes apparent to the organism, it's outraged—and cures itself. The medicine actually has very little to do with it."[14]

Enslin also described how, when the symptoms drop off, they go back in time:

"In the treatment of a condition, a conditioning which has gone on for many years, sometimes it is not possible to cure with one shot; it's not a miracle at all. That's one reason a good prescriber wants to know as much about the patient as possible: everything. So you begin a reverse process. You begin, very practically, with what is exactly there. When those symptoms are cleared, very often you will find that that patient has symptoms that are prior, of things that happened before that. And you keep on going. You go back to childhood. And there are many stories about the actual walking off of the last symptom. You get to the point where it will go right off a finger, the last wart or pain. There are many case histories like that. Sometimes this process can take a number of years."

Homoeopathy is a system that, at first, to most people seems totally opaque and impenetrable, and they doubt that they will ever understand it. When they gain a basic understanding of the principles, their response is often that it is perfectly clear—bizarre but clear. Then contradictions appear and new difficulties develop, as in the homoeopathic cure itself. The process of clarification must go through many such confusions and resolutions before one has any real sense of the system. At this point, we will introduce the two most common questions: Why does it sometimes require many remedies and sometimes only one to cure a disease? How can homoeopathy explain the obvious facts of contagion, germs, and epidemics? These questions appear together because they are related. In homoeopathic terms, diseases are layers, patterns imposed upon each other. Or, if we are to call disease a single phenomenon, then the disease of any one person is built up of historically successive miasms. These miasms, at any given moment, describe a totality; since the person is a unity, the disease is a unity. There is perhaps one medicine which expresses the base of the miasmatic pattern more profoundly than any other, but that medicine cannot be prescribed unless the present symptoms call for it. The doctor must begin by prescribing for the current miasmatic layer, as he perceives it, ignoring temporarily the deeper levels contained within it. If he removes one miasmatic level, the pattern will change like a moiré wave, presenting a new picture.

The number of prescriptions necessary is determined by the miasmatic depth of the disease, which is not the same as its intensity or pathology. These may well be minimal in a deep miasmatic disease because the defense mechanism is not strong enough to produce a curative response. The systemic apathy is too great. Likewise, an intense disease does not mean a deep miasmatic condition. Usually it means a healthy defense system, except in the final throes of long chronic disease before ultimate demise.

Acute disease is then nothing more than a stimulation of the defense mechanism by a pathogenic agent. Chronic conditions seize upon agents to which they are responsive in order to provoke an eruption and with the ultimate aim of feeling better. Pathogenic bacteria increase and decrease in the organism according to the disease level and its requirements. Very contagious ailments (i.e., agents) affect large numbers of contiguous people, but not all people and not all people in the same way. It is the defense mechanism and disease level that determine the nature and meaning of the response. The morbific agent, on which standard medicine focuses in its interest in the common symptoms and relationship of cases, is secondary to the limitless individual responses of organisms. Each organism will use the occasion of the "bug" to express its particular chronic needs. Thus, each organism still requires individual treatment in an epidemic. Furthermore, not everyone becomes sick (so-called Legionnaires' Disease, which gained attention in 1976, affected a limited number of people).

The pathology is not as important as the miasmatic pattern. Sometimes the morbific agent itself is so severe as to be life-threatening. It may also be powerful enough to impose consistent symptomology on a large number of people. In such circumstances, homoeopaths may well use a small number of remedies or even a single remedy for all people during an epidemic. This is not ideal. It is an admission that the disease itself is too powerful a "medicine"—a stimulant—at this stage of history for a people in a society. Even though an epidemic is potentially exteriorizing and cleansing (as the Hippocratic coction), its workings are life-threatening and must be removed if the organism is to survive the lesson. A homoeopath may agree to antidote this "medicine" with an allopathic drug. He recognizes that the person is not ready to handle such strong cleansing. Treatment may fail, and the patient may still be lost—but history has never been kind and disease as an adjustment is real. Homoeopathy can no more cure all conditions by similars than it can negate death. It can only engage the organism in the most creative and curative response of which it is capable. Since the organism's own defense mechanism is already the first remedy, the homoeopathic medicine is chosen as a continuation of its working. If the most creative response will destroy the organism, the homoeopath can make his single use of allopathic pharmacy—to antidote. He can use an allopathic drug to antidote a bad homoeopathic prescription, so he can certainly use it to "antidote" a bad disease. The relationship between the two systems (from a homoeopathic standpoint) is set clear by this: homoeopathy is a creative use of disease to bring about human transformation and, ultimately, health; allopathy is a means of antidoting the dangerous and creative disease process and, at worst, limiting human potential to what can be achieved in a drugged condition.

In esoteric homoeopathy—which deals with the religious, philosophical, and cultural aspects of disease—civilization, society, environment, and sickness are interlinked and homogeneous conditions. A morbific agent arises when the over-all civilizational process requires it at some level. If individuals die, it is as they die in nature: the disease itself is not their death knell—it is their opportunity, their civilizational opportunity, to escape a particular rut or stagnation through the deepest possible organic realignment. All other political and economic solutions must be palliatives, doomed attempts to make the law of contraries work.

For instance, the present economic crisis of the West and its energy dilemma are symptoms. If humanity were transformed (and disease is the most profound transforming agent), then the solutions emerge from within the actual crisis. In that sense, the present disease level of the world is a creative symptomatic response to its problems. And, from a Hahnemannian standpoint, these are diseases. Slaughter in Uganda or Cambodia or Guatemala is the work of disease driven inward to the mental plane on an epidemic level. Pornography, sexual violence, mayhem in the United States, and terrorism in Western Europe in the 1970s are diseases, attempts to resolve deep inner imbalances in the only way the organisms themselves know how. The murderer-rapist so little understands his deed because he *is* his deed.

This is why the decadence is so consistent and contagious and why, despite the horror it provokes in us, we almost expect it and would be disappointed without it. We would be disappointed because we know that our sensitivity is still great enough to respond to disease with profound pathology, and we are relieved by the pathology. In this way, the Vietnam war relieved the United States of the premonition of a far deeper disturbance; at the same time, it enabled that innermore layer to erupt into pathology, and it has. People intuitively understood that we were collectively sicker before the appearance of the disease.

Allopathy deals with society much as it deals with the body: circumstances are separate and unconnected; roles are temporary and circumstantial. An ailment of the liver is an ailment of the liver, and a job driving a bus is a job driving a bus. If a bus driver has a liver malfunction and cannot go to work, the allopath returns him to work. His liver is "improved," and he can drive the bus. He can return to his job, his family, his general social station.

Homoeopathic treatment changes the entire organism. Job and social station may be part of the disease; thus, when patients start to get better, they find themselves unable to fill the same roles in the world. If they do continue in old paths, the illnesses will return. So the larger treatment requires an adjustment of all circumstances, organic and environmental, in which the patient finds himself. The liver ailment and driving the bus are no longer interdependent circumstances, but *the same thing.*

We can propose something of a hierarchy. The deepest individual disease is genetic; an organism inherits the constitutional predispositions and weaknesses of its ancestors. Onto the genetic level are imposed the miasms of early childhood diseases and conditions suppressed by allopathic medicine or otherwise internalized. Onto this level are imposed perhaps another chronic disease, then an acute disease (which is simply the sensitivity of the chronic to external events), and then the exact environmental conditions to which the organism is exposed, including the social order, the economic order, the spiritual condition of the society, and the actual biochemical pollution. These different webs may be imposed onto each other in a variety of ways. The patient is an expression of all the forces that exist around him, which have brought him into being and which sustain his world.

Esoteric homoeopathy and practical homoeopathy are often different medicines. In the former, the deepest cure must always be sought, initially at the risk of the patient's balance, job, and relationships, and ultimately at the risk of his life. At the same time, the physician realizes that absolute cure is an impossibility because disease is *in* civilization, so he goes as far as circumstances allow.

Practical homoeopathy compromises on the level to which it will seek cure. The physician may decide not to treat an ailment if he feels that the patient has no space into which to expand and make room for the cure. If the disease and life situation are in a state of balance, the disease may be necessary for the survival of the patient. A strong remedy can have suicidal consequences if the patient cannot integrate the new implications. It is also possible that a remedy can be driven back onto the physical plane in a debilitating or life-threatening way. One homoeopath mentioned a patient who was chronically ill until she joined a very expressive religious sect. She was both fanatic and miserable and sought homoeopathic treatment through her new belief in spiritual medicine. Soon after taking the remedy, she lost interest in religion entirely and developed multiple sclerosis. There is at least the possibility, in homoeopathic terms, that the law of cure worked to return the ailment to its new corresponding point on the physical plane, protecting the mental plane.

Esotericism is a luxury for most practicing homoeopaths, and they must succeed with their patients if they are to continue to believe in the system. In fact, many doctors who use homoeopathic remedies dismiss the interpretation of disease and human history as nonsense and claim that even the medicines are impossible and unbelievable. They go on practicing *only* because it works. Of course, they are little different than any modern medical school graduates. They practice by precedent, not theory. They do not know how people get sick or why the trusted methods cure them, or even if the methods are the cause of the cure. Any intimate discussion with the allopathic family doctor will reveal this.

It is the *language* of conventional medicine that is socially acceptable. Its lapses are covered by a familiar jargon. Its enigmas have been integrated into our social expectations and cultural superstitions in a way that allows common discussion of ailments and cures without deep understanding. The allopathic disease names are still the common names for diseases, and, as names, they are half of the explanation and half of the cure.

The keynote of practical homoeopathy is the correct interpretation of sequential pictures from the administration of remedies. Kent, for instance, gives twelve very careful "observations," to use his idiom for them, to make after the medicine is given:[15]

The first is that when there is prolonged aggravation of the symptoms, followed by the final decline of the patient, it means too strong a medicine: the action was too deep for the degree of deterioration that had already taken place and the weakened vital force was unable to throw off the new attack. Since the medicine can work only through the vital force, the physician must assess how strong the vital force is before giving a remedy. The potency of the medicine can be harmonized, approximately, to the capability of the vital force.

In the second observation, there is also a long aggravation, but one leading to slow and final improvement of the patient. In this case, the disease was deep but deterioration was not as great, hence the medicine was appropriate. The aggravation was long because tissue change had already begun.

The third observation is that if there is a quick strong aggravation, followed by rapid improvement, the remedy was correct, and no serious tissue change has already taken place.

In the fourth observation, where there is recovery without aggravation, Kent wonders if there was any disease in the first place or if the disease was relatively new and superficial.

In the fifth observation, improvement and amelioration of the symptoms followed by aggravation indicate that the disease is deeper than the medicine and the medicine was acting only palliatively.

The sixth observation is slightly different: short relief followed by return of the symptoms might mean the patient has antidoted the remedy by coming into contact with substances that neutralize the potentization.

In the seventh observation, the symptoms are relieved, but the patient still feels sick. This means the wrong medicine because there are latent organic conditions preventing a cure.

In the eighth, there are patients that prove every remedy. This may be an idiosyncrasy; it may also indicate an incurable condition. Kent suggests using a higher potency.

The method of bringing on symptoms in a healthy person by giving a medicine is known as proving (the ninth). It is the procedure for discovering new remedies and is said to be beneficial to people who do it.

New symptoms might also indicate a proving, which would mean the wrong medicine had been used (the tenth). It is important, however, to distinguish between a proving and the reappearance of old symptoms. When old symptoms reappear in the reverse order of their original occurrence (the eleventh observation), this confirms that the healing process is moving in the natural direction.

In the twelfth observation, the symptoms move from without to within, driving the disease deeper. This indicates the doctor prescribed only for a peripheral condition, and in so doing hastened the disease process.

The vital force expresses the organism as a whole. Since it is unitary, it insures the singleness of the disease and the single effect of the medicine: each plucks its modulation like a string. Disease is a distortion of the vital chord that is then transferred to the physical body as susceptibility. When the medicine is given, the vital force recognizes it. Homoeopathy does not confer the power of dynamic readjustment on the organs themselves, only on the vital force. Dissections even of the living cannot reveal the disease or the curative process because they show only the flesh, and the flesh is animated in another plane. Hahnemann writes:

"This *dynamic* action of medicines, like the vitality itself by means of which it is reflected upon the organism, is almost purely *spiritual* in its nature. . . . This dynamic property is so pervading that it is quite immaterial what sensitive part of the body is touched by the medicine in order to develop its whole action . . . immaterial whether the dissolved medicine enter the stomach or merely remain in the mouth, or be applied to a wound or other part deprived of skin."[16]

Homoeopathic medicines are "spiritual" medicines. Despite their elaborate chemical preparation by an overt pharmaceutical procedure, they are not drugs. The final product, the actual pill, is such a high dilution of the original substance that nothing is left of it; in some cases, an extremely tiny amount, not known to have any effectiveness, remains incidentally. The actual procedure is as follows:

The medicinal substance, which might be plant tincture, animal product, mineral, disease discharge, or, in fact, anything that one chooses, is diluted in nine parts neutral medium. If it is a liquid or soluble in alcohol, then alcohol is used and the new solution is shaken vigorously after dilution. If it is not soluble in alcohol, then it is pulverized (triturated) in a mortar with milk sugar. This operation is used for silica, animal charcoal, graphite, sulphur, crude antimony, gold, platinum, zinc, copper, silver, tin, a variety of carbonates, and other alcohol-insoluble materials. The process, carefully defined by Hahnemann as to the amount of milk sugar and the technique of cutting at each stage, apparently changes the original material in some unknown way. But the preparation is so tedious and so different from anything in standard science that chemists do not even bother to test it.

To form the next decimal potency, one part of this dilution is then mixed with nine parts more neutral medium and shaken or triturated. The third decimal potency is made with one part of the second decimal and nine more parts neutral medium. At this point the original substance is only one thousandth of the final pill.

There is another common scale in which the dilutions are made, with one part substance and ninety-nine parts neutral medium; in fact, this, and not the prior scale, is commonly used in triturations. The third centesimal dilution produces a pill with one-millionth part of the original medicine. If poison nut were the tincture for its tendency to produce symptoms like the symptoms of a disease, then the nut juice would constitute one millionth of the actual medicine at the third centesimal dilution. By the twelfth centesimal dilution (or twenty-fourth decimal dilution), there is almost certainly no trace of the original substance in most of the medicine, no trace at all (!).

No poison nut juice in the remedy called "poison nut," no cuttlefish ink in the remedy called *"Sepia,"* no mercury in the *"Mercury,"* no gold in the *"Aurum,"* no dog's milk in *"Lac Caninum."*

To assume that there is any original substance left would be in violation of either Avogadro's Law or some other law of physical chemistry. Avogadro's Law itself is a mainstay of physical science. Proposed originally by the nineteenth-century Italian physicist Count Amadeo Avogadro, it states that the number of molecules in a gram molecular weight of a substance is 6.0225×10^{23}. The 6.0225 is not the key here, but 10^{23} is. For, if a substance is diluted beyond 10^{-24}, with uniform mixing at each stage, there is nothing left of it. Each dilution reduces the number of molecules of the substance, which begins at the unimaginably high figure of, roughly, six followed by twenty-three zeros, until by the twenty-fourth decimal dilution (one to nine each time), there should not be a single molecule remaining in any one pill. No doubt, if one or more hung on from irregular mixing, they would be in mortal jeopardy in the passage from the twenty-fourth to the twenty-fifth decimal. Yet the preparation has just begun.

This process continues, usually to the thirtieth decimal, but often as far as the one-millionth centesimal, and there is no reason to assume it should stop there. This amount of dilution is beyond comprehension. There is nothing left at the twelfth centesimal, and yet that substance continues to be diluted, one to a hundred, one to a hundred, one to a hundred, almost a million times more to produce the millionth centesimal. Furthermore, there is another scale, called the millesimal, in which substances are serially diluted one part to fifty thousand of neutral medium up into the hundreds of thousands of times. It is worse than putting a sugar cube in the ocean. A bewildered Abraham Lincoln called it the "medicine of a shadow of a pigeon's wing." Yet we are in the "other" science and a different law holds.

Each dilution, according to homoeopaths, increases the effective power of the original substance. One would not think of using the ten-thousandth decimal, let alone the one-millionth centesimal, except in the case of severe long-standing illness. It is no wonder that homoeopathy finds little acceptance in mainstream medicine. Convinced homoeopaths have expressed such dismay at the bizarre principles of their own pharmacy that one doctor regularly treated animals, with the same success, to reassure himself that his treatment was not just suggestibility plus placebo.

In the physical world, some substances are poisonous, some are nutritious, some are virtually inactive in the human body. After homoeopathic "potentization," the majority of these physical properties disappear and new properties occur that are unknown in chemistry. Although there is a rough resemblance between the behavior of a potentized substance and its raw physical base, the differences are great enough to establish a whole new system of hermetic medicinal chemistry.

The potentized form of matter, as described by homoeopathy, is a unique and stable state, different from gas, liquid, solid, or plasma. Thus, it is theoretically possible to potentize any substance. In actuality, some substances are preferred, for they were in herbal and medicinal use for centuries before homoeopathy was formulated. But experimental homoeopathy continues to examine the possibility of potentizing new substances and learning their full properties as medicines—from their toxicology in material doses to their spiritual vibration in microdoses. This is done not only in the search for materials with unknown therapeutic qualities, but in the adjustment of the basic pharmacy to a world in which both human and environmental chemistry is changing. The philosophy of esoteric homoeopathy demands that the world continue to produce new forms of illness and simultaneously new medicines to treat them. Furthermore, as homoeopathy was practiced in new regions, different local substances were available. For instance, after a disciple of Hahnemann brought homoeopathy to India at the middle of the nineteenth century, local provings contributed panther, tiger, and leopard to the medicine chest.

A new class of medicines, prepared from bacteria and pathological tissue, was added in the early twentieth century. The bowel nosodes, as these are called, include such initially dismaying substances as gonorrheal and syphilitic discharges. More recently, homoeopathic experimenters have potentized cat hair, tobacco, their own sperm, sulphur dioxide, and LSD—in each case following the loose homoeopathic rule that a substance which brings about an imbalance or pathology in material form is a possible remedy in potentized form.[17]

Clearly, the original physical substance is diluted into nonexistence and passes from the picture. In the case of bacteria and strong poisons, this is fortunate and reassuring. If anything remains after the physical substance is gone, it must be in the form of a message, a message that has already been passed to the neutral medium before the dilution destroys its source. Perhaps the tincture transfers something like a template of itself or some of its properties to the surrounding solution, much in the way DNA and messenger RNA exchange information in the duplication of living cells. The succussion (shaking) of the tincture after each dilution may "hammer" the message in, and then each successive dilution, with continued succussion, would serve to charge the message, increasing its volume, potency by potency. We seem to be left with tiny, white, chemically neutral balls, but if anything like the above occurs, we would also have the record of a potency. That record would contain not the chemical properties of animal, plant, or mineral, but something that precedes their manifestation and generates it, even as the invisible core disease precedes the visible symptomology.

In any case, the medicines cannot be considered drugs: they are parallels, vibrations, spiritual entities, intelligences, messages—they are any of these images we use to understand their action. They are qualities of substance, not quantities, however we understand that. In 1900 Kent wrote:

"Vital disorder cannot be turned into order except by something similar in quality to the vital force. It is not similitude in quantity that we want, in weights and measures, but it is similarity in quality, in power, in plane, that must be sought for.

"Medicines, therefore, cannot affect the high and interior planes of the physical economy unless they are raised to the plane of similarity in quality. The individual who needs Sulphur in the very highest degrees may take Sulphur sufficient to move his bowels, may rub it upon the skin, may wear it in his stockings, can take Sulphur baths, all without effect upon his disease. In that form the drug is not in correspondence with his sickness, it does not affect him in the same plane in which he is sick, and so it cannot affect the cause and flow from thence to the circumference."[18]

I asked Theodore Enslin about this phenomenon[19] and he chose to emphasize the high potencies, the nonmaterial dilutions, which, he said "are a division of energy in the sense that the low ones are not. Up to six or seven ✕, there is a recognizable amount of molecular structure left in the pill. In the high potencies, it's not substance at all; it depends entirely on a release of energy. Energy is divisible, but it's not divisible in the same sense that molecular substance is.

These potencies are really quite dangerous. A good physician prescribing can give a high potency and in one dose clear up something that has resisted all kinds of prescribing for years, and it seems miraculous. Anyone handling that had better be pretty competent. I mean, there are things, that no good physician would deny, that are not known so far as those things are concerned. Substances that have absolutely no effect in low potencies suddenly have a very high one in the high potencies. And they usually are far more marked mentally than any other way. The one that is the old warhorse of the thing is *Silicea,* which is nothing more than flint. In a low potency you can take flint, you can eat rocks until they make a hole in your stomach, and it will have no medicinal effect whatsoever. But suddenly you get *Silicea* at 30× or higher; you can take it to the CM [the one-hundred thousandth centesimal], which is the ultimate, and it has a profound mental effect, something that is not present in the lower potencies."

Nowadays, the tendency is to present this issue in quasi-pharmaceutical language, as a 1974 publication of the American Institute of Homoeopathy demonstrates:

"The homeo-discipline is concerned with the specific, the individual, the distinctive. In order to achieve that goal, the homeo-medical discipline endeavours to study the reaction of the organism to an incitant and not the action of the drug itself. In doing so it reverses the roles of organism and drug and places emphasis on the vital response. . . .

"The point we wish to make is that the homeo-discipline denies that the drug possesses any power or virtue, but postulates that contact between the drug and the living organism sets in motion an influence. The drug is not injected, digested, assimilated, or transported physically. In and of itself it can do nothing except under the highly specific circumstances: when the properties of sensitivity, irritability, idiosyncrasy are exquisitely developed, the vital reaction—which is a function of the host and not of the agent—takes place."[20]

The meaning of homoeopathic pharmacy has been a much discussed issue. The best people have been able to manage are models of the transfer of virtues from substances to potencies. Edward Whitmont, a practicing Jungian therapist for several decades, is also a trained homoeopath. Beginning in the 1940s, he has written many speculative articles on the various remedies, arguing, in essence, that the same vitality that gives rise to the shape and character of the entity from which each one is extracted also gives rise to its cohesive healing virtue.

Whitmont acknowledges that pharmacy and psychology are linked on a profound psychosomatic level, but he also makes the point that they are linked on an even deeper level by a rule of identities we intuit through myths and archetypes. "False" and imaginative associations speak only a deeper truth. When we make subjective associations or intuit relationships, we are realizing material that is already *objectively* associated in the world of nature. The dynamic totality of nature brings together events and images according to their own essential natures. According to Whitmont, "Even as the symbol is the image and expression, in terms of form and appearance, of specific psychic energies, so is the morphological manifestation or appearance of an objective function in nature the expression and image in the world of sense perception of its intrinsic functional dynamism."[21]

This system recalls the Doctrine of Signatures, of which the Doctrine of Similars was a singular refinement. Dog's Milk, Poison Oak, White Cedar, and Silver are medicines for reasons we may intuitively grasp both through the mute psychology we share with them and through the morphological qualities expressed both in them and us at different levels of structure. Neither their shape nor our shape is accidental; thus, the connections are, in some sense, correct as associated. Our discovery of their intrinsic virtues, like our discovery recently of the DNA helix and the meiosis of cells, is not accidental, for we are intrinsic, imbedded, and morphological by the same order and under the same terms of nature. Ancient herbal and animal medicines come from psyche, but a psyche which is large and collective and includes the structure of botanical and animal forms in its meaning even if these seem to lie outside the more limited mind-psyche of the organism.

Carl Jung himself writes: "The assumption that the human psyche possesses layers that lie *below* consciousness is not likely to arouse serious opposition. But that there could just as well be layers lying *above* consciousness seems to be a surmise which borders on a *crimen laesae majestatis humanae*. In my experience the conscious mind can only claim a relatively central position and must put up with the fact that the unconscious psyche transcends and as it were surrounds it on all sides. Unconscious contents connect it *backwards* with physiological states on the one hand and archetypal data on the other. But it is extended *forward* by intuitions which are conditioned partly by archetypes and partly by subliminal perceptions depending on the relativity of time and space in the unconscious."[22]

To Jung, any one source of energy, like mayapple or carbon, was still an energy in nature. The objective psyche could transcend space and time and embody the full meaning of that energy, not just its imagined medicinal virtue. But Jung never translated pure integers or morphologies into the biological and genetic realms as absolutes; only the archetypes were absolutes—any given manifestation was fluid. Whitmont tries out a more fixed system of relationships in combining Jungian analysis and homoeopathy.

The potentized medicines embody archetypes that express themselves morphologically in the phenomena of nature. If one can tap the essence of an animal, plant, or stone, not its procreative seed or crystal per se but its elemental source, then a medicine can be made on the same plane. Plants, animals, stones, stars, diseases, metals, even human artifacts are equivalent on this level. The impulse which gives rise to the precise form of an oak tree or an eel, under highly individual environmental-embryological blueprints, gives rise, under different matrical circumstances, to an ulcer, a virus, an art style, a myth, a phobia, a potency, etc.

The homoeopathic remedies are taken from the tinctures of plants, animals, minerals, and other formations, reduced to the archetypal plane, and dematerialized so that they are in tune with the disease as archetype rather than as pathology. The intuition is that each substance will naturally reflect some aspect of its potential healing archetype in its habitat and growth patterns.

Whitmont calls these things "psychosomatic wholes," "dynamic totalities"; they exist simultaneously in nature and psyche, meaning they exist complementarily in medicine and myth. Some characteristic of the plant, animal, or mineral must persist in the character of its disease and its remedy. In discussing *Sepia*, for instance, he draws our attention to "the dynamic meaning of the shell-enclosed jelly".[23] This has a symbolic relationship to the alchemical vessel of prima materia, which is also the uterus, and the feminine receptacle of the self in both sexes. It may then have a healing function for its equivalents in personality or physiological process.

Whitmont writes: "Even as a half of the cuttlefish's body must remain within the enclosing shell, in spite of all attempts to break loose, so also the temperamental, sexual and emotional tendencies which one would disown cannot simply be cast off; they can only be slowly and gradually transformed by developing a conscious understanding with which to complement the world of instinctive feeling which is woman's primary expression and experience. Wherever the gradual expansion gives way to a violent, protesting attitude, suppression takes the place of gradual transformation and pathology arises. Challenge to and suppression of the quiet, contemplative and receptive feminine qualities, symbolized by the 'creative vessel,' thus become the keynotes of the *Sepia* pathology."[24]

This is not necessarily itself the *Sepia* illness, but it is, conceivably, the underlying somatic message which precedes, in the meaning of the objective psyche, the onset of pathology. Whitmont mentions the irritable, faultfinding, spiteful quality of *Sepia*; the movement from antagonism to gentleness and affection, the oversensitivity, the premature aging. These come from the suppressed unconscious personality, which must also have a concrete somatic reflection.

The *Natrum muriaticum* patient, the one whose disease is "salt," is inconsolable for a reason having to do with failure of basic assimilation of vital energies, hence disintegration of life forming in the seed.[25]

The *Phosphorus* patient is ecstatic but terrified of a coming darkness, speedy but easily exhausted, somehow stunted in growth and anemic.[26] But then *Phosphorus* also contains within it an extreme brightness, a luminescence that is not radioactive but oxidating.

Rudolf Hauschka writes: "Phosphorus . . . shines and pours out light, but is also a condensing agent. . . . Nerves are built of protein high in phosphorus. Indeed, the nervous system as a whole is as clear a revelation of the phosphorus process as the circulatory system is of the aluminium process. Phosphorus flames give light, but are cold. Our nervous system endows us with the cool, clear light of consciousness; but it is also the transmitting agent for the formative impulses that shape the body's plastic organs.

"The phosphorus process co-operates on the one hand with the silica in our skin, on the other with lime in our bony structure. The skin contains innumerable nerve-endings, which convey impressions of the world around us. Though silica creates skin surfaces, it is the phosphorus process that gives them surface sensitivity. It is to phosphorus that we owe awareness of our bodies and a bodily consciousness of selfhood. The skin, with its nerve inclusions, thus forms a boundary between world and individual."[27]

The diseases treated with homoeopathic *Phosphorus* include many of the nervous system, especially left-sided symptoms, which suggest the unconscious part of the brain; gastrointestinal irritations, including lightheadedness and desire for cold water which is then vomited; liver cirrhosis; diabetes; and general tubercular conditions. The person suffering from *Phosphorus* is nauseated by the fragrance of flowers when too strong; he is extremely jumpy, sensitive to touch, and disturbed by thunderstorms.

With *Lycopodium*, Whitmont focuses on its habits as a creeping moss whose spores "do not moisten as they repel water . . . are extremely hard but burn with a very bright flash when ignited . . . germinate only after 6–7 years."[28] The *Lycopodium* patient has high nervous tension, is developed mentally but with a weak body. He craves open air and loosens tight clothing; he is dry, constipative, and noneliminative, with kidney and urinary symptoms. His diseases progress slowly and inwardly, with a tendency toward cancerous growth. He is bloated and does not digest well; he has bad circulation and lacks inner heat. Is this symptomology then the form taken by club moss spore when its archetype is realized in a disease and its potentized substance is used as a remedy?

Whitmont emphasizes, alternately, the physical manifestation of the substance, its makeup as a plant or animal or mineral, and its meaning in human symbolism and myth, as if these were related to the same function. For instance, with *Lachesis*, rattlesnake poison, he marks the serpent as the dark, underground function, the figure which, in Gnostic tradition, replaces Christ on the Cross: "The serpent pathology is the unintegrated life impulse, the unintegrated libido, the unintegrated instinct split off and split in itself. . . . *Lachesis* is the penalty of unlived life."[29] Thus the *Lachesis* patient is egotistic, vicious, and mean, all in frustration for the actual self not lived. The person has intense pain everywhere, cramps, pressure, sensitivity, swollen gums and toothache, extreme excitability with irritation and disease in the sexual organs, especially the ovaries.

Sulphur is decayed and putrefied earth, but in alchemical terms, it is the ferment which is the source of fire and gold and can be transformed by the mutative process into spirit and soul.[30] The *Sulphur* personality is characterized by skin eruptions, general congestion and stagnation; it contains raw uncomplicated psora, with a tendency to dirtiness, distraction, unfocused genius, and mental brilliance with disregard for personal being. Whatever meaning these relationships have, the doctor uses his tools to grasp their underlying unity. In a sense, club moss and sulphur have personalities too, expressed in both diseases and medicines.

The homoeopathic doctor, operating in the terms of Western culture, in general tries to communicate the level of integration the remedy entails. One older physician in California closed a diagnosis with the following announcement:

"Gold is an interesting thing in the history of man. It has been hoarded as wealth. People have worn it as jewelry and struggled for possession of it. It is associated with the sun. It is found often in quartz, and near the surface of the ground. Pans in rivers trap gold particles. It is purple in the colloidal state and used for staining glass in cathedrals. Gold anchors the value of money systems. Without the anchor, value disintegrates. You have a disease called *Aurum*, gold. And I will give you the medicine."

In terms of the conscious mind or of any usual system of mind/body, the remedy is ridiculous. In terms of the belief in an underlying relationship between nature, the organism, and civilization, it is a powerful characterization. But we must put all this in deeper perspective. What is left for us here, as in all mysteries, is to return to the birthplace before the actual birth in order to understand better what was born.

XIII

The Life and Work of Samuel Hahnemann

Samuel Hahnemann was born at midnight, April 10–11, 1755, in the town of Meissen (now in East Germany, near the Polish and Czechoslovakian borders). Curiously, the history of alchemy and homoeopathy cross there. The Hahnemann family had migrated from the west a generation earlier so that Samuel's father could work at the local porcelain factory. So-called Dresden china had been originated by Johann Böttger, an alchemist, in 1710, only as a distraction from his search for gold, and the Saxon porcelain industry was located at Meissen, on the Elbe River, close to its rich clay beds. A factory was established at Albrecht Castle and in 1743 an art school was added. Writing in his journal at the age of thirty-six, Hahnemann describes his beginnings:

"I was born on April 10th, 1755, in the Electorate of Saxony, one of the most beautiful parts of Germany. . . .

"My father, Christian Gottfried Hahnemann, together with my mother Johanna Christiana, née Spiess, taught me how to read and write whilst playing. My father . . . was a painter for the porcelain factory of [Meissen], and the author of a brief treatise on water-colour painting."[1]

Hahnemann was born also into the centuries of German war. The Seven Years' War, during which the Prussian King, Frederick II, raided the Saxon porcelain factory, ended in his eighth year, leaving his family impoverished. His life's work reached its zenith during the reverberations of Napoleon throughout Europe. More obscurely, Hahnemann was born into a German occult tradition, not by personal study or inclination so much as by the time and place of his birth and the nature of his quest. All his life, he worked explicitly to establish himself in a lineage of physical scientists and, instead, he fulfilled a hermetic prophecy. To the south, in Switzerland and Austria, Paracelsus, two hundred and fifty years earlier, and Carl Jung and Rudolf Steiner, one hundred and fifty years later, challenged the mysteries of spirit in matter with the same ambiguous results. Each time, out of the original riddle, a new riddle formed, but, for a moment, to which one can return, the mist cleared, and a single sparkle shone on an unknown sea. Hahnemann did his work in the name of matter, and, like the Austrian physician Wilhelm Reich, also a century and a half later, he came to spirit, to vital energy, only inevitably and by default.

Hahnemann emerged from his adolescence a learned man. It is not clear how he came to know all he did, for it has a momentum that transcends quantitative subject matter. When his boyhood studies were interrupted by war and his father's demands he learn a trade, he studied on his own, and, at age sixteen, was taken into the Prince's School in Meissen by the rector, tutoring pupils in Greek and Latin in exchange for tuition. He graduated at twenty with a dissertation (in Latin) on the construction of the human hand, after which he attended Leipzig University.

"By teaching German and French to a wealthy young Greek from Jassy in Moldavia, as well as by translations from English, I procured for myself for a time the means of subsistence. . . ."[2]

The translations were no small matter. They included physiology texts, descriptions of experiments with copper, a work on hydrophobia, two volumes on mineral waters and warm baths, and various writings on practical medicine. Hahnemann's own earliest work merges with the translations themselves. For instance, at twenty-seven, as an amateur chemist, he translated a complex French work on industrial chemistry, correcting chemical errors and adding additional techniques in footnotes.

The intellectual impact on Hahnemann of his own prehomoeopathic work is underestimated because its direct historical impact was so small. There is a reason, though, why homoeopathy spoke clear and advanced words from the beginning. Its fluency came from somewhere. Out of the labyrinth of ancient languages and remote peoples, and the ignored work of obscure botanists and physicians of different nations, Hahnemann made a synthesis utterly different from any of its parts.

From the age of thirty to thirty-four alone, he published over two thousand pages, most of it translation, with a few conventional articles of his own on sores, ulcers, and drugs. The translations are not only scientific; almost a third of that work was his translation of the French classic "The Story of Abelard and Heloïse" from English into German.

We might ask, How could this translating have had an impact? It's not medicine. But homoeopathy was not "medicine" either in any usual sense. Translation involves a highly scientific and disciplined meditation on the structure of language, the roots of meaning, and the transformations between codes. Homoeopathy resembles these codes and structures more than it does standard medicine. The rigor and symmetry of Hahnemann's thought is primitive and classical, not nineteenth century.

He did not plan to spring homoeopathy on the world, but he had the classics in his head and he knew from experience that contemporary medicine was a failure. Greek alchemy, European herbalism, Arabic chemistry, native pharmacy—even though we cannot show their exact contributions to homoeopathy—are there, transformed through Hahnemann's intellect.

He worked with traditional and archaic texts, but he did not attempt to reapply them to "modern" medicine. He had a new grid by virtue of his time in Europe, and he did much more than bring back olden wisdom. In that brief and almost silent hiatus between the end of academic hermeticism and the birth of professional science, Hahnemann coaxed a single child from their unrecorded union.

As we earlier noted, Hahnemann was also surprisingly practical, and he laid down rules of hygiene that were almost totally unknown during his era. For instance, he insisted on scraping clean a wound and in bandaging with alcohol-soaked cloths; he prescribed fresh air, exercise, cheerful company, warm and cold baths; he recommended that doctors prepare their own medicines and be personally responsible for the entire continuity of the treatment. Throughout his career, Hahnemann remained a mixture of the erudite and simple, the dreaming magus and the efficient nurse. He stumbled from the wisdom of his books into a hodgepodge of doctors all "born yesterday" and knowing nothing of their classical tradition. That doctors should prepare their own medicines seemed to him ethical and practical, for he had already trained himself in sophisticated laboratory techniques and in the history of botany and medicine, and he naïvely assumed others would be willing to do the same. When he first realized the pitiable state of the medicine of his time, he refused to practice it, out of fear of doing more harm than good, and he supported himself only by translating.

From age thirty-five to thirty-eight, his translations included a group of significant medical, agricultural, and chemical books, notably materia medicas from English, French, and Italian. His last translation, fourteen years later, in 1806, was the Swiss physician Albrecht von Haller's *Materia Medica of German Plants, Together with Their Economic and Technical Use*, from a French version of the original Latin. Hahnemann's mind, by this time, must have been an encyclopedia of plant names, medical uses of plants, chemical compounds, and various European-language syntax systems. When, in 1810, in his fifty-sixth year, he was required to give a public lecture in order to get permission to teach at the Medical Institute in Leipzig, everyone expected a passionate defense of homoeopathy. He surprised and overwhelmed his audience with a lecture on the ancient medical uses of hellebore, quoting from German, French, English, Italian, Latin, Greek, Hebrew, and Arabic sources, including doctors, herbalists, and natural philosophers. It was a *tour de force* not only in medical theory, but also in botany, etymology, and comparative mythology. From this brain, which had so long been coalescing bizarre and discontinuous elements, came the resolution of homoeopathy.

Homoeopathy was Hahnemann's self-initiation. It made the difference between a fragmented and eccentric intellect and a charismatic system builder. Hahnemann, in his middle years, escaped from the interminable factual knowledge and its scholarly tyranny. From the thousands of separate sources and types of knowledge, he formed a new alloy. Then it rested on the plains of German science like a meteorite fallen from the greater heat of another world.

It is in Hahnemann's 1790 translation of the Scottish physician William Cullen's *Treatise on Materia medica* that this emerges.

Cullen had a typical, mechanical view of the body and its diseases. He believed that disease was caused by the variation in the "flux" of nervous energy through the system. As primary organs, like the heart and brain, become blocked and irritated, they communicate this information to other parts of the body, leading to general debility. Nervous ailments were equally mechanical. They might come from the direct pressure of agitated blood, which could be relieved by bloodletting. Pure physical inflammation was treated by acid or alkaline medicines, the former to counteract an alkaline abundance and the latter to counteract an acid abundance.

Since the body was something like a fat, irritable jelly, the role of medicines in general was to stir up that jelly, stimulate its irritability, and set it into corrective spasm. On the surface, this is not strikingly different than homoeopathy, except that Cullen's medicines were always contraries, in order to irritate, and his "body" was a relatively simple solid. His tendency, then, was to reduce the number of diseases to inflammations and blockages and to classify any varying forms as subcategories of the major ones. That way, the number of medicines could be determined by the types of spasms necessary to clear the system of disease. The resemblance to homoeopathy on the general issue of irritability is not entirely accidental, for Cullen was a follower of Georg Ernst Stahl and the early Montpellier school of Vitalists. It was necessary only for him to replace Stahl's *Anima*, a natural, harmonious, self-corrective healer and regulator, with a more fleshy kind of irritability, to arrive at "Solidism." Cullen and Hahnemann collide in the notes to the latter's translation of the former.

Cullen rejects the notion that Peruvian bark (quinine) can have a specific (i.e., unexplained) effect in the treatment of intermittent fever; he says it is just a composite tonic, bringing together the bitter and astringent qualities which combine to give it a power. The translator balks here, and, in his notes to page 108 of Volume II of Cullen's work, he offers a different solution:

"By combining the strongest bitters and the strongest astringents we can obtain a compound which, in small doses, possesses more of both these properties than the bark and yet in all Eternity no fever specific can be made from such a compound. The author should have accounted for this. This undiscovered principle of the effect of the bark is probably not easy to find. Let us consider the following: Substances which produce some kind of fever (very strong coffee, pepper, arnica, ignatia bean, arsenic) counteract these types of intermittent fever. I took, for several days, as an experiment, four drams of good china [cinchona, a quinine source] twice daily. My feet and finger tips, etc., at first became cold; I became languid and drowsy; then my heart began to palpitate; my pulse became hard and quick;

an intolerable anxiety and trembling (but without a rigor); prostration in all the limbs; then pulsation in the head, redness of the cheeks, thirst; briefly, all the symptoms usually associated with intermittent fever appeared in succession, yet without the actual rigor. . . . This paroxysm lasted from two to three hours every time, and recurred when I repeated the dose and not otherwise. I discontinued the medicine and I was once again in good health."[3]

The debut of homoeopathy in a footnote suggests that Hahnemann intended scholarship more than invention. Healing by medicinal similars was one time-honored way of treating disease. Certainly he had come across it hundreds of times in his reading and translation. To that, he was adding a forceful, almost anti-intellectual experiment. The implication was obvious: forget categories and philosophy and test things personally and empirically. His confidence and zeal were such that he usually forgot others had neither his learning nor his purity. He meant to be helpful, but he sounded self-enamored and peevish. Other doctors complained immediately: of what use is idiosyncratic personal data? Are we to test all medicines on ourselves at mortal risk?

Hahnemann took a number of medical positions in his early life, but he always gave them up and returned to translating and research. In 1781, when he was twenty-six, he married the seventeen-year-old daughter of the local apothecary in Gommern, and after serving as Medical Officer of Health in Dresden, he moved to Leipzig to be near the university. It was here that Hahnemann translated Cullen, but the real controversy he stirred up was not homoeopathic at all.

In 1792 Emperor Leopold II of Austria, an important figure in the strategy between Germany and Napoleon's France, died under emergency treatment by three doctors. Because of the political delicacy of the situation, the doctors involved issued for publication a full description of Leopold's illness, its treatment, and the ensuing death of the patient. Hahnemann responded in a Gotha paper:

"The bulletins state: 'On the morning of February 28th, [the Emperor's] doctor, Lagusius, found a severe fever and distended abdomen'—he tried to fight the condition by venesection [bloodletting], and as this failed to give relief, he repeated the process three times more without any better result. We ask, from a scientific point of view, according to what principles has anyone the right to order a second venesection when the first has failed to bring relief?

As for a third, Heaven help us!; but to draw blood a fourth time when the three previous attempts failed to alleviate! To abstract the fluid of life four times in twenty-four hours from a man who has lost flesh from mental overwork combined with a long continued diarrhoea, without procuring any relief for him! Science pales before this!"[4]

Hahnemann originated homoeopathy, but he was, by inclination, a pragmatist and a holist already. He opposed untested precedent; he proposed reevaluation of every remedy and technique. His Christian and medical ascetism made him scrupulous about life-style and diet. In a time of poor ventilation in houses, fear of fresh air, and contaminated food and water, he prescribed exercise, nutritious meals, clean running water, and open windows. His spiritualism did not interfere with his sense of bounteous, living nature, and his intuition of invisible disease did not keep him from discerning the great danger of microbes and infection.

It is a telling irony of medical history that the man who seems to stand most against modern germ theory as a primary hypothesis of disease was an early advocate of boiling the utensils used by patients with contagious diseases and isolation of those patients from others, either in a hospital or a private house. He criticized hydrotherapy (cold-water treatment) and mineral baths as ineffective and standard pharmacy and bloodletting as excessive and unhealthy. He just as strongly criticized the standard modes of treatment of mental patients, which combined crude cranial surgery and criminal punishment. Doctors often took the provocative language of mental patients seriously and responded to insults with insults and to asocial behavior with punishment. Hahnemann argued that aberrant behavior was a disease, no different than physical disease. This mind/body unity was to be a touchstone of homoeopathy.

Hahnemann took public health as a personal responsibility and wrote educational books and pamphlets, in one of which the following exegesis appears:

"In order to save fuel and high rents, several miserable families will often herd together, frequently in one room, and they are careful not to let in any fresh air through window or door, because that might also let in the cold. The animal exhalations from perspirations and the breath become concentrated, stagnant and foul in these places; one person's lungs do their best to take away from the others all the small amount of life-giving air remaining, exhaling in exchange impurities from the blood. The melancholy twilight of their small, darkened windows is combined with the enervating dampness and musty smell of old rags and rotting straw; fear, envy, quarrelsomeness and other passions do their best to destroy completely what little health there is; all this can only be known by one whose calling has compelled him to enter these hovels of misery. Here contagious epidemics not only go on spreading easily and almost unceasingly if the slightest germ has chanced to fall there, but it is here that they actually originate, break out and become fatal even to more fortunate citizens."[5]

During the years preceding the writing of his *Organon*, Hahnemann was unsettled and unable to come to terms with professional medicine. After an unsuccessful attempt at a mental hospital in Gotha, he spent ten years moving between city and country, attempting to earn a living. His career itself was marked with brilliant cures but incessant controversy. His insistence on making his own medicines and practicing in an unorthodox manner alienated both apothecaries and physicians. In one much-publicized case, a certain Prince Schwarzenberg died after leaving Hahnemann's care for the bloodletting of his own physicians. Hahnemann walked in his funeral procession to show respect and to dramatize his conviction of his own innocence in the death.

These were painful times, in which he witnessed the illness and death of his own children. He searched the existing system of medicine for the missing remedies and finally concluded, in despair:

"After 1,000 to 2,000 years, then, we are no further!"[6]

What was critically missing was a system that explained the variety of disease and offered a consistent strategy of treatment. The Hippocratics had discovered important medicines, but their system was a mass of contradictions. And medicine since that time had only answered its own questions in nonproductive circles. No one knew why one disease expressed itself in fever, another in chills, and what the heat of a bath or the spirit of a tonic actually did to a disease. Hahnemann could not accept Paracelsus either because he did not believe that nature expressed itself in occult signs. Yet he realized that Paracelsus practiced the Law of Similars with conviction and from experience, and he considered, as a chemist, the possibilities within alchemy while rejecting the specific formulas.

More than any of his contemporaries, Hahnemann realized what a serious matter disease was and how unequipped science was to deal with it. The depths of disease were like the depths of history itself, the depths of a marvelous and terrifying nature. It *was* the invasion of an unconquerable army, spreading war and poverty and threatening to put all mankind under its dominion. Compared to this enemy, Napoleon was a schoolboy. The invading army was not alien, against man, either; it was the substantial corruption of man's own nature. The devout Christian in Hahnemann led him to associate that corruption with original sin. We no longer use this kind of language, but in the twentieth century we talk, for the first time in scientific terms, about how man is his own enemy and how the illness and "physician" collaborate through the ages to produce the society. Hahnemann warned that man no longer wanted to be well nor knew how to be and that planetary survival was at stake. He demanded of the doctors that they come to their senses before it was too late.

While he was writing the *Organon*, Hahnemann reflected on his path in a letter to a close friend who was a professor of pathology:

"For eighteen years I have been deviating from the ordinary practice of the medical art. . . .

"My sense of duty would not easily allow me to treat the unknown pathological state of my suffering brethren with these unknown medicines. If they are not exactly suitable (and how could the physician know that, since their specific effects had not yet been demonstrated?), they might with their strong potency easily change life into death or induce new disorders and chronic maladies, often more difficult to eradicate than the original disease. The thought of becoming in this way a murderer or a malefactor towards the life of my fellow human beings was most terrible to me, so terrible and disturbing that I wholly gave up my practice in the first years of my married life. I scarcely treated anybody for fear of injuring him, and occupied myself solely with chemistry and writing.

"But then children were born to me, several children, and after a time serious illnesses occurred, which, in tormenting and endangering my children, my own flesh and blood, made it even more painful to my sense of duty, that I could not with any degree of assurance procure help for them. . . . Whence then was certain help to be obtained?—was the yearning cry of the comfortless father in the midst of the groaning of his children, dear to him above all else. Night and desolation around me—no sight of enlightenment for my troubled paternal heart."[7]

In 1796 there appeared, under Hahnemann's authorship, "Essay on a New Principle for Ascertaining the Curative Powers of Drugs, and Some Examinations of the Previous Principles." Cure by contraries he rejected as dealing only with symptoms. He dismissed all exciting, inciting, cleansing, heating, and cooling actions of medicines: these were the results of alleviation. He identified the healing power of medicines *solely* as their ability to produce specific illnesses. The organism had two responses to such medicines: aggravation from the similarity, followed by stimulation of the vital force. In his definition of homoeopathy as the only scientific medicine, Hahnemann got the burden of fear and doubt off his own shoulders and transferred it to mainstream medicine, which has continued to wrestle with it just as ungracefully in the century and a half since.

In the same essay, Hahnemann proposed a basic theory of disease interaction. A severe chronic condition would, he said, prevent an acute disease of less severity from getting a hold on a system, but this was not healthy even if it reduced troublesome symptomology. An acute disease of greater severity might take, and, in the process, "cure" chronic disease, but the older symptoms would always return. Hahnemann noted the similarity between vaccination and homoeopathy; for instance, inoculation of smallpox not only protected against smallpox but often cured other diseases, including deafness, dysentery, and swollen testicles. Indiscriminate vaccination of large populations, however, took no account of individual defense mechanisms and was dangerous. He felt that an individual who could successfully be inoculated against a disease would likely be immune anyway or cured easily homoeopathically, whereas a person responsive to the inoculation in another way would develop chronic disease from the presence of this foreign substance in his system, or, more precisely, its initial effect on his internal equilibrium.

Hahnemann began the science of homoeopathy by testing substances on himself and recording the "artificial" diseases they induced. He preferred deadly poisons because of their inherent power. Of course, his provings of small doses of aconite, strychnine, and belladona astonished and dismayed the medical profession.

It is wrong to assume that Hahnemann fully adopted homoeopathy in 1796 and never looked back. He was tentative in his reliance on the new insight; for instance, he mentions, in one case of tapeworm, using more than sixteen allopathic medicines before, in desperation, trying white hellebore for its ability to cause a colic like the patient's. The result was such a violent colic that the person almost died, but afterward improved rapidly and permanently. From this Hahnemann learned that the artificial disease can be as dangerous as the original one.

In order to get a milder response, Hahnemann tried diluting his medicines even further, hoping to find the point at which they still had an effect but their aggravation was least. As expected, he found that substantial dilutions had the least aggravation, but also the least medicinal value. Then he tried shaking the vials very hard at each dilution. It is uncertain what caused him to try this, and there is no one explanation in Hahnemann's known studies, although many different hermeticisms, including alchemy, urged creative interaction with substances. Later ethnographic literature shows that primitive peoples prepare medicines by pounding, grinding, blowing on, aiming at the Sun or stars, scraping with coral and ivory, punching once with the fist (in the case of leaves), and (in the case of pollen) suffocating a bird in the medicine before its use—all to wake the spirits in the medicine or bring spirits to attach themselves to it. African doctors have claimed that medicines contain no power in themselves but gain it from dynamic contact. The well-read Hahnemann may have been aware of some of this lore.

In any case, with his new shaken dilutions, Hahnemann took the same steps and approached the threshold of effectiveness again. The results were startling, and are still startling: the smaller the dose, not only the less the primary aggravation, but the more profound the secondary healing. He had no reason not to pursue this phenomenon to the limit. The original homoeopathic doses were at times as high as seventy grams of substance, but commonly five grams. From 1799 to 1801 he began using notably smaller doses, mentioning 1/5,000,000 of a grain of opium and 1/432,000 of a grain of dried belladona berry. During his lifetime, he only went as far as the thirtieth centesimal ("It cannot go on to infinity," he writes,[8] but he was already at infinity, and he had opened a Pandora's box).

More than anything else, however, microdose would undo homoeopathy from without and within, taking the testing of remedies out of the realm of conventional chemistry and dividing Hahnemann's followers inexorably on the meanings and limits of dilutions. The criticisms of microdose were absolute and scathing right from the beginning. Dr. Hermann Schnaubert of Cahla wrote satirically:

"Death has no further power over man, the homoeopaths have

taken away his sting! For, if shaking and rubbing a dead medicinal substance, reduced to an unimaginable size, can give an effective power passing all comprehension, surely nobody can be surprised if he sees dead men brought to life by shaking and rubbing, sustained appropriately."[9]

The dilemma was posed by the inability of homoeopaths to place a limit on dilutions that was anything more than personal predilection. If each dilution were, successively, more powerful, the ultimate promise was awesome. It is more likely that there are different ideal dilutions that respond harmonically to different planes of illness, and that continued potentization by dilution and succussion makes some medicines ineffective while bringing others out. Such high dilutions may have particular relevance for modern diseases. Specific potencies may also contain subtleties and unknown properties but not greater absolute power. Since remedies work through the defense mechanism and the vital force, they can hardly raise the dead.

When microdose first came to America with immigrant European physicians, the full meaning of the system was not grasped in this country, partly because of the foreign language of the original texts. But as the American doctors began to see what was proposed, the response was derisive. In his history of American medicine, Harris Coulter notes:

"One doctor estimated that a volume of water 61 times the size of the earth was needed for the 15th dilution. Others talked in terms of the Caspian or the Mediterranean, of Lake Huron or Superior. One man calculated that 140,000 hogsheads of arsenic were dumped every year into the Ohio and Mississippi Rivers from the poisoning of rats in Pittsburgh and St. Louis, that this raised the Mississippi water to the 4th dynamization, but that it apparently had no effect on those living downstream."[10]

He quotes from two other attacks:

"According to this view it is the spiritual influence of the sabre that pierces the body, not its material form. It is the spiritual influence of the club that breaks the skull. It is the spiritual influence of fried onions that causes an attack of cholera morbus."

And: "This spiritualizing of matter by trituration is an insult to modern philosophy, and in reference to this spiritualization and tendency to mysticism, it is the mere adventitious result of habitual modes of thinking in Germany [where] science is as much pestered with spirits as poetry is."[11]

The difficulties raised in the above comments have no resolution. Homoeopathy was practiced in the ensuing years because it apparently worked, not because it could be explained. While Hahnemann the doctor produced thousands of disciples who tried the remedies with the same results, Hahnemann the philosopher and metaphysician produced only great riddles and controversies that his own temperament and background did not prepare him to handle.

From 1805 until 1812, he lived in Torgau, near his own birthplace on the Elbe, treated patients enthusiastically, and wrote his *Organon*, the book that was to be the foundation of homoeopathy. It was published in 1810.

Given the radical proposition of the text, the book was reviewed generously by the medical profession, the common opinion being that the author had much of importance to say about the Law of Similars, a well-known and ancient doctrine, but tended to extend it into areas where it was inappropriate and not indicated. Doctors were smug enough not to realize that Hahnemann's attack on medicine was total, so he was treated as an eccentric with a specialty.

Hahnemann's anger at being, in essence, ignored, changed his life. He returned to Leipzig to seek a public stage, and, with the paper on hellebore, delivered in 1810, won the right to lecture to medical students, as described above. In the winter term of 1812, the founder of homoeopathy, fifty-seven years old and nearly bald, awkward but dressed elegantly, presented his new-age medicine. As word spread, the audience grew. But he was considered an entertainment, with his raging at and blaspheming the whole profession. For the most part, he was not taken seriously, and he was belittled and quietly mocked by his colleagues. It was not their acceptance he sought anymore. At the university he finally acquired a group of loyal disciples from among the medical students. Together with them, he organized the first controlled provings and spread homoeopathy to the world.

Writes one: "We lived very happily together, caring very little for the hostile glances and remarks of our colleagues. We stuck to our studies faithfully and honestly and gathered together occasionally in our teacher Hahnemann's household some time after eight in the evening.

"This was then the little circle formed round Hahnemann which even under the best of circumstances had to tolerate much mockery and irony and in malicious cases, hatred and persecution, not only during the student years but far beyond them. I can always re-

member very clearly how Hornburg was worried in his Final Examination by the old pates and only just managed to escape being
plucked, whilst miserable thickheads, not fit to wipe Hornburg's
boots, passed cum laude and are now flourishing aloft here—narrow-
minded but successful physicians."[12]

Homoeopathy was a totally new concept, so Hahnemann taught
his disciples to prepare medicines from scratch, collecting the plants,
minerals, insects, and so on, and doing the dilutions and succussions
by hand. Despite the growing popularity of the system and Hahnemann's fame as a healer, homoeopaths never won more than temporary and conditional rights to dispense medicines in Leipzig. The
local apothecaries fought to maintain their control over all pharmacy
in the city, though they in no way understood what was involved in
microdose.

As it became more clear that he was not being understood, Hahnemann grew bitter and, in 1821, retreated to Köthen, in Anhalt,
north of Saxony, where he lived under the protection of Duke Fer-
dinand whom he had treated successfully. There he wrote his last
major work, *The Chronic Diseases, Their Peculiar Nature, and Their
Homeopathic Cure*, which appeared in 1828. Like Freud's *Civilization and Its Discontents*, also a late book by the founder of a system, it is a pessimistic reevaluation of the diseases of mankind and
the possibility of any widespread or lasting cure. Freud exposed the
miseries, wars, and crimes of mankind as indications of man's collective inability to deal with the essential biophysical condition of life;
since civilization had suppressed man's true nature, no psychoanalytic
system could offer more than superficial relief. So with Hahnemann.
Years of practice had shown him that disease was not as curable as
he once thought, even with the Law of Similars and microdose. He
explained this persistent pathology as the collective and accumulated
disease of man in civilization. Furthermore, he understood the failure of homoeopathy to be a symptom of the pathology itself. Early
homoeopaths often overlooked this volume in the optimism of their
own practices, but later generations have drawn the desperate conclusions. If the *Organon* is the text of practical homoeopathy, *Chronic
Diseases* is the bible of esoteric homoeopathy.

The book explains the original meaning of disease. Psora, or itch,
was the primary malady, with leprosy being its unchecked florescence. External symptoms of itch—rashes, pimples, sores, boils—were
often readily cleared up, but the internal itch persisted. Deprived of

its outlet on the skin, itch penetrated and weakened the inner organs. It was inheritable at the level to which it had been suppressed. Thus a child is born healthy only insofar as it has no external manifestation of the disease, but it carries within it the psoric potential accumulated in the generations of its flesh.

All history is rewritten as mankind's internalization of surface disease. These internalizations are integrated as symptomatic predispositions, eventually penetrating the mental plane, from where they are exteriorized as the products of civilization—not only its warfare but its arts, not only its hate and despair but also the quality of its love and vision, not only the "sick" who lead but the "healthy" who must follow. We have internalized something that was never meant to be inside us. Once there, it becomes us. By then, we have lost our destiny.

The individual patient must now be treated not only for the ailments he has or those of his lifetime but for the disease level into which he is born. This is the scenario:

"Mankind . . . is worse off from the change in the external form of the *psora*,—from leprosy down to the eruption of itch—not only because this is less visible and more secret and therefore more frequently infectious, but also because the *psora*, now mitigated externally into a mere itch, and on that account more generally spread, nevertheless still retains unchanged its original dreadful nature. Now, after being more easily repressed, the disease grows all the more unperceived within, and so, in the last three centuries, after the destruction of its chief symptom (the external skin-eruption) it plays the sad role of causing innumerable secondary symptoms; *i.e.*, it originates a legion of chronic diseases, the source of which physicians neither surmise nor unravel, and which, therefore, they can no more cure than they could cure the original disease when accompanied by its cutaneous eruption; but these chronic diseases, as daily experience shows, were necessarily aggravated by the multitude of their faulty remedies."[13]

The more practically oriented homoeopaths see *The Chronic Diseases* mainly as a statement of the importance of skin ailments, their relationship to other organic and mental conditions, and the danger of repressing them. Yet this is a new apocalyptic Hahnemann, standing at the turning point of the centuries, offering mankind its first chance in thousands of thousands of years to break with a prehistoric scourge. The next paragraph continues:

"So great a flood of numberless nervous troubles, painful ailments, spasms, ulcers (cancers), adventitious formations, dyscrasias, paralyses, consumptions and cripplings of soul, mind and body were never seen in ancient times when the *psora* mostly confined itself to its dreadful cutaneous symptom, leprosy. Only during the last few centuries has mankind been flooded with these infirmities."[14]

Hahnemann goes on to ascribe seven eighths of all chronic diseases to suppressed psora—psora so deeply suppressed that a succession of remedies are needed to unravel the archaeology of the disease in any individual.

The other two chronic miasms, syphilis and sycosis, are relatively modern, according to Hahnemann; they form as complications of psora and are usually treatable with homoeopathic *Mercury* and *Nitric Acid* (syphilis) and *Thuja* (sycosis). On one level syphilis and sycosis (from Greek, *sykosis*, from *sykon*, fig, not *psyche*, hence figwort disease, i.e., gonorrhea,* not psychosis) are the venereal diseases. Their relationship to psora is complexly tied in with their inheritability and genital expression. They overlie psora and are the field in which it is hidden and expressed. In one sense, they are nothing more than venereal-genetic complications of basic psora. In another sense, their complexity suppresses even the natural pattern of the psora and shifts it into a more erratic vibration. While psora abounds and is infectious on an unimagined level ("the hermit on Montserrat escapes it as rarely in his rocky cell, as the little prince in his swaddling clothes of cambric"[15]), the germination of these other miasms requires direct genital contact or genetic transfer through offspring. They are extremely deep emotionally and spiritually, and their individual and venereal symptoms interact with prior psoric disturbances to increase pathology and lead to insanity. They make the psora incurable until a remedy is used against their overriding miasm.

As a book, *The Chronic Diseases* is mainly a voluminous list of psoric symptoms followed by sixteen hundred pages of antipsoric remedies and their indications. Later miasms have been announced since Hahnemann's time, and their appearance atop the previous three levels is taken as an indication of the continued deterioration of man. Ostensibly we are now more miasmic than human, and a

---

* Sycosis generally describes barber's itch and scrofula, neither of which are venereal or gonorrheal. Hahnemann's special usage reveals his opinion of the source of this itch.

current homoeopathic homily claims that it was the syphilitic predisposition in Beethoven that allowed him to create beautiful music—and the syphilitic miasm in us that hears it as beautiful.

While Hahnemann's earlier writings emphasize disease as a constitutional disturbance, curable through a stimulation of the vital force by a single correct remedy in low potency, the later Hahnemann not only believed in high potencies but paradoxically invented the most dilute scale in the history of physical science as an expression of them: the millesimal.

Many homoeopathic movements sprang up, not only in Leipzig where the seeds were sown, but throughout Europe and America. Hahnemann himself continued to have medical success, and his fame spread, in part because of his cures during the European cholera epidemic of 1831–32. In a perception that predates microbiology, he describes certain minute but discrete disease entities. He names the "cholera miasm" an "organism of a lower order" and later speaks of an "invisible cloud of perhaps millions of such miasmatic living organisms, which, first brought to life on the broad and marshy shores of the tepid Ganges, are continually seeking out man to his destruction."[16]

His researches had carried him well past the original proposition, but, when he came down, like Moses from the mountain, he found his disciples worshiping the idols, and he cracked the tablets. Homoeopathy survived the split for a long time, but eventually it proved fatal.

"I have heard for a long time and with displeasure," he wrote angrily in a newspaper, "that some in Leipsic, who pretend to be Homoeopaths, allow their patients to choose whether they shall be treated homoeopathically or allopathically. . . . let them . . . not require of me that I should recognize them as my true disciples . . .

"Blood-letting, the application of leeches and Spanish flies, the use of fontanels and setons, mustard plasters and medicated bags, embrocations with salves and aromatic spirits, emetics, purgatives, various sorts of warm baths, pernicious doses of calomel, quinine, opium and musk, are some of the quackeries by which, when used in conjunction with homoeopathic prescriptions, we are able to recognize the crypto-homoeopath, trying to make himself popular. . . . They swagger in the cradle of homoeopathic science (as they choose to call Leipsic) where its founder first stepped forward as a teacher. But behold! I have never yet acknowledged you; away from me, ye medical ———!"[17] (The newspaper chose not to print the word.)

In the last years of his life, Hahnemann was not only purist but totally unpredictable. He renounced doctors and hospitals he had initially blessed and helped found. As his fame spread, he charged great sums of money for his services while continuing to work in isolation on later editions of the *Organon*. He was already surrounded with controversy and myth when a singular and unexpected event whisked the doctor away from his disciples and German practice with the suddenness of an angelic entry.

Hahnemann's wife of forty-nine years died in the spring of 1830, and in 1834, a French woman, thirty-two years of age, having been inspired by the *Organon*, arrived in Köthen, ostensibly to meet the famous author in person and seek his aid. They had a spirited dialogue, and she stayed on; their friendship continued, Hahnemann proposed, and they were married in June of 1835. Hahnemann was eighty. He had always prescribed marriage, on one occasion just before remarrying calling it "a general specific for body and soul."[18]

With Marie Melanie Hahnemann, he moved to Paris, where she presented him in triumph to the French homoeopathic community, as though after a secret journey to the land of the dead, she had recovered Hippocrates himself.

Hahnemann lived in Paris until his eighty-ninth year, practicing medicine, continuing his revisions of his books, and preaching against the ravages of allopathy and the half-breeds. He was cared for, admired, and pampered. The controversy that surrounded his departure from Leipzig, however, grew in his absence. Reports from Paris indicated that his young wife had taken over his practice, that no one could see Hahnemann except through her, and that she did the diagnosis and prescribing while he sat, impassive and observing, approving her work.

Apparently, Madame Hahnemann did take over her husband's practice, but no easy conclusion can be drawn from this, and certainly not that the old man was bewitched and corrupted by her. He chose this particular form of retirement and discipleship through her. Perhaps he saw in her a strength, for she did become a homoeopathic physician of renown.

From his Paris outpost, Hahnemann was able to aid the spread and advancement of homoeopathy. His instruction of an English physician from India led to the founding of a separate Indian ho-

moeopathic tradition. If it was a decline or senility, it was an energetic one, as if Hahnemann sought to prove his system by his own vitality.

There is a dark side also to this affair. He dropped out of touch
with former associates and abandoned his family in Saxony, even in
his will. His death, on July 2, 1843, went unannounced for many
weeks, and his burial was absolutely private, unknown to his friends
and family, either in France or Saxony. Marie Melanie Hahnemann
buried her husband above the two other spouses she had already
outlived by the age of thirty-two, at the same grave site—and she
kept the sixth revision of the *Organon* unavailable during her lifetime.

Hahnemann was, all his life, a puritanical Christian. Obsessed
with keeping himself healthy, he punctuated his scholarship with
regular exercise. Although his first marriage shows some romantic
tendency, he was a nonromantic almost to the end: a stern father,
unyielding teacher and master—and absolutely blind to any other
psychological or spiritual system. He had the kind of mind and attention that bores to the center of things, through all the diversions
and eccentricities of an era. But he never turned that analysis back
on his own condition, either his psychospiritual condition or the cognitive intelligence from which he formed the system. He was a mystic by ideology only.

So homoeopathy comes to us from Hahnemann as a system of
concrete events in a spiritual world. There are plants, animals, minerals, flesh and blood people, pathologies; beneath that is a pattern
of oscillations and energies. While Hahnemann's original loyalty was
to physical science, botany, and industrial chemistry, by the time the
system was completed and he was an old man, spiritual potency had
replaced matter. It was Hahnemann's stubborn blindness that led
him to keep calling this system medicine and science, and to attempt
to deliver it to the world as that—a stubborn blindness that made
the clinical practice of the system possible. Even today, we lie within
that definition of homoeopathy. For as Blake showed, physics, too, is
a dream from which we have yet to awake.

The only way back into matter for Hahnemann would have been
through mind, but he never admitted mind into his system, hence
homoeopathy's nonintersecting, parallel course with psychiatry. Jung
later put spirit back into matter through mind. The merger occurred

in geometric shapes, laws of science, myths, etc., simultaneously in flowers, starfish, and galaxies, as we saw in Whitmont's theories in the last chapter. The "archetypes" are the mind behind matter which mind in matter recognizes in itself and all things.

Hahnemann's "archetypes" were instead imprinted on balls of milk sugar and alcohol—each ball inert, but each containing a universe to be manifested through a living system. By ignoring mind, Hahnemann was forced to find intelligence behind matter. The homoeopathic medicines *are* the Jungian archetypes.

In the end, it would appear, the undiagnosed spirituality of Hahnemann's life took over. His rigid puritanism condemned mankind to the chronic diseases and renounced the very movement he had spawned. At the same time, he fell before the attractions of the Anima and was lured from family and disciples into a foreign country by a young and playful pixie skilled in such escapades, who concealed his final work and buried him unnamed in a tomb with her earlier lovers.

It seems almost planned. His renunciation of his disciples and his self-imposed exile are the same event. His discipline and rigor are seemingly "proven" by this last escapade. It was a far prouder and heroic statement of homoeopathic vitality, to flee in that way rather than to stay in Leipzig and squabble until death.

The last fling with Marie Melanie is convincing. Hahnemann had long ago cast his lot in strange lands with unknown voices, and, in his eighties, with his scholarship completed, he finally got to follow them home. He knew it was over. The system was already a mongrel. So he returned to the pagan forces whose system it was. Homoeopathy had been his destiny and release, but it took him almost a lifetime to get there. In the end, he was freed. But no wonder homoeopathy has sought a founder and a clarification ever since.

XIV

The Homoeopathic Tradition in America

The American medical profession of Hahnemann's time was a small part of the general healing arts in the New World. Midwives, Indian doctors, and lay practitioners flourished, and other regional systems, such as chiropractic and osteopathy, arose during the nineteenth century. The alternative medicine scene today is a fulfillment and florescence of the original multicultural diversity. Ground roots and ethnic medicine challenged the establishment from the beginning.

The original North American naturopathy was, of course, the heritage of native peoples. These remedies had been tested for centuries and generations, and they were adopted by the Europeans. A specific steam bath and herbal treatment of the New Hampshire farmer Samuel Thomson was immensely popular, and his followers, running their own hospitals, drug manufacturing houses, and drugstores, had three million adherents in 1839 when the whole population of the United States was estimated to be seventeen million.

The system of the "irritable mechanism," developed by William Cullen and John Brown in England, was the fashion in orthodox American medicine too. The body was portrayed as a machine made out of flesh, with membranous pipes, pullies, levers, strainers, its hydraulics maintained by the breath and the heart. Medicines were given either to provoke or relax spasms. For an overactive system, vomiting was provoked or blood drawn off and cold baths administered. Opium, liquors, hot baths, garlic, mercury, and wine by the gallon were used as stimulants for phlegmatic ailments. This theory lingers even today in the laxatives that "break up" stalled matter in the bowels, the magnesias, milks, and vegetable antacids given for an overactive stomach, and even, in a sense, the antibiotics that attack the viruses.

Theories of Solidism must always lead to a reduction in the number of different recognized diseases, with a corresponding reduction in the number of medicines used. Solidism simplifies explanation and categories. The categories are arbitrary, set by precedent, yet prevail over chemical and physical reality. Bleeding was a relaxant; yet some doctors bled to stimulate, with a suitable mechanical image to explain the contradictory effect.

Oversimplification, reinforced by fad, finally settled on one mercurous chloride medicine, originally a stimulant, as the absolute cureall. It was called "calomel," after the Greek for "beautiful black," though its final form was a white powder. It was used daily and in high doses for current illness and as a general preventive for future ailments. Benjamin Rush, the most respected American physician of the late eighteenth and early nineteenth century was a strong advocate of mercury and bloodletting. Harris Coulter describes a scene from the 1793 yellow fever epidemic in Philadelphia:

"'The story is told that Rush was surrounded one day during the epidemic by a crowd in Kensington, north of Philadelphia. All implored him to come and treat their families.

"'There were several hundred. Rush, without stepping down, threw back the top of his curricle, and addressed the multitude 'with a few conciliatory remarks.' Then he cried in a loud voice, 'I treat my patients successfully by bloodletting and copious purging with calomel and jalap—and I advise you, my good friends, to use the same remedies.'

"'What?' called a voice from the crowd, 'bleed and purge every one?'

"'Yes!' said the doctor. 'Bleed and purge all Kensington! Drive on, Ben!'"[1]

Mercury poisoning was common during this era; many people suffered from undiagnosed chronic disease caused by calomel. Mothers often clutched their children in the presence of the doctor and would not let them be treated, despite malaria, croup, and often severe respiratory and intestinal diseases.

Historians of medicine usually admit that homoeopathy came

onto a corrupt scene and unwittingly exploited peoples' fear and anger. If they had been giving out placebos only, as most doctors claim, they would have been doing more good than most of the calomel and bloodletting hacks.

At the beginning, though, the medical profession did not have a clear sense of homoeopathy. Some assumed it was just orthodox German medicine, and they accepted it. Others lumped it together with Indian medicine and Thomsonian treatment as another botanical. The first homoeopaths began to practice in the United States in the mid-1820s. Most of them were immigrant doctors, but a few were American-born and learned the new system by correspondence, reading, or visits to Europe, as many are learning it anew today. A graduate of Leipzig University, Constantine Hering founded the first American school of homoeopathy, the Nordamerikanische Akademie der Homoeopathischen Heilkunst, in Allentown, Pennsylvania, in 1835, with instruction in German. It lasted six years, and seven years after its closing, he replaced it with the Homoeopathic Medical College in Philadelphia. Students from this college carried homoeopathic practice into the Middle Atlantic and southern states, while fresh homoeopaths from Germany appeared in all the states, especially the Midwest. As early as 1844, significantly before the establishment of the AMA, the American Institute of Homoeopathy was founded in order to license physicians and maintain standards of practice. This body also served as a clearing house for the provings of North American native plants and other new remedies. The AMA was formed in reaction, and as a business guild, to protect the interests of its physicians.

As homoeopathic works were translated into English and homoeopathic doctors became more ubiquitous, the nature and weight of the threat began to sink in. Homoeopathy was the prince of the underground—it appealed to the vast audience of the naturopaths and Thomsonians, yet provided doctors trained in medical schools who gave pleasant-tasting sugar pills (in contrast to the high doses of foul-tasting mercury), heard out one's full symptoms and life history, and were learned without being irrelevant. Professional medicine reacted to this popularity by denouncing homoeopathy as a European scam intended to hoodwink backwoods Americans. "Sane men," doctors said, "could hardly be fooled by such patent nonsense."

The formal counterattack began slowly, but picked up steam as the confidence and seeming arrogance of the newcomers incensed the entrenched practitioners. The first shot was fired in 1842 when the New York State Medical Society ruled that homoeopathy was a form of quackery, not science, and "a departure from the principles of a well defined system of medical ethics."[2] Committee members argued that homoeopathy should *not* be granted immunity as another medical system with its own licensing because it dealt in pretentiously named sugar tablets under the guise of pharmacy. Four years later, when the National Medical Convention met in New York to review the problem, the members concluded that the success of homoeopathy was a result of their own bad marketing and public relations. Since many of their own medical schools gave bogus degrees and it was often impossible to tell the difference between a pseudomedical college and a legitimate training program, they decided to police their own ranks, define who they were, and isolate the rest as quacks. Their long-term goal was the improvement of medical education, but their short-term goal was the ostracism of the homoeopaths. This was the birth of the American Medical Association.

In the AMA charter, the association withheld membership from state and local medical organizations unless they assured the national organization that no homoeopaths any longer belonged. Only Massachusetts balked. In 1856 the AMA banned any discussion of homoeopathic medical theory in their journals and threatened the expulsion of any doctor who consulted with a homoeopath. Allopaths married to homoeopaths were also expelled.

The AMA has historically argued that its stance was against all quackery, in an attempt to professionalize the medical occupation. Documents make it clear, though, that homoeopathy was the main target. The homoeopaths had their own medical societies, journals, and courses in the medical schools, and they were the only serious competitors from the middle of the nineteenth century until the current rebellion.

The strategy failed initially because most people considered medical philosophy an esoteric issue and continued to use their favorite local physicians regardless of affinity. Doctors were also used to cooperating with each other and taking each others' patients in emergencies. The public could only be offended by a new rule that seemed arbitrary. The moral authority of the AMA is a relatively recent event.

Many medical schools bowed to the tightened regime, but some, the University of Michigan school in particular, retained a homoeo-pathic curriculum and forced a compromise on the AMA. In Michigan, as elsewhere, members of the Board of Regents were patients of homoeopaths and members of the legislature were more sympathetic to homoeopathy than to the AMA.

More significant, ultimately, was the merger of the two systems. Most homoeopaths, as we pointed out, practiced allopathy, too, as part of the "new" medicine. Innovative procedures were, in a sense, nondenominational and adopted by both. Even as homoeopathy survived the attack at first, the number of pure homoeopaths declined.

Meanwhile, homoeopathic procedure had a major impact on American allopathy, which not only changed it permanently but made it more palatable for homoeopaths to adopt. If the Old School did not learn to give spiritual doses, they gradually came to the conclusion that their own heroic doses were at the very least unnecessary and that sheer mass of medicine did not equal amount of healing power. Professional acceptance of specifics returned, and the standard medicine chest was completely remodeled. Calomel, quinine, and jalap passed out of fashion, and, with them, bleeding. Doctors experimented with different natural remedies and compounds from the drug companies. Even if a doctor did not accept microdose, he could prescribe the same substance in material form. If he liked the medicine but not the Law of Similars, he could explain its action mechanically, i.e., that *Kali nitricum*, or St. Ignatius' Bean, had the power to stimulate the system. Since homoeopathic pharmacy came from Classic, Mediaeval, and Arabic sources, allopathic pharmacy was also returning to its own origin in adopting homoeopathically used substances.

The cholera epidemic of 1849 in the South had an enormous effect in promoting medical change. The medical establishment admitted freely that it had no cure for this condition. Hahnemann had used *Camphor* early in the disease for its similar alternating diarrhea and constipation. The American school tried this remedy with ostensible success. In Cincinnati, homoeopaths claimed a 97 per cent cure rate in over a thousand cases and published a daily list of their patients in the newspaper, giving the names and addresses of those who were cured and those who died. Bleeding was of little use, though it remained the allopathic standby. Nonhomoeopathic doctors had a hard time believing the *Camphor* results. Elaborate explanatory hypotheses were concocted: late-acting allopathic remedies, hypnotism, and power of suggestion or even the wrongness of their own techniques, hence the advantage of no treatment at all. Perhaps the commonest interpretation was that the unusually high cure rate of the homoeopaths came not from their medicines but their rules of hygiene and diet. This belief literally changed allopathy from within, without turning it into homoeopathy. By comparison, the AMA was heavy-handed and flat-footed in dealing with the real situation.

The cures also won converts. One prominent allopath, William H. Holcombe, wrote of his guilt and sleeplessness the day of his first homoeopathic remedies:

"The spirit of Allopathy, terrible as a nightmare, came down fiercely upon me and would not let me rest. What right had I to dose that poor fellow with Hahnemann's medicinal moonshine?"[3]

Another reason for the popularity of homoeopathy was the seeming simplicity of the system. A lay practitioner need know nothing about physiology or chemistry; it was a matter of matching actual symptoms with lists of symptoms in a repertory. The medicines were given by clergymen, housewives, and other lay practitioners. Hering himself put out a kit for simple and common maladies, with instructions, and the medicines identified only by numbers. A certain condition might require number 8, but if the fever was higher, number 3 was used, number 12 if the ailment was primarily on the right side, number 18 if it turned into a rash. It was not uncommon for the wives and children of allopaths to treat their families in this way while the sire himself failed even to notice. The stern pessimistic decrees of Hahnemann in Germany became a playful American fad. It freed people from medical bills and from the general fear of medicine that existed in the nineteenth century.

Wrote one doctor: "[The] whole art is reduced to the precision of a game of nine pins."[4]

Another: "The system may be practiced by persons totally ignorant of the structure and functions of the human body."[5]

And another: "The entire range of diseases, the entire range of therapeutics, converted into Chinese puzzles; the phenomena of diseases and the effects of drugs upon them treated as algebraical equations."[6]

The serious weaknesses of homoeopathy were exposed by these responses, but the homoeopaths generally ignored them. They were at the height of their success through the 1870s and 1880s, doing three to seven times the business of allopaths by region, with the editorial support of the Detroit *Daily Tribune* and the New York *Times*, the backing of powerful politicians and business interests, and a strong lobby in the Republican Party. During the yellow fever epidemic of the 1870s in the South, homoeopaths not only used microdose successfully, but recommended specific sanitary corrections in the canals, sewage systems, dry wells, and bogs around Savannah and New Orleans. Homoeopaths were appointed to state medical boards and federal pension examination boards. They were supported by government funds and covered by insurance companies. There were hundreds of homoeopathic hospitals, clinics, insane asylums, nursing homes, orphanages, and schools.

Nowadays people shrug and smile if one suggests that homoeopathy ever represented enough of a threat to bring the powerful AMA into being. How quickly whole stages of history disappear! Major institutions collapse, and a generation is born into a different landscape. No doubt one day children will find the century or two of professional sports leagues an oddity of the past, hardly likely to spur the attention claimed for them. The remains of the old homoeopathic "empire" are scattered throughout the whole of the United States, especially in the eastern half. The hospitals and other buildings have been taken over by other parties. The patients have drifted to other doctors or back into the silence of their untended conditions. Libraries have moved out of the science section into storage facilities or been sold at a quarter a copy as rare books (I found an incredible wealth of homoeopathy books hidden in a corner of the University of Michigan Medical Library). No doubt, with growing interest in homoeopathy, they will now go the way of the alchemy collections in these same libraries: the rare book room for those not already stolen by the time the library realizes the trend. New, young homoeopaths are presently "liberating" these volumes on the claim that they are political-industrial "prisoners."

Homoeopathy is a blink of the eye away, and it can be found by those who are looking for it. It is like the old names on buildings, chiseled in stone and then covered by a temporary wooden sign announcing a new clinic or a multimillion-dollar health facility. The former patients, still alive, in their seventies and eighties, patronized the last of the homoeopathic doctors, until they also died, with no one to take over their practice. It is difficult to believe that something so fervent ended so abruptly.

Homoeopathy, in fact, was doomed to failure from the beginning.

It was an uncompromising, rigorous system, demanding a kind of commitment and purism few could maintain, especially in light of very sane demonstrations that the whole thing was impossible and unscientific. Hahnemann demanded strict adherence to the Law of Similars to find the correct remedy; there was no compromise on this; either one was discerning enough to work through the symptoms and come to a clear picture of the disease or one was not.

A few of Hahnemann's early students were purists, but most simply used homoeopathy as another tool. If homoeopathic procedure failed, there were many other systems of remediation to fall back on. Hahnemann viewed these hybrids as "worse than allopaths . . . amphibians . . . still creeping in the mud of the allopathic marsh . . . who only rarely venture to raise their heads in freedom toward the ethereal truth."[7]

If doctors felt there was an alternative to the strict de-layering of disease, they would never follow their cases through to the psoric base and homoeopathy itself would be faulted for their inability to produce a lasting cure. Furthermore, it made little sense first to heighten and then to reduce the same symptoms and call each an attempt at cure.

Many homoeopaths, however, took the old position: the Law of Similars was just one law of nature, and should be used along with other laws. They preferred low potencies because these still had some physical substance in them and were compatible with general American pharmacy. For the pure Hahnemannians, however, the high potencies were the most effective tool for getting at deep-seated disease and the core of their practice. The argument of their colleagues against nonmaterial doses was the identical argument allopaths had used against homoeopathy from the beginning.

At this point, too, the ranks of homoeopathy swelled with newcomers and converts from the yellow fever and cholera epidemic days. These doctors were poorly trained in the repertory and materia medica and probably practiced allopathy with a homoeopathic bent. They were attempting to follow the current and would be swept along with it into general medicine as the times changed.

Homoeopathic literature reflected the change in attitude. Homoeopaths themselves heralded the new pathological knowledge as a basis for genuinely informed prescription and saw the days when they had to rely only on the totality of symptoms as a kind of dark age, a groping in the dark. They developed a new language of "important symptoms" and streamlined the repertory, giving all the remedies an active explanation.

Social changes cannot be underestimated. Homoeopathy was buoyed by the basic life-style of the mid-nineteenth century, but allopathy benefited from twentieth-century demographic shifts. Specialization became as popular and necessary in medicine as in other areas of industrial society, and suddenly the homoeopathic general practitioners seemed as old-fashioned as they had once seemed modern. Their books were outdated; they were isolated from general science. At one point, they caused less pain than the allopaths, but with better palliative and first-aid drugs, allopathy had at least drawn even —and without the long period of trial and error and ensuing aggravation.

A homoeopath needed more time with his patients, so he charged more. Suddenly he was in competition with cut-rate medicine. He also needed continued contact with not only single patients but families over generations. Mobility robbed him of this. Mobility cried out for a standardized medicine. People could not move their doctors across the country, so they came to count on a repetition from locale to locale. Shifting clientele led to quick prescribing and brought out the worst in homoeopathy. Trapped by economic and social circumstances, some homoeopaths cheated and used any medicines that would get quick results.

The most orthodox group of Hahnemannians, who represented the power within homoeopathy, became something more than healers and scientists. They were fundamentalists, with the *Organon* as their Bible. They continued to use Hahnemann's language of symptomology even after it became dated and less useful diagnostically. The style of the *Organon* became required not in place of the substance but as well as the substance. They forgot that Hahnemann had written in the language of *his* day, adapting contemporary disease terms to explain actual disease processes.

The fundamentalism went even further than this. As long as homoeopathic philosophy opposed the notion that disease could be known, it opposed experimental science and medicine. Following an obvious rigidity in the master himself, homoeopathy became a religion—an antiscientific fundamentalist sort of Christianity. For the believer, research into disease cause was equated with research into the evolution of man and the origin of life. It was original sin with a psoric impulse at the root. Curiosity had been man's undoing once.

The disease cause was unknown because it was meant to be unknown, contained as it was in God. Much was made of the obvious affinity of the miasms with "unclean sexuality."

The purists were condemned by their history to moralism. They inveighed against the shoddiness of practice, but they made no attempt to understand it. They were like church fathers from the Old Country who stood against progress and democracy and who had no sympathy for difficulties a young doctor faced in trying to practice homoeopathy. They may have been creative doctors, but they were not creative elders. Before the progress, or seeming progress, of standard medicine, they stood as stagnation. Fooled by their own rigidity and antimodernism, they missed the point.

They attacked modern science as if it were uniform and atheistic, but the attack was from the perspective of Hahnemann's eighteenth-century German theism. Homoeopathy, or at least Hahnemannian homoeopathy, missed the branch of science that was to discover untold, greater mysteries at the depths of what could be known, and that was to rediscover a more powerful and generous God at the base of matter—a science that, in fact, would one day rediscover homoeopathy. Hahnemann was a literalist, and homoeopathy bowed out on the side of literalism, even though the microdose principle and the theory of miasms could not be applied literally. It was a strategic error, but it was unavoidable. The *Organon* suggested a deeper dialectic of mystery and reversal, but it did not honor it. Hahnemann's personality contained seeds of a genius he kept to himself, a core of wild inspiration that came out in his biblical rages and seeming last apostasy. As against a medicine of unnecessary bloodletting and general poisoning, homoeopathy was an angel and guardian of the sick. When the issues became more subtle and the gap between purisms greater, orthodox homoeopathy resorted, unaware, to rhetoric alone. Loose homoeopathy was no better, for it resorted to the jargon of progressive liberal science. In so doing, it abandoned the principle that alone made homoeopathy distinct.

From this point on, there were individual gifted practitioners, but professional homoeopathy was doomed. Only the purists could maintain the science, and only the "half-breeds" could maintain cultural relevance. Born on the other side of this divide (with two World Wars and the full transmutation of the twentieth century in the middle), we often miss the impact of what happened. When we "rediscover" pure homoeopathy, we assume that its principles, somewhere down the line, come into harmony with physics and biology. We have lived long enough past Newton, Darwin, and Cullen to accept the truth of their work, while excusing the remaining gaps and errors. In the nineteenth century, the purists stuck to their Christianity and did not imagine that anything would survive atheistic science, let alone an active God. Their God, however, was as much a cultural artifact as their science, and a larger "process" deity appears to have survived the tumult. The "half-breeds" saw no way to stick to homoeopathic principle and also participate in new science, so they were eventually absorbed into allopathy, priests who literally forgot their own ceremonies.

The purists went even further: they maintained Hahnemann's dated politics, allying themselves with the most conservative positions in American thought, often taking racist and ultracapitalist positions that reflected more the cultural conventions of Hahnemann's time than their own world. Homoeopathy, unfortunately, was identified with these positions. Radical, or for that matter mainstream, progressive ideas were defined as "disease complexes" by strict homoeopaths. One homoeopathic journal of the late 1960s, during the war in Vietnam, departed from medical issues only to urge a return to Christ and the immediate bombing of Hanoi, the enemy capital. It is all the more ironical that homoeopathy was finally rescued by creative post-Einsteinian scientists and the radical counterculture. But this explains the conflict that is frozen like a mask on the face of current homoeopathy.

To summarize the above: homoeopathy had triumphed and then burst from within. The pharmaceutical revolution completed the process, and the AMA later sealed the original crack.

When the powerful and unpopular calomel-style drugs of early allopathy passed into disuse, they were replaced by a mixture of Indian medicines, substances suggested by homoeopathy, and new laboratory compounds. Harris Coulter has done a survey of medicines taken from homoeopathy during the late nineteenth century. These include: Hellebore, Bryonia, Cactus (as a heart medicine), Poison Ivy (homoeopathic *Rhus toxicodendron*), *Cocculus indicus, Drosera rotundifoila* (for whooping cough), Cannabis (for gonorrhea), *Pulsatilla nigricans,* Conium (for cancer and paralysis), *Apis mellifica* (bee poison for rheumatism).[8]

The common use of other medicines was extended by homoeopathic proving. *Camphor* for cholera is one example. Homoeopathy used *Thuja occidentalis* (the Arbor Vitae) for secondary illness caused by vaccination and gonorrhea. Poison Nut and Red Pepper came to be used in paralysis and hemorrhoids, respectively; *Ailanthus glandulosa* for scarlet fever and Coffee for headaches were also homoeopathic extensions.[9] They, along with all the other herbal medicines, are lost in the synthetic mélée of modern pharmacy, but they lie at its base. Coulter writes:

"Sharpe and Dohme, E. R. Squibb, and Frederick Stearns got their start during the Civil War and were later joined by William R. Warner (1866), Parke-Davis (1867), Mallinckrodt Chemical Works (1867), Eli Lilly (1876), William S. Merrell, H. M. Merrill, E. Merck, Abbott Laboratories, and others. For the first decade these firms competed in terms of the traditional medicines used by the profession. In the 1870's, however, it became clear that this was too narrow a channel for disposing of the production of an ever-growing industry, and the outcome was an invasion by these 'ethical' drug companies of the patent-medicine field."[10]

That is, drug companies changed from the production of simple medicines whose ingredients were familiar to physicians and whose uses were established by tradition to the invention and marketing of new synthetic compounds, whose basic chemistry was unknown by doctors and whose uses had to be determined by chemical-mechanical assumption and research. These new medicines were known as "proprietaries." Their ingredients were the trade secret of the drug company producing them, and their application was no more than a designation on the label. These could be marketed directly through the pharmacies to the clients, who would be "informed" by advertising rather than medical prescription. Even if a doctor were to intercede between the drug company and the pharmacy, he would be as ignorant as the patient, since he did not either know the make-up or effects of the compounds.

As Coulter points out, the AMA was wary and critical from the beginning:

"The first stupendous error, one which is so vast in its influence that it hangs like a withering blight over the individuality of every man in the profession, is the dictation of innumerable pharmacal companies, the self-constituted advisers in the treatment of diseases about which they know nothing, to the entire profession. . . . They are so solicitous that they flood your office with blatant literature, full of bombastic claims and cure-alls, and I am sorry to say, too frequently with certificates or articles used by permission from physicians who call themselves reputable."[11]

In 1900 the American medical profession was still at war with every system that threatened it, and Squibb, Parke-Davis, et al., were as dangerous as the disciples of Hahnemann. The moment was seized by both businesses. The drug companies and doctors recognized each other as natural allies, sensing, perhaps always, that the homoeopaths were their common enemy, both in terms of medical-chemical principle and commercial ethics.

Parke-Davis and Squibb began publishing medical literature. Never openly propagandist, seemingly historical and scientific in intent, their pamphlets and periodicals (given away at national and local doctors' conventions) rewrote history in favor of the proprietary medicines, in essence congratulating the medical profession for being in the vanguard of new science.

Parke-Davis alone was responsible for a startling number of "respectable" medical journals: *New Preparations, Detroit Medical Journal, American Lancet, Therapeutic Gazette, Medical Age, Druggists' Bulletin,* and *Medicine.*[12] In some cases, they purchased existing journals and renamed them; in other cases, they expanded house organs into scientific publications, with the addition to their staff of professors of medicine and well-known doctors. Other physicians advanced professionally by their association with the journals.

But patronage did not stop with the direct issuing of publications. Virtually all other medical journals, at least all the major ones, including the *Journal of the American Medical Association* (JAMA), were supported by the advertising of proprietary medicines. Doctors were solicited as successfully as the public had been. And the journals, which gave the drug manufacturers their necessary legitimacy, at the same time raised the AMA from the status of another political party to a scientific and professional body representing the whole medical profession. Gradually, the resistance to proprietary medicines quieted, and the drug companies, under protection of the secrecy of their products in a market economy, were held only to the most perfunctory disclosure of the contents of drugs advertised in medical journals.

Medicine gradually passed into a modern era in the United States. A phase came in which both allopathy and homoeopathy seemed to disappear into archaisms. A new system arose, with controlled experiments, advanced machinery, vast facilities, and a microbiological pharmacy. A fellowship of science in the coming age was proclaimed: "We are all now professionals," the argument went. "No more schools and sectarian positions, only general universal objective medicine." It was a compelling argument. But since homoeopathic and allopathic principles are opposed, the new system had to work by one principle rather than another, and it was allopathic in its allegiance.

From 1899 to 1911 George H. Simmons was general secretary of the American Medical Association and editor of the *JAMA*. He remained editor until 1924. Notably, he was once a homoeopath in Nebraska, and, according to Coulter, an ardent one. After his conversion to allopathy, he was well qualified to handle the thorny homoeopathic issue. Instead of continuing the long-standing attack, he went against precedent and against some of the AMA membership in welcoming not only homoeopaths but all sectarian practitioners into the AMA. They were offered entry in general celebration of the end of sectarianism. A great number of homoeopaths accepted, especially low-potentialists, who felt more cut off from their Hahnemannian brethren than their mainstream opponents. Homoeopathic pharmacies became regular American drugstores, carrying proprietaries and patent medicines because the public, uninvolved in the philosophical issues, demanded them. These drugs were widely advertised and advocated. They continued to carry homoeopathic remedies until they were no longer in demand.

The passage of so many homoeopathic doctors into general non-homoeopathic practice severely weakened the homoeopathic movement. Mainstream medicine constantly advanced the position that the aim of medicine was to effect cures of the sick and not to hold to any rigid positions at the expense of that. The *JAMA* declared:

"It is a favorable sign to find a faithful follower of Hahnemann who acknowledges the natural tendency of which most medical men are aware, and it causes us to renew our hope that the time is not so very distant when the believers in the efficacy of dilutions will cease to shut themselves up in a 'school' and will become a part of the regular medical profession, the members of which are ready and anxious to employ any and every means which can be scientifically shown to have a favorable influence upon the course of disease."[13]

The American Institute of Homoeopathy began a countermovement in 1910, but individual homoeopaths were not interested in anything that smacked of either unionism or hucksterism. They held onto the nineteenth century as firmly as to any principles. They guarded their practices like hawks, not preparing any newcomers to replace them. When homoeopathic doctors died out, the practice died with them. Even the homoeopathic medical schools were taken over. The lower-potency prescribers felt quite at home with courses in anatomy, physiology, and pathology. Those who taught materia medica were kept on in acknowledgment of the school charters, but were looked on as relics and virtual "historians" of medicine. These events proved that Hahnemann was right when he denied the possibility of half-homoeopathy. Half-homoeopathy is nonhomoeopathy.

The field secretary hired by the American Institute of Homoeopathy could do nothing to turn the tide. Homoeopaths had been so spoiled by the recent mass conversions that they expected history to deliver them whole. He wrote in his final report:

"He who sits comfortably in his easy chair in his smoking jacket enjoying a genuine Havana bought with the silver earned by means of a successful homoeopathic prescription, grunting a 'Cui bono?' when called upon to do his share toward the perpetuation of the homoeopathic doctrine, and he who vainly asserts that 'Similia is a mighty truth and cannot die, no matter whether I get busy on its behalf or not!' letting it go at that, are likely to awaken some wintry morn to find themselves undeceived."[14]

Meanwhile, mainstream medicine, with its organizing body, the AMA, and the JAMA, had a new authority in relation to the sectarian medical schools. Having taken the sectarians into their mainstream, they now could claim a right to have their say in such medical education. They represented the new syncretist medicine, and they sought to develop its standards and criteria for practice. As long as there were two medical traditions with two theories, the homoeopaths were immune to interference from the allopaths, immune legally unless they were declared to be quacks by a recognized government scientific body. When a significant proportion of homoeopaths accepted general nonsectarian medicine—many of them innocently, thinking it was an inroad for homoeopathy to be heard and tested in wider circles—the basis for a separate homoeopathic training had disappeared.

In preparation for a grading of medical schools, the AMA developed a series of criteria for a good medical facility. These were terribly biased against homoeopathy, for they required nonpracticing research doctors (a contradiction in homoeopathic terms), extensive laboratories (meaning pharmaceutical laboratories), and a balanced curriculum. The balanced curriculum was a spider's final web from which homoeopathy could not extricate itself as long as it advanced its own superior methodology handed down by Hahnemann. It had isolated itself from both the American scientific tradition and professional etiquette.

In association with the Carnegie Foundation for the Advancement of Teaching, the AMA prepared a working paper on medical education in America and Canada. This study, issued in 1910 under the name of Abraham Flexner, the Carnegie representative, gave the AMA a basis for refusing licenses to the graduates of low-ranking institutions. Although ostensibly a temporary survey, the Flexner Report, rightly or wrongly, became the new basis on which medical education was organized. Modern medicine was recognized as the nonsectarian collection of the methods and theories that had proven accurate and scientific. The sectarian schools were not immediately forced out of business, but they were permanently identified as "sectarian schools" rather than medical schools. Their attendance dropped, and, at a period of time that orthodox medicine received substantial foundation funding and government support, they were left to their own fate. Over the years since, the gap has merely increased. Funding of mainstream medicine has spiraled; the sectarian schools have dwindled and all but disappeared. The Flexner Report said:

". . . now that allopathy has surrendered to modern medicine, is not homoeopathy borne on the same current into the same harbor?

"For everything of proved value in homoeopathy belongs of right to scientific medicine and is at this moment incorporate in it; nothing else has any footing at all, whether it be of allopathic or homoeopathic lineage."[15]

Seven homoeopathic medical schools were left by 1918; the Hahnemann Medical College of Philadelphia lasted until the 1920s, when it changed its orientation to allopathy. Homoeopathic experiment, even were there a simple way to pose the problem of microdose, became as irrelevant and on the same basis, as the alchemical experiment in transmutation of metals. The Flexner Report was reasonable to a fault in its assessment of the situation, but it was not a reasonable situation. Homoeopathy could not be merged with allopathy in a new medicine. Standardization required that homoeopathy be left behind.

The decline of homoeopathy not only brought an end to the Law of Similars and microdose in general medicine; it also changed the popular perception of disease categories. The emphasis fell away from chronic conditions, which were virtually untreatable anyway, onto severe disease and the demography of health, illness, and health care, where allopathy had the greatest success.

Chronic diseases were either passed on to specialists or declared undiagnosable and treated symptomatically. The kinds of fees doctors have come to expect, after years of medical training, are not possible from the treatment of headaches and digestive difficulties; many doctors have found it demeaning to be asked to solve these personal cases, so they are dealt with in depth only by psychoanalysis, where they are linked with neuroses and other personality disorders that are prestigious and lucrative enough to treat. Only by becoming mental illness can chronic disease get respect. Even then, it is treated physically by psychotropics and turned back to the fashions and progress of the drug industry. If there were anything significant in Hahnemann's progression of chronic ailments, modern medicine is in no position to discover it, let alone test it.

From, roughly, 1910 until the late 1960s, few new homoeopaths entered the ranks in the United States and Canada; as the last classes of homoeopaths graduated from American medical schools in the 1920s and 1930s, only European-trained physicians were available. It was generally agreed that homoeopathy in North America had been consigned to the history of medicine. The homoeopathic community tended to accept their martyrdom; their mission was to keep the flame alive during these dark ages, to keep it from being blown out by the inexorable winds of materialism.

Ostensibly, during this time, the situation in Europe has been far more promising. Homoeopathy has continued as a viable medicine, with its hospitals and medical schools, throughout Western Europe and in the countries once part of the defunct British Empire, notably India. But it never achieved the dominance in these places that it did in America, and it is now a secondary medicine at best wherever it is practiced. Standards have deteriorated; far worse, there is controversy from country to country, and even from doctor to doctor, as to what constitutes acceptable homoeopathic treatment.

From a Hahnemannian perspective, we have a homoeopathic landscape of small national practices of mediocre and stagnant homoeopathy, with a handful of dying exiles in the once-vibrant North

American center, and individual prescribers of merit scattered throughout the world. Of course, the same landscape, from a twentieth-century mainstream scientific perspective shows a successful universal medicine with some minor pockets of ignorant and superstitious resistance.

Developments of the last ten years have altered the landscape significantly. There has been a resurgence of homoeopathy in the United States; it is not yet significant in terms of absolute numbers, but it is unexpected in the context of the prior unchecked decline. It is also notable that in the last ten years, perhaps as many as a hundred new M.D.s have taken up homoeopathic practice. A visible homoeopathic clinic in Berkeley sees a rapidly growing number of patients, now at two thousand. In April 1978 a conference brought together homoeopaths from around the United States, but mainly from west of the Rockies, and George Vithoulkas interrupted his practice and flew in from Greece to deliver fifteen hours of lectures to five hundred people at the California Academy of Sciences. At the end of this conference, the formation of an International Foundation for the Promotion of Homoeopathy was announced, with the explicit intention of raising standards of homoeopathic practice and publicizing homoeopathy throughout North America and the world. The founding directives included "strict scientific research on homoeopathic potencies and their clinical application" and the establishment of full-time four-year homoeopathic schools in Athens, Greece, and California.

Vithoulkas himself came to California with great misgivings. On the one hand, he was moved and intrigued by the energy and attention, some of which he had seen in the increasing flow of visitors to his clinic in Greece. Bill Gray, a young Mill Valley physician, educated at Stanford, had temporarily abandoned his practice to spend two years in Greece studying with him, during which time he helped him edit and write his major three volume work, *The Science of Homeopathy: A Modern Textbook* (1978), perhaps the most significant new homoeopathic text in some fifty years.

In California Vithoulkas spoke of both the enthusiasm and the superficiality of the new homoeopathy. He did not want to encourage it in its present form, and he certainly did not want to be viewed as an avatar of world homoeopathy. His message to interested practitioners was "discipline and practice." "If," he said, in essence, "we cannot cure every difficult case brought before us as a challenge, and turn away with confidence that which is incurable, then we will never gain credibility in the eyes of the establishment, and homoeopathy will never find its place in the world." Anything less than perfection in this fragile time, he argued, would jeopardize the very existence of homoeopathy. He announced that he would no longer receive lay practitioners at his seminar in Athens, not because an average M.D. was better qualified to learn homoeopathy but because he alone could practice medicine within the law.

The appearance in the Bay Area of the most internationally renowned homoeopath raised all the ambiguities that presently exist both in American homoeopathy and homoeopathic practice in the world. The audience was made up of local Bay Area students and practitioners of homoeopathy, older homoeopaths from across the United States, and hundreds of previously unknown doctors, lay prescribers, nurses, and patients, many of them practicing homoeopathy in isolation. One had the sense that the underground movement was perhaps even stronger than was believed by the more public homoeopaths and members of homoeopathic groups. When Vithoulkas spoke at the University of California Hospital in San Francisco, he received a five-minute standing ovation from the medical personnel despite the fact that he had demolished in his lecture everything that the medicine practiced in that building stood for. At the Academy of Sciences, he was interrupted with applause frequently, sometimes for almost offhand descriptions of outdueling an allopath in a difficult case. At the high points of his talks, he was serenaded with "right on's," as people stood and shook fists and gave V-signs.

For the older homoeopaths there, it must have been a both deeply disturbing and elating event. It challenged their own strategy of fifty years. Never in their lifetime did they expect to see such an audience in praise of homoeopathy. But it was not the audience they would have wanted. M.D.s had their hair in braids and wore turbans and robes, and country enthusiasts came down from parts of Oregon, Idaho, Washington, Nevada, Utah, New Mexico, California, etc., dressed for the road or the farm, bearded and long-haired. It was the social and political order Hahnemannian homoeopathy had always stood against. In fact, the American Institute of Homeopathy fears that an awakening of this sort will bring down the wrath of the AMA and Food and Drug Administration (FDA), which, to this point, have been content to let homoeopathy quietly die out without challenging the older practitioners. The policy, up to now, has been the safe one of nonconfrontation because the obvious result of an FDA study of homoeopathic remedies would be a ban on practice.

Vithoulkas' lectures themselves presented the same paradox. Even as he was cheered, he warned the audience of their attitude. "Faddism," he said, "will give the momentary illusion of success, but it will lead even more swiftly to the end of this wonderful science than any amount of isolation."

During the conference, I spoke to people from other parts of the holistic health community and heard a certain amount of criticism. Vithoulkas himself was seen as rigid and authoritarian by some. Others questioned the usefulness of such a volatile, rooting audience. One could almost see the event two ways. It was obviously an epic moment in the history of homoeopathy, no matter what followed it, and the excitement was warm and epochal. A specially woven banner hung on the curtains behind the podium with the homoeopathic logo (SIMILIA SIMILIBUS CURENTUR) stitched between two yellow daisylike flowers. It was a medical lecture and ceremony both. On the other hand, one could see that the audience sought a charismatic healing figure and Vithoulkas both filled and was willing to fill the role, his warnings notwithstanding. Furthermore, Bill Gray seemed anxious both to promote and to protect his teacher, and an inevitable inner circle tried to predetermine the mood of the event. The audience at moments seemed anti-intellectual and threatening, especially when they appeared to cheer for the demise of specific allopathic patients. Humanity had disappeared and been replaced with an almost desperate wish that this be the path to the abstract ideal of health and the full realization of human potential.

Adding to the mystery, as well as the mythology, was the publicly oft-repeated statement that Vithoulkas was seriously ill and had come to America at great personal risk. This could have meant a whole number of things, but disbelievers tended to offer "Physician, Heal Thyself" retorts whereas the most devoted believers claimed that the doctor had worked his way so far back through the miasmatic history of the human race that he was experiencing the oldest sicknesses in Western civilization and was transmuting through his own body the protean spores of man's plight. Since this is a myth, it need not be confirmed or denied, but it does show the strongly Christian, even Christlike undertones to homoeopathy.

It is sufficient for us to note that homoeopathy is presently at a crossroads in the United States. It is being practiced again by new professionals and is available to the public. What the political and legal consequences will be, especially of lay prescribing, one does not know. Different levels and types of homoeopathy are inevitable as long as basic contradictions within the system and the practice are unresolved. A person today seeking homoeopathic treatment truly enters a great metaphysical riddle, further compounded by historical and ideological variations. We are finally left without an absolutely clear sense of what homoeopathy is, without a sense that will allow us to judge practitioners and give clear advice to people seeking doctors. But what is clear is that, from the beginning, homoeopathy has been a process working toward something extraordinarily important. That process will press on through the different forms and versions until something is manifested. But it may be a very long time. Until then, we may have to accept what we have and live within the mystery and paradox in order to live somehow in the future that is alive in our own time.

XV

Sigmund Freud and the Origin of Psychotherapeutic Healing

The missing key to the twentieth century is Sigmund Freud (1856–1939). All other major components have been accounted for in one way or another. Psychiatry drove a wedge through Western medicine, and the different parts have been struggling to realign themselves ever since. It emerged from pre-Freudian intimations and passed, through Freud's systemization of it, into a territory beyond his imagination, offering the beginnings of solutions to problems that had previously been poorly conceived and thus insoluble. Everything else was sucked into its opening, twisted and otherwise deformed to fit the space.

New medicines change the basic relationship between the art of healing and the science of medicine, and psychiatry is no exception. On the side of healing, it invented roles for the shaman and "word doctor" so they could join the Western physician as equal colleagues. But, on the side of science, it extended the mechanistic model to include language and psyche and thus further isolated the spiritual healer as a nonprofessional. Back on the other side, it dislodged the major functional basis for a physiological mechanism and thereby forced scientific medicine to abandon much of its core, including territory it had seized from the shaman and the spiritualist over the centuries. In that sense, psychiatry lays the groundwork for a return to "native" medicine, but, by setting the terms for that return in psychosomatic language, it makes it into a new event entirely.

Coming a century later and equally the grand synthesis of one
man, psychiatry runs on a parallel track to homoeopathy—not in its
cultural destiny but in its concern for the simultaneity of mental and
physical symptoms and its attempt to establish a code for the psychosomatic expression of the whole organism. The difference between them is crucial. Homoeopathy is like a mad saint on the
outskirts of civilization, preaching in a wilderness where paradox tri-
umphs over reason: few can survive its message, and no one can
carry it back into cities without abridging and distorting it. Psychiatry is like a well-bred and educated statesman, translating the hidden
messages of an era into a workable government.

In order to understand and unscramble the complex lineage of
psychiatric thought in this century we must go back to the father,
Freud. His absolute paternity is perhaps challengeable, but there is
no other single pretender. Even those radical therapies that arise in
direct defiance or complete ignorance of the Freudian tradition share
in the basic kinship. The psychoanalytic mode of thought has permeated our culture and influenced our institutions, from labor relations to philosophy.

It is not only a matter of psychology and medicine. Decades after
his death, Western science has been extending his model to include
all human phenomena. In fact, "human" is an understatement. Animal psychology owes at least as much to the Freudian influence:
psychological terms like "behavior," "instinct," "dominance," and
"learning" have their roots in psychiatry and psychological thought.
Anthropology, ethology, ecology, and computer science inherit parts
of their structure from a system which began with the treatment of
mentally ill patients. This in itself is an insight into how fragmented
Western civilization *had* become. Psychology now lies at the center
of modern aesthetic theory, linguistics, and art criticism—but equally
physics, corporate management, criminology, and strategic warfare.
Who-we-are has been redefined from square one.

Of course, one man is not responsible for all of this. If it was going
to come in such legion, it would have come anyway. But Freud was
the one who recognized the new set of meanings and made it into a
text. His text stands, though its fine clarity has been blurred by secondary issues, his own excesses, and sometimes the excesses of others
claiming him. He is a feminist target because of his development of
a psychology of women out of and subsidiary to a psychology of

men. He is a political target because of his initiation of the privileged and exploitable role of the therapist. Modern social scientists exile him to history for his mystical theories of evolution and his "subjective" use of data. Humanists disown him for his cynicism and pessimism about human potential.

But Freud could hardly do everything, and he certainly could not transcend all of his own cultural biases. These mistakes, so-called, are minor and sectarian and do not affect his over-all theory. So major and fundamental were his primary insights—in a sense the single insight—that they are without ideology and adaptable on a number of levels to a variety of different ends. No particular adaptations, including Freud's, describe, let alone discredit, the essential discovery.

First and foremost, Freud disclosed unconscious process. Or more accurately, he opened the door of Western rationalism to the hidden nature of its own mentality at exactly the moment it had chosen to explore the nonmental phenomena of the physical world. The new levels of organization it had discovered external to its being, Freud restated as internal analysis, changing both the phenomena themselves and human nature. What was new was the shape in which the unconscious was revealed, not unconsciousness itself which had had many earlier versions in the West alone. For all of human history, poets, shamans, magicians, scientists, and philosophers had explored the unconscious world and used its powers. But Western orthodoxy came to divide the kingdom of reality between concrete scientific types of things whose existence could be experienced directly and, to all intents and purposes, proven and other phantasmagoria which were ceded to vestigial primitive mankind. The two exceptions were the flights of fantasy allowed to artists and the disease of insanity granted to madmen. The only way this whole latter territory could be salvaged for science was by being proven to be "true," i.e., to exist in the same way all things exist, by the same natural laws.

Nowadays science and philosophy assume the reality of these things, despite disagreement as to their location and meaning. But this is Freud's legacy, not something to which he had access. He uncovered the laws by which the world of fantasy, madness, and nonsense was connected to the world of concrete phenomena, to the same world. Nothing could transgress these laws, no matter how excessive—no dream, no war, no state of delirium, no slip of the tongue. Freud saddled Western civilization with its unconscious for the duration, and perhaps he did it just in time, before the illusion of human grandeur had gotten totally out of hand. There was no longer any way to pretend that these things could be purged from reality by a golden age of reason.

The ideal of transcendent progress was so strong that it continues to dominate our modern world at least as much as Freud's correction. With the improvement of knowledge, all things should be brought under benign control; of course, this requires that all things be conscious, hence controllable. Those things that are not must be left behind, as trivial and childish and unrelated to the advancement of science, the spread of prosperity, the improvement of government, and the general progress of awakened humanity. Premeditated correct action will solve the scourges of the past: tyranny by laws; poverty, disease, and famine by scientific discovery; and human quarrelsomeness, at last, by collective recognition of the common good. Two world wars and a subsequent precariousness of civilization have done away with the sheen on that vision, but not the stuff of which it is made. Science continues to leap into the future, tearing away confinements of space, time, and energy and placing its golden-age promise against the current tyranny and pain. Communist and Democratic nations both claim a political judicial ideal, and certainly both ascribe to the view that government can give humanity a better lot. Most people still hope that reasonableness will prevail. Yet the discovery of the unconscious has shown man his own nature and placed his future hopes under entirely different auspices. We live during a transition of power.

Our conscious cities and industries stand under continuous threat of collapse from the forces they contain. Progressive nineteenth-century science, which built them, wanted all of reality to be conscious. Freud gave back to the unconscious its clear deed to much of the world, including those same cities and industries. Or, we might say, the unconscious claimed it anyway, and Freud named and predicted it at a moment when it had no name and was an enemy within of uncertain size and composition. Freud showed that it was very powerful, that it could not be suppressed or defeated, but he gave us a more distant hope that is sometimes forgotten: it is not the enemy— it is who we really are. The other thing threatens us only because we deny its existence. It is the fact that it already *is* that propels it to claim, by law, its place in reality.

By proving the unconscious, Freud established its priority. Once we acknowledge that living organisms carry the full potential of what they are, in psychoembryological formation, the weight and persistence of the inner process and the fragmentation must overwhelm the small amount that can become conscious. According to Freud, the events that go into shaping a person are internalized and reenacted throughout life—and the earlier less rational impressions dominate the later reasonableness. The desires one is born with (and through), the instincts for survival and satisfaction, merge with actual being. So no matter what a person's attitude or expressed moral position, it is formed only of raw instinct. The ideological avoidance of sexual acting out, for instance, does not end the matter. The desire stays within the organism unconsciously and is expressed in some other activity which compensates exactly even though it may not have specific sexual content.

Civilization, with its etiquettes and repressions, offers no sanctuary against primary desires and original pain. A later life of ease and pleasure does not alleviate the terrors and agonies of childhood; unexperienced pain limits pleasure without the person even being aware of it. Humanity can no longer offer science and progress as its sole credential. Mankind is responsible for the raw data of living systems and the conversion of that, through psychic data, into the ongoing world—responsible under the threat that it will happen anyway.

Freud's proposal of the unconscious, with its associative dynamics, was a major event. Since then, we have been trying to figure out what it includes and how it shapes and changes known things. Initially it is a reservoir of psychological memory, containing the events of a lifetime cognized and symbolized in the way that they occurred and generative of habitual behavior. The organism is subject to its early learning, and it continues to formulate new situations in terms of the first events it experienced.

The unconscious is also the nerves and muscles and tissue in which psychological existence is recorded. Their locations are intuited as mind itself, whose contents then become memories. Pulses of information pass out of unconsciousness, creating a worldly environment, the very thing which was once thought to be an exclusively external phenomena. In fact, the spatial quality of existence—our seeming existence in space and with space around us—is an original experience that organisms have of their own inside, its contour and depth of tissue and information which is projected onto the world.

These emerging pulses give rise to styles and artifacts of existence.

They have their own language. If they seem to speak in clichés, that is because we already have adopted them by the time we hear them. They control us; yet they are also the modes through which we express our freedom and our very being. Language, for instance, is a collectively arising unconscious system—whether one takes it from Benjamin Lee Whorf, that our syntax shapes our philosophy of the universe, or from Noam Chomsky, that unconscious syntax and language interact dynamically with thought processes to make ideas. One step removed from language are art, politics, economics, and the rest—all once the prized arenas of human creativity and now also languages that tell people what they think even as people try to think *in* them. Physics and philosophy, the twin rulers who buried the unconscious before Freud's time and laughed at its fledgling attempts at reemergence, have now been forced to admit that they are opposed by a vast unknown, right in the center of human thought and knowledge; that they are only languages; and that they too must acknowledge their origin and form every step of the way toward objective reality if they are to have even a shred of it by the time they get there.

This hidden mind was an encumbrance and diversion not counted on a century ago, and certainly one that has bogged down a glorious quest for utopia. The poor sister to philosophy, psychology, now owns the West, and we have radical new philosophers whose primary gestures are to rediscover Freud himself more deeply in the process he unveiled and to apply to his system the circular laws of which his system is made.

A new French school, for instance, has reconstituted Freud in terms of the history and set of cultural symbols that gave rise to him as well as them and their thought of him, a Freudian complication itself. One doesn't have to understand Jacques Derrida completely to feel weight of this against the history of Western thought and its contemporary dilemma:

"Thus are perhaps augured, in the Freudian break-through, a beyond and a beneath of that enclosure we might term 'Platonic.' In that moment of world history 'subsumed' by the name of Freud, traversing an unbelievable mythology . . . , a relation to self of the historico-transcendental scene of writing was spoken without being said, thought without being thought: written and simultaneously erased . . ."[1]

The Freudian system even contained the terms for its own erasure.

It naturally evolved to the point where it was translated into French and derived again through structural and linguistic philosophy. But, even as that happened, the excavation went beneath its very existence and developed meanings that preceded and subsumed Freud. His intention, as it was written into the history of thought, disappears into the paradox he was portraying. By bracketing, for a moment, the affective emotional aspect of Freud and giving it a context but not their literal acceptance, the French "post-modern" philosophers transformed the old doctor into the spiffiest member of their own society. For them he had freed philosophy to consider itself, to consider its dreams, its unconscious, *its* philosophy in the making of true things. To all that would be spoken in the world, he gave an unspoken, and a dream.

Psychiatry has taken Freud's theory of the unconscious in a number of ways. The simplest interpretation was the one developed through rational psychoanalysis and typified by the confident therapist who tells his neurotic patient: "You don't know what you are doing, but I do because I can see your thought process through your manifest behavior." In many parts of his work, Freud himself was this confident, and he defended this rational orthodoxy against his more radical followers.

Dark Freud, though, was in awe of the power of the unconscious, and he diagnosed humanity's situation as hopeless because of it. The species would eventually be dragged down into its own creationary darkness, the thin veneer of civilization and consciousness crumbling around it.

Carl Jung, Freud's immediate disciple, added a cosmic and spiritual aspect to the basic unconscious, suggesting that not only chaos and fragmentation, but also the most creative and curative of human powers were contained there. Freud himself realized the healing function of dreams and other psychic material, but he placed a strict limit on how much was stored there—very little, in fact, beside the already vast and bloody desires and terrors to which nightmare is our closest encounter. Jung's unconscious was collective and preembryological. He found in it the beauties of geometry and mathematics, the original forms of the gods and mythological heroes, and the blueprint for civilization itself—for temples and poems and cities, all of which existed as unrealized seeds in the human psyche and to which mankind was heir. Freud saw civilization as the product of distorted instinct thrown up around himself by a frightened creature, but Jung insisted, no, it too is a true and prophetic realization of the psyche and the inner mind of nature. He did not return to the golden age of science, but he did propose a healing psyche/soma as an aspect of the unconscious depths, and he gave the creations of humanity an equal claim to primary structure and tissue.

Jung proved what Freud no doubt feared: that by opening a Pandora's box, he had let out everything. Derrida would later show him to have let out the nothing that everything is and so sent Western philosophy back to the bare rocks of its beginnings. Freud discovered the inevitability of war and misery in uncontrollable instinct, but Jung showed Freud to have also rediscovered the hermetic arts and sources of magic, not as second-class citizens, but with the same living integrity as DNA and electrons. Thus, Freudian psychology became, through Jung, the lost ancient hermetic psychology, but only partially, for it located all these things now in a bounded secular space. Freud revealed, if only in rough semblance, the archaeology of a vast healing system, like an underground city inhabited by Navaho medicine men, Australian shamans, and African voodoo priests. As our sense of the unconscious has grown in the decades since Freud, it has come to exist outside of the system that spawned it. The alternative medicines rely, post-psychiatrically, on the intuition that great and primeval energies dwell inside us and that the forces which lead to our sickness and destruction are also the forces of our revivification.

Freud's second major achievement was the development of a theory of sexuality. Before Freud, there was a general preference to consider sexuality only an overt series of activities and to separate it ontogenetically from other behavior. In fact, there was a tendency to isolate all behavior and consider each facet of it somehow self-explicit; sexuality fell under this common assumption.

Following the plan of the unconscious, Freud extended sexuality to cover a swath of human activities not previously considered sexual. Beneath the usual range of genital activity and fantasy, he proposed a larger network of feelings, structures, and capacities for pleasure and pain which were reflected not only in genital behavior but all aspects of the organism's life. He said: "Genital being does not arise spontaneously with puberty, but is an aspect of the over-all sexual orientation of the human animal."

"Why sexuality?" people asked. "Why not hunger? Why not money? Why not power?" Many considered Freud sex-obsessed because of the priority he gave sexuality, though, of course, the critical objections indicate more the obsessions of the critics than those of Freud himself, even if in a negative (i.e., sexophobic) way.

The criticism misses the point. Freud actually advanced a theory of the interrelationship of behavior. All activities of the organism reflect internal dynamic components. The organism's life, as it is lived, is a process of connecting its single hungers and instincts to the various activities in which it participates. All these other things— not only power, money, territory, and security, but also games, music, plans for cities, etc.—are equivalent expressions of the underlying biological drive. They reflect symbolically in each other.

Sexuality is singled out because it is a direct concomitant of the life force. That is, it expresses primary hungers, undiverted by cultural sublimations; it is an original component of the unconscious; and it is developmentally linked to the emergence and maturity of the organism. We might also note that Freud's emphasis on symbolic sexual masking was, implicitly, a cultural diagnosis. It is possible to imagine a culture in which sexual development would not be symbolized in language considered "sexual" in Western terms. No doubt much of the "sexy" behavior reported by observers of the primitive world was sexy only by European standards, having other individual meanings in local customs and rites. Freud may have carried the Western model too far, but his prior intent was to arrive at a theory of formative bodily drive. The sexual difficulties of his patients led him to recognize this drive in repressed sexuality. Western culture had genitalized its experience of the body's life force and had created a network of fantasy and taboo about it. Freud's terminology developed from unraveling this network. Just beneath the fabric of neurotic and psychotic activity he found a zone of twisted sexual imagery. When he followed this curatively, he was successful, for he was, in essence, de-layering the biological rigidity of the organism. By enlarging its notion of sexuality, he was enlarging its sense of its own being, teaching it that it existed in a world of symbolic layers reflecting a process of energy rather than in a frozen patterning of its own self-image.

Phrased differently, we could say that Freud stated a new relationship between social behavior and biopsychological intention. The former attempts to establish itself and maintain its self-image and the latter tries to burst through, so the former tries harder to keep its boundaries. Sexual repression is actually repression of the full psychic contents of the unconscious. Thus, Freud could disclose the origin of behavior by uncovering the roots of sexuality.

Freud's analysis of the development of sexuality is crucial both as a description of how nonsexual behavior supplants sexual behavior without supplanting the sexual drive and as a model for the development of the social and symbolic capacities of the organism as a whole.

He calls the basic drive, or pulse, "libido": this is the presexual condition of the sexual drive, or, more accurately, the life force itself which gets shaped into "eros" through human biology. It appears first in the lips, as the desire for suckling but also as thumb-sucking and general lip and mouth contact with external things. Eventually, in the developmental process, the oral phase, without being overridden entirely, passes into an anal phase, in which the feeling from excreting and withholding feces serves as libidinal expression. With social and biological maturity, the oral and anal phases are translated into genital sexuality with oral and anal components. The adult personality often seizes on sexuality and stylizes it, forgetting its origins in oral and anal eroticisms, even as the man forgets the boy and the woman forgets the girl. They become committed to the "adult" quality of their sexual behavior. Freud cut through, as it were, the displays of sex and got to its substance.

Of course, "libido" is just a word, and Freud used it to describe the developmental patterns of human behavior because they seemed as if they were being shaped from such a source. He intuited underlying energy patterns. He did not mean libido to be synonymous with loving contact, despite its role in the formation of eros. Libido was the drive itself, which the organism expressed in whatever way was open to it. If libido ran into resistance of various sorts, it could find expression as aggression, denial, or sadism. Freud described sadism as "an instinctual fusion of purely libidinal and purely destructive urges, a fusion which thenceforward persists uninterruptedly."[2] What might have become love is no longer perceived comfortably as love by the organism, but it does get satisfaction from inflicting pain, so it does this from the same energetic source as it would express love. The desire to hurt is, morphologically, the desire for contact.

Libido allowed Freud to explain the functional relatedness of differing activities. Fetishism and other forms of sexual deviation might not be sexual in the usual sense, but they *are* libidinal. The oral and anal activities of the infant and child are not sexual in the genital mode but they are stages in the dynamic process which unfolds into adult sexuality at puberty.

In addition, Freud emphasized that sexuality (i.e., libido) was a pure function for "obtaining pleasure from the zones of the body" and that it was "brought into the service of reproduction" only subsequently in the life of the organism.[3] There were a tendency to assume that sexuality not in the service of reproduction was either nonfunctional or purposeless, even immoral. But Freud showed that it had a substantial role in maintaining health. Sexual atrophy or deviation led to a variety of mental and physical diseases. Conversely, restoration of sexual function led to an improvement in general health.

In general, Freud demonstrated an enlarged sphere of sexuality, its ebb and flow in the living system and its etiology in the development of personality and psychosomatic disorders and abnormal manifestations. He showed that these could be described not only from the point of view of their abstract phenomenology, but "from the point of view of their dynamics and economics [and] the quantitative distribution of the libido."[4] This was the basis for a general theory of the body as a quantum of energy expressed through a process rather than as the old-fashioned solid with its mechanics and sensitivity.

Freud developed a theory of energy for human thought processes. The theory itself is Darwinian, but it is not as simple as a psychological metaphor out of biology. So far as I know, Freud did not credit Darwin with a contribution to his own discovery. However, as we are heir to Freudian thought without acknowledgment, Freud was heir to general Darwinian logic—i.e., life is not a special case. Nothing occurs unless there is real force behind it—physical force, electrical or magnetic force, biophysical force. Psyche, too, must be explained as a product of the underlying natural world.

Once upon a time, mind might have been taken differently. Thought is apparently weightless and free to roam about a limitless territory, providing laws everything else must obey. Thought must also obey, Freud declared, Freud the neurologist. Thought is another layer of biochemical activity. It is not an ethereal counterpart to personality. It is not the human species' gift from a higher creation. It is a residue of biological process, reflecting the collective capacity of cells, organs, nerves, and muscles. Its content, like its physiology, is given in advance by the quantities and distributions that make it up.

The Darwinian laws of nature define the survival of the few—the "fittest," meaning only those who, by chance adaptation to change, persist when everyone else has succumbed. Just as animals cannot demand the longevity of their species on the basis of their own beauty, intelligence, or uniqueness, so thoughts cannot demand to exist by any property except the somatic context in which they exist already. The human being can claim no real creativity or latitude of meaning; he is stuck with the initial properties of mind. Where Darwin saw natural selection and extinction of whole lines, Freud saw the generation of thoughts from the unconscious into the conscious mind through the selective matrix of resistance, memory, and association. Crabs and algae in the pond, lions stalking zebras at the waterhole, dreams and insights—these (to quote Melville) were obedient to the same volition.

By "quantitative distribution," Freud meant "natural selection." Cognitive and emotional material operates on the nervous energy with which it was originally stored or cathected; it can be reordered by experience, but its capacity does not change, and, in any case, the new patterns are as indelible as the original distribution. Thus mental illness or trauma is a specific physical-emotional quantum which would require an equal and appropriate charge of energy to dislodge it.

Psychology is, by heritage, biological. Where Freud used subjective images for neuromuscular and mental processes, modern psychology has replaced them with neurons and hemispheres of the brain. Although Freud was headed in this direction anyway, the completeness of the dehumanization would have appalled him as much as Darwinism would have appalled Darwin. Freud was a remarkably gifted healer. His theories arose from his ability to heal. Those who came after him were often mere machinists and hacks.

Darwin, Freud, and Lévi-Strauss represent a sequence in the history of European thought, in which the law of quantitative distribution of energy was applied to phenomena ranging from species of animals to bodies of folklore and marriage systems of human groups. Darwin showed that the living were simply a special case of the nonliving and that no form came into being with outside help; he showed that there was no outside. Freud then demonstrated how dreams, madness, and fantasy were not only continuous with logical thought, but the basic materials from which logical thought was formed; likewise, there could be no thought from outside the original neurological environment. Lévi-Strauss then explained the exotic customs of non-Western peoples as the sociological source of all mankind, operating by the same laws as the most honored European mores; humanity was a single planetary condition subject to the same mechanisms. He opens his analysis of totemism with a description of Freud's work on hysteria:

"The first lesson of Freud's critique of [Jean Martin] Charcot's theory of hysteria lay in convincing us that there is no essential difference between states of mental health and mental illness; that the passage from one to the other involves at most a modification in certain general operations which everyone may see in himself; and that consequently the mental patient is our brother, since he is distinguished from us in nothing more than by an involution—minor in nature, contingent in form, arbitrary in definition, and temporary— of a historical development which is fundamentally that of every individual existence. It was more reassuring to regard a mental patient as belonging to a rare and singular species, as the objective product of external or internal determinants such as heredity, alcoholism, or mental weakness."[5]

The notable thing about psychiatry, then, and what it transfers to the rest of medicine, is not that it deals with mental disease rather than physical disease, but that it deals with the inevitability of disease, i.e., internal chemical change. It demands, as well, that every environmental and social influence be processed as a corresponding change within the organism.

There is no way to destroy anything and there is no way to lose anything, Freud wrote, so man is literally the realization and accumulation of his own biological existence:

"It is quite true that the unconscious wishes are always active. They represent paths which are always practicable, whenever a quantum of excitation makes use of them. It is indeed an outstanding peculiarity of the unconscious processes that they are indestructible. Nothing can be brought to an end in the unconscious; nothing is past or forgotten."[6]

Freud's work on dreams and dreaming was so fundamental that it has not been made obsolete by later studies on the subject. In fact, twentieth-century thought has merely sharpened its insights and developed an oneiric science from them. Yet *The Interpretation of Dreams*, one of Freud's earliest works, was substantially completed before he was forty and published in 1899 (post-dated, prophetically, to 1900 as a statement on the coming century).

Dreams, to Freud, typified the dynamics of mind and nervous system. They were exposed to view, perhaps more than any other part of the unconscious process, so he used them as insights into the basic structure of thought and mental illness.

But when the book first came out, Freud did not fully realize its import. His preface was modest and professional: he hoped that the study of dreams would give clinical insight in other areas of psychology. In the ten years it took for a new edition to appear, he began to realize the scope of the work and to regret its disuse in clinical circles. He notes that the second edition was made necessary by a general reading audience. Thereafter, though, new editions came rapidly, all with extensive additions and footnotes, so that each current edition was not only a compilation of the original research on dreams but a decade-by-decade reevaluation of specific issues and an ongoing yearbook of new insights into the dream process. His preface to one edition, dated March 15, 1931, shows Freud's ultimate assessment of this original intuition of a paradigm for a psychological theory. Looking back, he writes:

"This book, with the new contribution to psychology which surprised the world when it was published (1900), remains essentially unaltered. It contains, even according to my present-day judgement, the most valuable of all the discoveries it has been my good fortune to make. Insight such as this falls to one's lot but once in a lifetime."[7]

Freud begins *The Interpretation of Dreams* by examining the state of dream theory in the late nineteenth century. The problem was that, in enlightened European circles, dreams were considered insignificant and arbitrary, more likely the effect of a bad meal than an important part of the mind or personality. The belief that dreams were messages was considered archaic and superstitious because people did not understand the possibility of biological messages. Dreams were assumed not to be diagnostic because they were taken as superficial occurrences. Whereas Freud was to rediscover dreams as brilliant condensations and encapsulations of psychic states, the custom then was to see them as dispersing of meaning.

None of Freud's predecessors persisted long enough to realize that the difficulties and paradoxes of dreams were the result of the tremendous amount of information contained in their brief span. To the general observer, they were unpleasant, unfinished, primitive, and fragmentary; their bawdiness and absurdity further discouraged rationalists from looking more closely at what was already an embarrassment to the mature people who dreamed them. Freud summarized the attitudes of some of his colleagues toward dreams in the early part of his own book:

"It is as though psychological activity had been transported from the brain of a reasonable man into that of a fool."[8]

". . . it seems impossible to detect any fixed laws in this crazy activity."[9]

"What laughable contradictions he is ready to accept in the laws of nature and society before, as we say, things get beyond a joke and the excessive strain of nonsense wakes him up. We calculate without a qualm that three times three make twenty; we are not in the least surprised when a dog quotes a line of poetry, or when a dead man walks to his grave on his own legs, or when we see a rock floating on the water. . . ."[10]

". . . an archaic world of vast emotions and imperfect thoughts. . . ."[11]

Once Freud established the importance of dreaming in the psychic process, he had to explain its irrational form. There not only was an answer, but the answer explained the crucial role of unconscious process in human life:

Between the psychic sources of the dream in the nervous system and general tissue of the body and their representation as images in the mind of the dreamer is a vast network of quantitatively charged psychosomatic material that strives both to use the dream to get at the basis of its own organic energy process and to disguise by means of the dream the painful truth of its existence. Dreams, said Freud very early, are brief mental disorders and psychoses that prevent major disturbances of long duration. They are medicines, as we have since come to realize more completely, in both the biochemistry of their occurrence and the attempt to recall and make coherent imagery out of their basic psychosomatic impulse. The individual not only dreams his exact energetic circumstance; he has also the images and feelings arising from that dream by which to organize his waking life-process.

The so-called deceptions and circumventions of the dream do not diminish its curative thrust; they *are* that thrust, for they include, by their existence, the contradictory elements of psychohistory and the personal blocks of the organism. After all, by Freudian-Darwinian dynamics, a person in his dreams cannot be involved in creative freelance deceit. Every dream (like every psychosis and neurosis) has a cause in the quantitative distribution of the material demands of life. The resistance of a person to the expression of that quantitative distribution as well as his serving as a vehicle for it, are equally contemporary states of his mind/body. The paradoxes of dream are the paradoxes of life which, if uncontacted, become disease. The dream is there because another expression of the material would be more dangerous.

Freud's analysis of "dreamwork" is significant for the rest of twentieth-century healing, so we will summarize some of its aspects:

The meaning, in the sense of the energetic rationale, of a dream comes from the latent material, which endows the imagery of the mind with profound psychic contents. The state of sleep is what makes the formation of the dream possible, by breaking down resistance to latent material and forging a connection between it and the superficial energy. Without sleep, the psyche is dormant under unremitting censorship by the conscious mind.

Dreaming works by extreme compression, distortion, and replacement. The latent material, which has the deepest psychological meaning, forges itself with the relatively superficial and recent material of the conscious mind to make the language of the dream, which is marked by puns, rebuses, and associative logic. Freud writes: "If in the course of a single day we have two or more experiences suitable for provoking a dream, the dream will make a combined reference to them as a single whole; *it is under a necessity to combine them into a unity.*"[12] The emphasis is on the underlying psychic energy, not on the peculiar imagery: "The greatest intensity is shown by those elements of a dream on whose formation the greatest amount of condensation has been expended."[13] Logical relations become illogical when they are combined and when simultaneity in time is used to express what is actually association of meaning. Since the dream cannot choose between two equally charged streams, it must fulfill both of them instantaneously, even if they are contradictory. The illogic of the dream is the logic, i.e., the logos, of the organism.

A person, in the act of dreaming, has no choice but to express the real state of his being. If the conscious mind is closed to certain psychically significant material, the material will associatively merge with a familiar and innocent event and insinuate itself into the dream without contradicting the mechanics of the dream imagery (and so disturbing the dreaming), yet also without weakening its impact by compromising its importance. The mental apparatus of dreaming takes external and present bodily stimuli into the dream, incorporating them in the same way it incorporates present events: it uses them to contact hidden material while keeping the person asleep. "*Dreams are the* GUARDIANS *of sleep and not its disturbers,*"[14] wrote Freud. Powerful guardians indeed, for they keep things out of the dream only by changing them into the dream:

A recent acquaintance is suddenly dreamed of with features and feelings about her that seem old and important. A house down the block is dreamed of as having the eerie haunting quality of another place and time. The *images* occur because they are current, but their weak charge is taken over by *ideas* which were intensely experienced but have been lost or suppressed and which now achieve enough strength to force themselves through the censorship. The very elements that might have had the highest charge are the ones most drained of intensity by the dreaming, for the association of a high charge and an appropriate image might shock the dreamer into waking. On the other hand, materials of low psychic valuation are suddenly overdetermined in a transference of psychic charge which, in itself, is the process of dream formation.

The trivial events which seem to clutter the dream landscape are born of this displacement. There are no weak or innocent dreams, Freud insists. Dreams are too important to be wasted on "trivialities and trifles."[15] They afford priceless opportunities for the organism to reveal its secrets and establish its psychic balance upset by censorship.

Dreams do not discuss abstract matters. Everything represents the dreamer in some fashion or other. Relationships within the individual are translated, in the dream, into relationships between different individuals and things. Physiological components become part of the dreamed scenery. For instance, the dreamer is walking in a flower garden, and the flowers become more and more colorful and aromatic. These flowers may be the dreamer's own genitals which, as they penetrate consciousness, intensify the imagery. Even a gap in the dream sequence may represent a physiological fact which presents some problem to the dreamer. There is no possibility for a break in imagery because the imagery reflects the energy directly, and the energy is a pulse whose amplitude and quality may change but which never ceases. At one point Freud presents, despite his own reservations, an approximate dream code:

"The Emperor and Empress (or the King and Queen) as a rule really represent the dreamer's parents; and a Prince or Princess represents the dreamer himself or herself. . . . All elongated objects, such as sticks, tree-trunks and umbrellas (the opening of these last being comparable to an erection) may stand for the male organ. . . . Boxes, cases, chests, cupboards and ovens represent the uterus. . . . Rooms in dreams are usually women. . . . Many landscapes in dreams, especially any containing bridges or wooded hills, may clearly be recognized as descriptions of the genitals. . . . Many of the beasts which are used as genital symbols in mythology and folklore play the same part in dreams: e.g. fishes, snails, cats, mice (on account of the pubic hair), and above all those most important symbols of the male organ—snakes."[16]

Every dream expresses a latent wish, though the manifest content may be anxious and distressing because of the organism's censorship of the wish and fear of its consequences. The wish is the source of the dream, the primary and inevitable response to life energy in the nervous system; the manifest imagery is the secondary agency of the dream and the dreamer's defense against the full implication of that energy. It is his individual personal part (which Freud called the "ego") set against his cosmic undifferentiated part (which Freud called the "id").

To deny something is to express it, to give it form. Denial in a dream is part of its resistance to emerging material, producing the moment of fear/desire in which most dreaming occurs. For instance, a dream may seem to be anything but a wish fulfillment, but this is simply another form of desire. When one dreams of being unprepared for or failing an exam that was actually passed years ago, it would seem to be a needless anxiety. Not so, said Freud. The person is reminding himself that the fear of failing was groundless the first time, so it might be also in the future. Of one dream that seemed obviously not to be a wish fulfillment, Freud remarked that it fulfilled the secret wish of his friend who dreamed it to prove him wrong since he had been unsuccessfully competitive with Freud during their years together in school.

In one dramatic case reported by Freud, a father goes to sleep after the death of his son, while an old man watches by the body with a candle, saying prayers. The father dreams that the child is standing by his bed, then catches him by the arm and says, "Father, don't you see I'm burning?" The father awakes to a bright glare from the next room: the watchman had fallen asleep and a lighted candle fallen onto the wrappings, setting the body on fire.

Freud points out that the glare is what disturbed sleep and awoke the dreamer, but why, he asks, at this crucial moment, did he remain asleep long enough to have the brief dream? Freud explains: "For the sake of the fulfillment of [a] wish the father prolonged his sleep by one moment. The dream was preferred to a waking reflection because it was able to show the child as once more alive. If the father had woken up first and then made the inference that led him to go into the next room, he would, as it were, have shortened his child's life by that moment of time."[17]

Another subtle case involves one of Freud's own dreams. At a time he had a painful boil the size of an apple at the base of his scrotum, he dreamed he was riding a horse. The answer to this anomaly, obscure at first, becomes obvious on close scrutiny. Horseback riding was something he never did, but under these circumstances it was unimaginable. "It was," he wrote, "the most energetic denial of my illness that could possibly be imagined."[18] If the pain from the boil was threatening to disrupt the dream, the dream answered by having the dreamer engaged in an activity he could not possibly do with a boil. Thus reassured, he continued to sleep.

Freud's brilliance was displayed in his discovery of the dynamics of unconscious thought and their relationship to daily life. His attempt to translate these into a clinical methodology ultimately failed, though he himself was a successful doctor and began the basic lineage of psychoanalysis.

The problem with this system of therapy was that it lacked a clear set of rules and indications and had no charismatic initiation to compensate. In individual cases, doctors have been able to use Freud's healing style successfully and even to initiate others in it, but these are members of rare lineages of true post-Freudians; the bulk of other post-Freudians practice the *form* of Freudian insight without any of the incisiveness the system requires. They imitate the methodology without real understanding. Much of contemporary psychoanalysis is a scandal and a fraud. A relatively small number of wealthy patients attempt to reconstruct their illnesses out of the materials of dream and free association to gain insight into their behavior; this process is protracted and without any clear goal or consistency of method. Psychiatrists explain to patients the traumatic events of their past, their Oedipal relationship to their mothers or fathers, and the general psychohistorical source of their present unhappiness, but without a careful assay of what these things mean in terms of the quantitative distribution of libido or the precise body/mind balance. Early professionalism institutionalized forms of analysis before they had a fair test. Almost from the beginning, doctors were forgetting that Freud salvaged the Oedipal image as a temporary cue to a more remote form and that the image cannot be applied indiscriminately, and certainly not without some understanding of the thing he was groping toward as well as the thing he said. Freud, in fact, spawned many of the problems that followed him, for he was quite anxious to institutionalize his findings and establish a psychological profession, and this led him to compromise his actual insights. Even though he realized, in theory and by deep conviction, the priority of the unconscious biological process, the civilized doctor in him demanded that the rational mind attempt to control this beast. The system he evolved suffered from the fact that he never actually believed in it. He saw civilization as the ultimate repression, and psychoanalysis as a medicine of that civilization, enabling the individual to mediate between his primal needs and the chains into which he was born. Society would always be in conflict with the individual's basic drives, leading either to the ultimate breakdown of society or the complete enslavement of the human animal. Either way, it was a desperate trap. "Anatomy is destiny," he wrote, meaning "No way out."

"Do you see any joy for the human being?" the narrator of a documentary on Freud asked his British disciple and biographer Ernest Jones. Standing in front of a bust of his subject, Jones said solemnly: "Life is not to be enjoyed. Life is to be endured."[19]

Nothing could more fully express Freud's own pessimism.

In practice, psychoanalysis is based on the belief that if the unconscious "meaning" of a neurosis, character disorder, or even psychosis can be made conscious, the pathology will then be less necessary in the general economy of the organism. The doctor educates the patient, gradually gaining his trust and breaking down his resistance and denial, leading him to discover his pattern of distortion and self-abnegation. The patient is the only source of meaning, since it is contained uniquely in him. His symptoms are his behavior, including his dreams and language patterns, both of which the doctor tries to "decode" by a system of "free association" whereby latent meaningful links between materials are supplied in place of logical conscious ones.

There is no doubt that people are helped by this process, but the reasons may not be the ones Freud thought they were and the help falls well short of restoring function. This was acceptable, in a certain sense, to Freud, because there was no cure for life. All the human animal could learn was how better to cope with his fate. Nothing distinguishes psychiatric therapeutics more than the length of the treatment, easily ten or fifteen years, commonly twenty-five, thirty, and longer. The patient inevitably enjoys it: the attention alone is like an elixir in a society of alienated individuals—but cure is another matter.[20] The neurosis or psychological disorder is a necessary defense which the organism has evolved in order to survive. The process reaches a stalemate when the cause of the illness turns out to be the life-style itself. Most patients cannot change their family, job, or marital situation without jeopardizing their over-all sanity and the source of income for the therapy itself. This is not a light matter, since it speaks to the failure of the medicine to integrate itself into the social conditions in which it is trying to heal people.

The above is the best of situations. In the Euro-American world, where this medicine is most practiced, patients are educated for and temperamentally suited to verbal analysis. These are the ones who can afford, in all senses, this long and sophisticated dialogue with a doctor. For the rest of the people, not only in the Euro-American regions but much of the rest of the world, the Freudian legacy has become a kind of behaviorism backed by military and penal styles of group control. Drugs and behavior modification of various sorts have been found far more efficient than psychoanalysis. They do not treat the underlying disease either, but then Freud laid the groundwork for that by indicating that "coping" was the best that could be hoped for. Seen from the position of beleaguered society, it was more efficient to bully and train people into submission and acceptable so-

cial behavior than to try to teach them the sources of their freedom
and humanity. And this, for the most part, is what mass psychiatry
has become. The causes of behavior are incidental; and the emphasis
is on how to generate the "correct" behavior in the present. The discovery is that men can be trained like rats and pigeons.[21]

Freud in his later years tended to go farther and farther afield for
explanations of the incurability of the species. He created a mythology of the pseudoanthropological origin of the Oedipal complex,
suggesting that mankind had implanted a self-destructive cycle in its
gene base. His disciple Sandor Ferenczi took this to its logical conclusion, to the protoplasm which, he argued, had been traumatized
by the arousal of life within its deadness.[22] Civilization was a psychological "catastrophe," as Freud had concluded, but it was preceded
by prior traumas, of which life itself was the first, disturbing the
eternal sleep of inorganic stone, forcing it to become protoplasm. In
the Oedipal sequence this was followed by the traumas of cell fission,
emergence onto dry land, and the development of primacy in the
genital zone, all of which we inherit and suffer. We cannot undo the
damage, nor can we return to any of these primeval wombs. There is
no bottom to this pessimistic regression, except, perhaps that the
men who formulated it themselves lived with fruitful lives.

When he saw that his system did not, with any consistency, cure
the mentally ill by insight, Freud proposed a specific instinct preventing health, an instinct which must now balance libido in the
psychosomatic economy, giving rise to the wars, suicides, and other
destructive acts. He called this "thanatos," Greek for "death," and
set its longing for self-destruction as the counterpart to the libidinal
longing for contact. Thanatos resisted cure, resisted therapeutic
work, and sought final cessation in lifelessness. It was mankind's
destiny.

This is the basis of Freud's split with his followers. He posited the
death instinct as a libidinal adversary instead of revising his methodology on the evidence of its own flaws. But not everyone was willing
to accept his gloomy prognosis, and if they were willing to accept it
philosophically, as a collective judgment, they were not willing to accept it as a limitation on the therapeutic potential of individual
cases. So they sought other definitions of the energetic proposition.

In the meantime, the unconscious was loose on the world and is
now globally accepted. The magnitude of what we are up against,
which we have lived with not only post-Freud but also post-Heisen-

berg, post-Einstein, and post-Club of Rome ecological doom prophecies, now no longer seems as great, even though it is greater, simply because we have lived with it for the better part of a century and through a series of wars and other encounters with our human nature that suggest the problem may be so great exactly because we have ignored it for so long. It is no longer a surprise and a shock. Freud's *Civilization and Its Discontents* contains a prophecy we are still in the middle of. And we no longer have reason to feel shame and disappointment for ourselves. We know the scope and the origin of our struggle.

XVI

Wilhelm Reich: From Character Analysis to Cosmic Eros

In the most commonly promoted views the twentieth century is defined by a variety of self-images: as an epoch of reality-transforming breakthroughs in science and technology but also of catastrophic destruction and global warfare; an epoch in which former meanings and models of reality have been transformed, in which alienation and existentialism have uprooted belief and knowledge. For both Marxists and Fundamentalists this century is the end of ordinary time.

The personae of our epoch include Albert Einstein, Adolph Hitler, Pablo Picasso, and Mao Tse-Tsung, each of whom translated latent images into actual forms. There are others, just as important, who have engaged our central archetypes but provided only labyrinthine puzzles. It is by them perhaps that we are most truly defined, for the contradictions they embody cannot be resolved in our lifetime. Almost axiomatically each of them must seem to have discovered (or rediscovered) a global energy, a paradoxical force with both positive and negative connotations; each must have challenged the basic social order, must have seemed a miracle healer to some, a demagogue and destroyer to others. Aleister Crowley and G. I. Gurdjieff represent this shadow side of the twentieth-century West, but Wilhelm Reich (1897–1957) almost prototypically defines it. His biography is a tour of boundaries that have repeatedly turned us back.

Early in his career Reich was one of the first and most successful practitioners of the Freudian system. Progressively, as he came to recognize the seriousness of what-he-called "the global plague," he abandoned conventional psychoanalysis as unequipped and inadequate. Over the next thirty-five years he developed a radical new paradigm of psychology and physics, encompassing both libidinal and cosmic energy. This was not just a series of clinical metaphors or literary symbols. Reich isolated and observed the "atoms" of his proposed energy in experiments and then crafted a technology for applying them medicinally.

His diagnosis of a collective ailment was almost Biblical in its portent, his prescription revolutionary. He felt that the human species needed not only healing but a metamorphosis—a job requiring a physician in the largest sense of the term. His medicine ultimately embraced the social, economic, and political realms and fused the etiology of fascism, protoplasm, and galaxies in a single science.

In order to map Reich, we need to examine the difficult seams in the Freudian logos. Later we may be surprised to find that much of the Reichian cosmos has its separate origin in other pre-Freudian materials, but that discovery means much more once we have taken Freudian history into account.

Freud's single brilliant act was the revelation of the unconscious by demonstration of its economic exchange with the organism. To everything that humanity had done or would do, he gave a different meaning; in fact, he gave a bottomless well of transformational symbolisms. Because so much has been based on the Freudian unconscious and its dynamics of shadow and light, we often forget that in and of itself, the theory has no therapeutic usefulness. This is a stunning shortcoming, for Freud is usually viewed as a famous doctor. In his own practice he was clearly a humane and creative healer. But his methods arose from his observations while healing; they did not, themselves, give rise to a technique.

Insofar as they did, that technique is known as psychoanalysis, in all of its many and varied forms. The practice of psychoanalysis was never as successful as its theory. We have already seen that Freud's insights changed Western thought and had a decisive impact on the philosophies, the social and linguistic sciences, and the humanities. We can hear his echo in Lacan, Derrida, and even Whitehead. Military and aerospace sciences have inherited a Freudian component: the enemy operates from unconscious as well as conscious motives, and combat strategies come from the "theory of instincts" and the "interpretation of dreams." Formal economic theory is a wish-fulfillment dream covering generations. Politics in both Eastern bloc and Western nations have become little more than a laboratory study in psychological manipulation and reprogramming. But Freudian clinical methodology never had an equivalent impact on healing and general medicine. It produced a profession, but the profession was unspectacular and common, except when it was re-animated by an individual therapist as humane and insightful as Freud. Many of these have practiced and continue to practice: Robert Lindner, Theodore Rubin, Erich Fromm. Freud gave them a language and an institutional framework for their basic healing talents. Everything else was a "maybe," a "let's-try-this."

Reich met Freud in 1919 while still a student at the Medical School of the University of Vienna. As a combatant in World War I interested in political change, Reich had originally entered the Faculty of Law but changed to medicine from the insight that pedantic legalism led nowhere. He was committed to pure science, but even that early he had the goal of uncovering essential human nature. Psychoanalysis presented him with the perfect blend of intuition and fact. Throughout his career Reich's orientation to the psyche and the emotions was concrete and scientific, seeking energetic bases for behavior.

His talent in the relatively new field surfaced quickly, and by the mid-1920s Freud considered him one of his most promising disciples. But Reich was troubled by the technical inadequacies of psychoanalysis, a criticism which extended almost sacriligiously to Freud's own clinical practice. From Reich's perspective, psychoanalysis had slipped out of medicine. As long as a doctor and patient shared, essentially, images and ideas, they were two philosophers engaged in a debate; neither of them could be wholly right or wholly wrong, and, in any case, the issues were irresolvable. Rather than admit defeat, therapists extended the period necessary for analysis or declared the patient cured, either one for arbitrary reasons. "A patient was usually considered 'cured,'" Reich wrote, "when he said that he felt better, or when the individual symptom for which he had sought therapy disappeared. The psychoanalytic concept of cure had not been defined."[1]

But, he pointed out, when the patient declares himself cured, that does not mean he is cured; it means that he has chosen to end the discussion, for whatever reason.

In this dilemma, psychoanalysts fell back on the semimystical dogma of "transference." Even though language in itself cannot cure, they admitted, the relationship between the doctor and the patient contains within it a shared identity, a moment when they are one and when the health and clarity of the doctor pass to the patient through the sanctum of mutual trust and assimilation of boundaries.

Transference is what transforms the dialogue into a medicine and provides the basis for internalization of the "verbal" cure.

Reich felt that a total reevalutaion of the therapeutic process was necessary. He did not challenge transference itself, but he questioned the ability of therapists to recognize it and employ it and he questioned its universal application as language. He mentions his own "successful" treatment, early in his career, of a waiter who had been totally unable to have an erection. During the third year of analysis, patient and doctor were able to reconstruct a traumatic primal scene: the patient had witnessed the birth of a sibling, and "the impression of a large bloody hole" between his mother's legs had been imprinted on his mind. After this breakthrough, the treatment was soon terminated because the patient was cooperative, well behaved, and accepting of the role of this childhood trauma in his present condition. The only problem was that he was still impotent.[2]

At the time, several of Freud's major disciples in Germany ran a seminar in psychoanalytic technique. When Reich presented this case to them, it was accepted and praised. Despite the patient's obvious functional problem, cure was said to be complete. Reich had followed standard methodology, established transference, and reconstructed a primal scene. By the rules of the system at that point, actual cure was not required.

But why not, Reich wondered, consider the patient's very acceptance of an unacceptable situation the contemporary form of his resistance? By this perception, Reich undercut the verbal bias of the Freudian movement. The patient's announcement of cure, in his own language, had always been considered a hopeful sign because it indicated a willingness to participate in society. But if verbal acquiescence were no more than another symptom, the rationale of the system breaks down. The therapist must now go against medical etiquette, denying the patient his right to a self-declared cure and keeping him in therapy.

To Reich, it was ludicrous that one could pretend to declare a truce with the unabated id on the level of a conscious exchange of albeit intimate material and a handshake. He assumed that Freud would go along with his objection and that psychoanalysis would reexamine its clinical tenets. When Freud rejected his ideas, Reich did not retreat but instead assumed that the founder had become another victim of his own hypothetical death instinct. Since Freud never subsequently pursued a clinical solution to neurosis, psychoanalysis was maintained as a middle-of-the-road therapy, neither scientific medicine nor charismatic healing, but uncourageously respectable.

Because of his own professional failures, Freud doomed mankind to misery, said Reich. He misread his own unhappiness. He settled on the death instinct in the 1920s, and after that, psychoanalysis stagnated, satisfied it could work no real cures, content to give palliative relief and help man through his "too many pains, disappointments, and impossible tasks."[3]

Speaking of Freud late in his own life, Reich acknowledged this moment: "I know, today, that *he sensed something in the human organism which was deadly,*" But Freud called it an instinct. "'Death' was right," says Reich, but not death as an instinct. *"Because it's not something the organism wants. It's something that happens to the organism."*[4]

Reich's initial break with classic Freudian analysis was his decision to treat the character of the patient rather than just the content the patient chose to give or produce by association. Politeness and softspokenness were no longer virtues; if the person was sick, these were part of the sickness. The enthusiasm of the patient for free association and the willingness to provide juicy material from memory were also suspect, no matter how insightful the material. The patient's actual behavior was the only clue to the illness, for this was the thing he could not help, no matter what he said. Of the impotent waiter, he wrote:

"At that time, I incorrectly assessed the total personality of my patient. He was very quiet, well-mannered, and well-behaved, and did everything that was asked of him. He never got excited. In the course of three years of treatment, he never once became angry or exercised criticism."[5] In the end, he accepted the failure of the analysis, even when described as success, with the same stoic equanimity with which he had taken everything else. "I was blind," Reich implied. *"That* was the disease!"

To Reich, dreams were no longer the cornerstones of therapy. The manner in which the patient comes to the treatment, his politeness or stubbornness, his mode of speech, his dress, the style and firmness of his handshake were all records of character. And character is real;

it can be treated. Reich directed attention to this and away from the complication of content and free association, which engage and distract the interest of the regular analyst.

Since the Freudian unconscious was basically latent sensations and impulses in the body itself, Reich saw no predominant need to go back in time to the traumatic moment or origin of the condition. He wrote *"The entire world of past experience [is] embodied in the present in the form of character attitudes. A person's character is the functional sum total of all past experiences."*[6]

The doctor does not need to reconstruct a traumatic moment; the traumatic moment continues to exist in every breath the patient takes, in every gesture he makes. This is not to deny the importance of clinical history, but to place it in context. It is accurate in mapping the disease, but it cannot affect the disease core. In fact, the collaboration of patient and doctor in recovering sources and implicitly sanctifying them is counterproductive in that it encourages the patient to focus on unhappy experiences and gives them an existential priority in explaining the rest of life. Initially the pain may be eased by having a lineal cause for compulsion and anxiety, but ultimately the patient becomes so fascinated with his own history, he loses contact with the present terms of his body. The conscious mind becomes its own trap. In place of "psychology," Reich proposed "somatology"—but since mind and body are a unity, these are the same thing.

Reich perceived that an "actual neurosis" lay at the energetic core of the symptomatic and verbally expressed neurosis. In asking what fueled that surface neurosis, Reich answered in classic Freudian terms: Compulsions, hysterias, and the like must derive from blocked sexual energy. By 1927 Reich had defined a *sine qua non* of psychoanalytic cure—it was not an imagined experience of ancient traumas but an actual capacity to express feelings of tenderness and sensuality in love-making.

Reich came to this insight only after a long process of clinical exploration, and he considered it a correct application of orthodox Freudian theory not the first axiom of a new system. He was not seeking a revolutionary answer to the problems of analysis, only a way past the obstacle of the sham cure.

However, despite his initial intention, Reich had begun to redefine Freudianism in more explicit energetic terms, perhaps in keeping with Freud's original theories but definitely at odds with the psychoanalytic customs of the time. In a sense he had returned to the roots and become the most pure "Freudian " of all. Reich interpreted the human organism in terms of its inaccessible reservoir of energy. Society was a mere artifact of this energy, blocked and frozen. Reich ultimately blamed such an outcome on economic and business postures, though he never satisfactorily explained why, or what the evolutionary alternative might have been. The function of analysis, he said, is somatic — to soften the neuromuscular blocks that have developed from suppression of energy. Verbal therapy does not accomplish this because language forms are always already somaticized. They reflect levels of feeling, breathing, and orgastic potential that have been blocked and bound, so their conscious play at insight can be only superficial.

"Every increase of muscular tonus and rigidification is an indication that a vegetative excitation, anxiety, or sexual sensation has been blocked and bound."[7]

The collective effect of these bound responses is a wall of nerves and muscles built up by opposing forces. The wall prevents the organism from its singlemost expression of biological unity, the discharge of inner tensions. The forces within long for contact, but the armor warns them of a danger and seals them permanently in a consistent character the person comes to identify as himself. Anything originating "outside" this character is a threat to the integrity of the organism, even if this happens to be the natural excitations of the organism itself. Reich identifies the paranoia of psychotics exactly as their perception of pulses which have no identity within the structure of personality, so achieve their meaning as outside oppressors. The excitation seems like spirits, diseases, or even witchcraft, for it originates beyond accepted personal boundaries. To Reich, the work of great composers, painters, and poets comes from their remote apperception of the same pulses psychotics fear.

He emphasized sexuality to a degree that was appalling to the Freudians and which became, as he feared, a matter of contention among his disciples. He stated his cure in exact words:

"Psychic health depends upon orgastic potency, i.e., upon the degree to which one can surrender to and experience the climax of excitation in the natural sexual act."[8]

If insight is offered to the patient while the armor is still present, he will automatically depreciate its meaning on a somatic level even while accepting it intellectually. Only when a healthy sexual function is restored can the patient make use of insights. Until then, he needs the therapist's aid in dissolving the armor. The reason why

Freudian analysis failed, Reich claimed, was that it did not restore function.

Almost from the beginning, Reich was forced to disown the misuses of his method. "Sympathetic" analysts jumped to the conclusion that sexual intercourse with ejaculation was all that was required. Reich pointed out that phrases like "I slept with my boyfriend" or "I made love everyday last week" mask a variety of events, more different than similar. For doctors to conclude that patients are experiencing orgasm because they are able to carry out the sexual act, or even worse, to carry out the sexual act *with* their patients in order to "cure" them, was, by Reich's standards, criminally naive. He complained openly that the majority of practicing psychoanalysts were so dissatisfied sexually themselves that they were projecting their own deviant desires onto their patients. Reich explained pointedly what he meant by orgastic potency:

"Until 1923, the year the orgasm theory was born, only ejaculative and erective potency were known to sexology and psychoanalysis. Without the inclusion of the functional, economic, and experiential components, the concept of sexual potency has no meaning. Erective and ejaculative potency are merely indispensable preconditions for orgastic potency. *Orgastic potency is the capacity to surrender to the flow of biological energy, free of any inhibitions; the capacity to discharge completely the dammed-up sexual excitation through involuntary, pleasurable convulsions of the body.* Not a single neurotic is orgastically potent, and the character structures of the overwhelming majority of men and women are neurotic."[9]

Reich does not mean any sort of forced and attentive excitation; he means a unified pulse that passes through the body after the body is given up to the experience. This is the singular event for animal life on the Earth. To be able to do it maintains basic health. To be unable to do it leads to a variety of diseases, none or few of which are ordinarily ascribed to psychological causes. In fact, Reich explains mental and physical pathology as equivalent symptoms of the disruption of the life current. What produces psychic diseases like frigidity, symptom neurosis, perversion, psychosis, and neurotic criminality equally leads to cancer, heart disease, emphysema, epilepsy, and peptic ulcer.

The involuntary submissive aspect of orgasm is key here. It is not the sexual act as it is generally understood in Western culture.

"The increase of the excitation can no longer be controlled; rather it grips the entire personality and causes an acceleration of pulse and deep exhalation.

"The physical excitation becomes more and more concentrated in the genital; there is a sweet sensation which can be best described as the flowing of excitation from the genital to the other parts of the body."[10]

This is the original natural medicine. The differentiation between male and female disappears beneath its unity. The organs may be different, but the same involuntary pulsing of energy passes through both. The unity that each of them represents is joined to the single unity of both of them. The inner tension, from which disease might accrete, is released. Western man, to Reich, debased this stunning healing principle, this primal bliss into a fake pleasure of flirtation, perversion, or conquest, on exactly the level of the fake life he was already living.

Insofar as he was a moralist, Reich (like Blake) exposed Christian morality as mere moralism. He conceived the sexual function so profoundly he interpreted love-making as a sacred act akin to birth. Religious dogma had denigrated sexuality to a necessary evil in procreation, and that notion, even though it had not been taken literally in the secular realm, had had an unconscious and seminal role in Western customs. Reich said, No—it is the life energy which endows the seed, not the seed which invents sexuality for its own transmission. We can extrapolate that it is only because of a powerful pulsing through the body, culminating in orgasm, that the sperm carries procreative potency. Living man and woman are functionally and morally prior to the continuation of humanity. The egg and the sperm express the same tension in their "embrace" as the individuals do, and the orgastic "resolution" of that tension is the embryo.

"Now, you know that Freud began as a somaticist," Reich told his interviewer years later, "as a man who worked with the body. Then he discovered the unconscious. So he switched over into psychology. But he never forgot that he was a somaticist. *The greatest thing that ever happened in psychiatry was the discovery that the core of the neurosis was somatic, i.e., the stasis, the libido stasis was somatic.*"[11]

As Reich saw it, the basic somatic drive of human beings has been abnegated, on a planetwide basis, by a false social ambition. Everyone is involved in an unacknowledged collusion with everyone else, agreeing not to notice that no one is real, that no one is having a real experience, as long as they are not exposed either. The smiles thrown back and forth mask the underlying pain and the evasion of biological necessity, which then expresses itself in character disorders.

"People are dull. They are dull, dead, uninterested. And, then, they develop their pseudo-contacts, fake pleasures, fake intelligence, superficial things, the wars, and so on."[12]

Reich listed the various observable symptoms: "loud, obtrusive laughter; exaggeratedly firm handshake; unvarying, dull friendliness; conceited display of acquired knowledge; frequent repetition of empty astonishment, surprise, or delight, etc.; rigid adherence to definite views, plans, goals . . . ; obtrusive modesty in demeanor; grand gestures in speaking; childish wooing of peoples' favor; boastfulness in sexual matters; exaggerated display of sexual charm; promiscuous flirtation . . . ; pseudo-exuberant fellowship; . . . bashfulness."[13]

His intuition was to challenge these poses therapeutically. Instead of talking to people *about* these habits, he talked *to* the habits in people. He encouraged the quirks and tried to draw them out. The stiff polite gentleman was asked to exaggerate his stiffness. The ever-smiling woman was encouraged to expand her smile and fully experience the flippancy of her gestures. The superior knowlegeable lecturer was told to go on lecturing, but with attention to how he did it — his breathing and the grip of his muscles. If the patient produced provocative associations that seemed right but with a smile that was aloof to them, Reich ignored the associations and asked the patient to bring out his irony, to increase his sarcasm. It was resistance Reich sought, not information. Information was simply the words the patient chose with which to buy time. Resistance was the living beast.

Psychoanalysts had been too smart for their own good. While they were outwitting the conscious (and even the unconscious) minds of their patients in a labyrinth of symbols, the psychosomatic intelligence of the patients was leading them back through their own maze:

"The patients readily divined what the psychoanalyst expected in terms of theory, and they produced the appropriate 'associations.' In short, they produced material to oblige the analysts. If they were cunning individuals, they half-consciously led the analyst astray, e.g., produced extremely confusing dreams so that no one knew what was going on. It was precisely this continual confusion of the dreams, not their content, that was the crucial problem. Or they produced one symbol after another — the sexual meaning of which they readily divined — and in no time they were able to operate with concepts. They would speak about the 'Oedipus complex' without any trace of affect. Inwardly, they did not believe in the interpretations of their associations, which the analysts usually took at face value."[14]

Reich mentioned trying unusual methods to shock the patient into awareness. With one person, he imitated for him his own sullenness and misery; he "lay on the floor and kicked and screamed."[15] The patient's initial response was astonishment, but then, according to Reich, he laughed fully and spontaneously which, in itself, was a breakthrough.

The traditional analyst was content to have the patient lie on a couch, turned away from the doctor. This, thought Reich, heightened exactly those feelings of remoteness, contactlessness, and alienation that the analysis was supposed to dissolve. "This procedure did not eliminate but rather reinforced the patient's feeling that he had to deal with an 'invisible' unapproachable, superhuman, i.e., in terms of the child's way of thinking, a sexless being."[16]

From this position, the detached and unreachable doctor reassures the patient and tells him he understands his problems. He encourages, even exhorts him, to produce material. If the patient is silent and remains silent, the analyst can only intensify his line of approach. He can tell the patient that he is resisting, interpret the silence as resistance, and hope to break it down by persuasion. But, argued Reich, the verbal pressure to produce material in fact intensifies the resistance. It arouses a "contemporary reason for being stubborn."[17] The alternative is to stun the patient with the precise character created by his own resistance. Then he can deal with a real and present event and is also relieved of the pressure for psychoanalytic performance.

Reich had considered himself politically left wing for a number of years, but his radicalism remained incipient until sometime after July 15, 1927, when he left a therapy session and went out onto the street to get a firsthand look at a strike march. The police fired on the crowd, leaving eighty-nine dead.

This was a watershed experience for Reich, and it gave expression to a number of old intuitions. Some coalesced almost immediately, most formed gradually over the years. Soon after the event, Reich described the rigidity, the mechanicalness of both police and marchers — a depersonalized condition like that of warring soldiers, a collective pathology not given sufficient attention in Freudian debate.

Reich realized that the same blocking of energy that lay at the core of individual neurosis led to mindless confrontation and destructiveness on a scale that dwarfed the patient on the couch. When he joined Communist Party in Germany, he was not satisfied with going to meetings and listening to speeches. These were further deadening activities, ineffective "therapy sessions." Instead he began to practice as a politically-conscious physician, organizing like-minded doctors and travelling the streets in vans with sex-hygiene clinics (as he called them), giving out literature, holding counselling sessions for working class youth, and in general trying to provide information about the sexual basis of true freedom.

This "sex-political" work was, to his new way of thinking, seminal to both community health and social change. As long as the masses were frozen in character defenses, they were not capable of using their energies to transform society, and they were particularly susceptible to the appeals of fascism, which at least provided an energetic charge and excited their suppressed sexuality. The workers had to be "healed" from the epidemic of social repression in order to be able to bring about an unneurotic new order.

Reich had integrated Freud and Marx—the psychological etiology with the economic dialectic.

He now took an active role in therapy, encouraging patients to break away from bad marriages, going to their houses to observe the role of living conditions in sustaining neurosis. He came to see the psychoanalytic hierarchy (with its laboratory of office and couch, the patient facing neutrally away from the doctor) as rigid, frightened, and isolated from the real causes of the disease. Recognizing the importance of contacting patients somatically, he turned them around to face *him* and replaced the dialogue of insight with an aggressive encounter of their resistance; he used physical exercises and touched them at the points of armoring (Freud immediately balked at this interventionist style, the replacement of free association with provocative confrontation).

Reich's accounts from this time of his visits to the homes of his patients recall those of another doctor equally at odds with a medical bureaucracy—Samuel Hahnemann. He mentions one particularly dramatic case in which a woman lived on the verge of starvation with three children, deserted by their father. She regularly had compulsions to push them into the water. As an orphan child she had been boarded with strangers, six or more people to a room, and raped by older men.

Reich did not ask her to make an office visit. He went to her apartment. There he was overcome by her survival in a world of such misery. "I had to grapple not with the exalted question of the etiology of neuroses but with the question of how a human organism could put up with such conditions year in and year out. There was nothing, absolutely nothing, to bring light into this life. There was nothing but misery, loneliness, gossip of the neighbors, worries about the next meal—and, on top of it all, there were the criminal chicaneries of her landlord and employer."[18]

Reich put this case before the collective psychiatric profession at a local gathering and asked them to square it with their complex and erudite theories of trauma and neurosis. He declared that it was impossible to have libidinal health under the existing social conditions (rushed intercourse often without the semblance of privacy). The Freudian movement had dealt only with the wealthier classes. Reich felt that its doctors were blinded by fake intellectualism and could not see the social conditions at the base of psychopathologies. Their kind of therapy was useless in the present social environment. They'd be better off forgetting practice until after the revolution.

Initially Reich was encouraged by Lenin's program of sexual reform, but when Stalinism followed, he quickly recanted. Over the years he moved further and further from his early left wing position. The emotional plague ran deep, he reasoned. Fascism had corrupted Communism. Mankind was too terrified of what lay within to advance sane political systems. People would always choose further symptomatic repression. Ultimately Reich turned against Communism as a fraud. The political radicals, he said simply, "*promise happiness without really establishing the mental-hygiene requirements for it.*"[19]

In a sense Reich had one of his great achievements in his negative outcomes. His twin banishments from the German Communist Party and the International Psychoanalytic Association exposed the limitation of both groups, one unable to handle sexuality except neurotically and the other unwilling to consider the societal underpinnings of neurosis. His critique remains as salient and unacknowledged today. Toward the end of his life he took an absolute position, without retribution and withour amelioration: "*There is no use in anything but infants. You have to go back to the unspoiled protoplasm.*"[20]

And elsewhere, about Freud:

"He gave up before he started. I came to the same conclusion, but only after much experience and failure. *Nothing can be done with grownups. . . . Once a tree has grown crooked, you can't straighten it. . . .* He was disappointed, clearly disappointed. And he was right. Nothing can be done. Nothing can be done."[21]

Long after Reich had been excommunicated from virtually every psychoanalytic and medical group he still proclaimed his commitment to initial insights of Freud: "I alone was true to the master," Reich said in effect. "Even the master was not true."

After fleeing Nazi Germany in 1933 Reich lived in various Scandinavian countries, but his "sex-pol" mode of treatment and rhetoric led to his being maligned as a debaucher. He was subsequently investigated by authorities who could not begin to fathom the complex evolution of his work; his medical license was continually under challenge.

Reich's rejection of the death instinct, an axiom of the Freudian logos, also led to his being unwelcome in all but the most radical psychoanalytical circles, and his resulting lack of professional backing exacerbated his civil difficulties. Eventually, in 1935, he settled in Oslo, where he had the most reliable support from a psychoanalytic community. It was during the Norwegian years that his investigations led him away from psychology (as it is traditionally understood) into experimental biology. He gradually abandoned Freud's model of neurosis as a social and environmental dysfunction revealed by language and replaced it with one of neurosis as a distortion of core energy manifested neuromuscularly.

Reich began his explicit move toward biology with a series of bioelectric skin measurements—he was attempting to concretize and quantify the libidinal energy of sexual pleasure, and, at the same time, to prove that intercourse itself was no guarantee of orgasm or sexual potency (as most Freudians were satisfied to claim).

The roots of the orgastic response lie as much in the metabolism of simple cells as in the psyche—there is a fundamental relationship between the pulsating of life and the structuring flow of cosmic energy through all of nature. In the simplest organisms primordial tissue generates a bodywide pulse of breath and movement, cohering finally in the emotional and cognitive rhythms of the mammals.

Psychology had limited itself, he claimed, by looking only at man. Pulsating head-to-tail motion was fundamental to wormlike creatures. If picked up, with resulting pressure against its sides from fingers, a worm exhibited exactly the twisting and blocked squirming of the torso of human character armor. Dropped, the worm regained its smooth and unified peristalsis. This was because the obstacle was external and superficial. But human armor comes from within and is earned through a lifetime. It cannot so easily be taken off.

The somatic circumstance of the human is not qualitatively different from that of the worm. When the worm is moving forward, with plasmatic waves of excitation, it is expressing itself as "wanting to," "saying yes to," to use Reich's words. After it is squeezed around the middle, the current is broken, and the animal twists and contorts itself, as if to say, "No, don't do that, I can't stand it." Likewise, people are frozen into permanent pain and discomfort by their armor. When it is dissolved, they express "yes" and "wanting to."[22]

In Freud the id and libido are metaphors, intuitions that biological currents flow through the personality. But Reich is not reinventing these metaphors; he is seeking their somatic source. Sheer protoplasm, he observed, responds pleasurably by radiating outward to its periphery, in the human cell as in the amoeba. Painful stimulation causes it to contract from the periphery to the center.

"The central nerve apparatus of the jellyfish is located in the middle of the back, as is the solar plexus in vertebrates. When the jellyfish moves, the ends of the body approach and move away from one another in rhythmic interchange. This is the heuristic substance of our mental leap: *the expressive movements in the orgasm reflex are, viewed in terms of identity of function, the same as those of a living and swimming jellyfish.*"[23]

These patterns are not remnants of past life, contained in memory traces of early evolutionary stages; they are the present basis for the more complicated emotional and intellectual structures that the human species has developed. When the jellyfish pulses rhythmically, it not only suggests orgasm; ontogenetically, it *is* orgasm, the same reflex allowing the animal to feed and swim. Likewise, a worm and a newt are contained embryogenically in our nervous systems. Even the great armored deflection of civilization must be an animal at its core, an expression of protean vegetative streaming. Man experiences cosmic dreams and oceanic fears, Reich said, not because he is in touch with another spiritual world but because his life force embodies the original pulsing.

Freud had developed psychology from an understanding of the quantitative economy of the soma and its translation into mental function: this, according to Reich, was his one and singular discovery. Freud was the first to understand that love and life are actual flows of current containing fixed quanta of electrical charge. Of course, Reich adds, "the libido which Freud talked about hypothetically and which he suggested might be chemical in nature is a concrete energy, something very concrete and physical."[24]

Furthermore, inorganic matter has the "same fundamental reactions of tension and relaxation, energy stasis and discharge, excitability, etc. . . ."[25] Bioenergy originates in atmospheric and cosmic energy. The "tension and relaxation" of the crystal or the cloud become the pleasure and fear of the frog which become the complex emotions and images of the mammals. All are "life" currents organized and differentiated in layers.

Reich made this one point very emphatically: the difference between his universal energy and that of the alchemists or the anthroposophists was that his was physically discoverable. That required him to go one step further; he had to find it in nature.

Since amoebas were primordial expressions of life energy, Reich interpreted their motility as the historical substratum of the nerves and muscles of more complex animals. But, in attempting to generate clusters of these protozoa from dead grass, he came upon "amoeba-like" forms that had never been reported. These "bions," as he called them, were vesicles that detached themselves from dead matter in solutions of sterilized organic materials. They resembled protozoa in their contractions and expansions, eventually gathering in clumps where they formed their own membranes, but they could not be ordinary microbes, appearing as they did when parched grass or moss was placed in sterilized water or in solutions of incandescent coal dust, rust, and sand. Reich assumed he was observing the discrete pulsing of "life energy." No mainstream scientist from the time of Darwin and Pasteur had proposed spontaneous life units, but Reich alone was seeking the quantitative basis of orgasm.

Further experimentation with bions revealed an energy of strange and unique proportions, a form of radiation with optical properties (emitting a haze or fog and spreading in blue dots and lines). It escaped confinement and expanded everywhere, penetrating even concrete and steel. This "bionic" force appeared to paralyze cancer cells on contact and was also naturally present in human beings, more strongly in healthy people. Reich later named this fundamental energy "orgone" and began to explore its applicability in healing.

In his mind, Reich had now taken Freudianism to its natural conclusion. Orgone was proof of libido; it was its "visible, measurable, and applicable form." Freud had grasped the essential pattern of psychosomatic disturbance, but had not gone far enough; he became stuck on the issue of "mind." "Are the 'electromagnetic waves' of Maxwell 'the same' as the 'electromagnetic waves' of Hertz?" Reich asked, comparing such terms as "id" and "libido" to an earlier intimation of the existence of an unknown energy. "Undoubtedly they are," he answered. "But with the latter one can send messages across the oceans while with the former one cannot."[26]

By 1940 Reich had fled the critics of Europe and was living in New York, but the city was not a suitable place for his grail, either environmentally or professionally, so in 1945 he moved to a farm near the small Maine town of Rangeley. It is here that myths and facts become confused and various Reichian personae are unveiled. To some, Reich transcended twentieth-century science and discovered and unleashed a force so powerful and far-reaching that the laws of Newton, Darwin, and even Einstein were challenged. To others, Reich lost his own sanity in the ancient quest for "vital energy" (the psychoanalytic establishment regarded him as a once-brilliant therapist lapsed into psychosis). In Rangeley, Reich experimented with a structure to contain and concentrate atmospheric orgone, an accumulator made of layers of alternating organic and inorganic material. The organic layers drew orgone out of the atmosphere, and the inorganic layers repelled it into the core of the accumulator.

By general Reichian definition orgone is a primordial, omnipresent substance that differs from all other energies in that it does not obey ordinary thermodynamic laws but expands and contracts and is transmuted *sui generis* into the building blocks of matter and life. Orgone provides rhythmic, pulsating energy for blood and bones, for generations of cells, and for clouds and rain; cosmic orgone provides the original energy of the rotations of planets, stars, and star systems. Orgone is the ocean-aura in which Earth floats — an aspect of the sparkle of the sky and the luminescence of galaxies. Though neither electricity, magnetism, nor light, orgone can be converted into any of these under appropriate conditions. In human beings it is replenished from the atmosphere, its natural pulsations turned into cell generation, free neuromuscular functioning, and the waves of emotions. Reich explains his new physics in these words:

"The 'bions' are microscopic vesicles charged with orgone energy; they are developed from inorganic matter through heating and swelling. They propagate like bacteria. They also develop spontaneously in the earth or, as in cancer, from decayed organic matter.

"Orgone energy is also demonstrable visually, thermically, and electroscopically, in the soil, in the atmosphere, and in plant and animal organisms. The flickering of the sky, which some physicists ascribe to terrestrial magnetism, and the glimmering of stars on clear dry nights, are direct expressions of the movement of the atmospheric orgone. . . .

"The orgone contains three kinds of rays: blue-gray, foglike vapors; deep blue-violet expanding and contracting dots of light; and white-yellow, rapidly moving rays of dots and streaks. The blue color of the sky and the blue-gray of atmospheric haze on hot summer days are direct reflections of the atmospheric orgone. The blue-gray, cloud-like Northern lights, the so-called St. Elmo's fire, and the bluish for-mations recently observed in the sky by astronomers during increased sun-spot activity are also manifestations of orgone energy.

"All cooked food consists of blue, orgone-containing vesicles or bions obtained through the heating and swelling of inorganic mat-ter also containing orgone. Protozoa, cancer cells, etc., also consist of orgone-containing, blue energy vesicles. Orgone has a parasympa-theticotonic effect and charges living tissue, particularly the red blood corpuscles. It kills cancer cells and many kinds of bacteria."[27]

Wilhelm Reich was not a single-theory radical. His life was a suc-cession of radical departures from territories that already seemed perilously experimental. Despite the consistency of his line of devel-opment, he abandoned and even contradicted coherent sets of prin-ciples at each new stage. No wonder his lineages are presently at war.

Despite these enigmas Reichian science has had an enormous im-pact on a variety of therapeutic schools. Gestalt and other forms of "direct analysis" are Reichian in their interpretations of body language and character. Many diverse styles of somatic work draw on Reichian exercises. Even Reich's physics and biology do not seem as exotic in light of recent developments, including the discovery of organic molecules in space.

Yet, without firsthand experience of Reich's experiments in biology and physics, one is left with only the contradictory literature about them. It is difficult to be precise and consistent when discussing descriptions of energies and entities that are outside of mainstream scientific discourse and were discovered under inexplicable and para-doxical circumstances. While homoeopathy and acupuncture are widely practiced, there are relatively few orgonomists; I am grateful to one of them, Jesse Schwartz of the Living Tree Center in Bolinas, California, for pointing out errors in an earlier version of this chapter and making suggestions for a new version. In addition, I have made use of a book published several years after *Planet Medicine*—Myron Sharaf's unflinching biography, *Fury on Earth*, which places Reich's different stages of development and apparent self-contradictions in perspective. This edition of *Planet Medicine* incorporates as much revision as was feasible without my rewriting an already-published work.

In particular, Schwartz pointed out that I have created a New Age Blakean version of Reich which is at odds with the man himself if not with meanings implied in his writings. Although Reich's text provided the material for my vision of galaxies as spiral organisms giving birth to planetary systems, he himself avoided such blatantly hermetic derivations. Because I have merged the archetypal Reich with the historical one, my chapter is a blend of biographical facts and the myths arising from them. After all, despite the limits he placed on his system, the crisis Reich precipitated still engulfs us.

A meeting with Albert Einstein in January, 1941, marked the end of Reich's attempt to merge his own science with existing physics. After Einstein answered a provocative inquiry with an invitation, Reich prepared a series of experiments, then drove to Princeton, and for five intense hours, presented his discoveries. Einstein expressed amazement at the flickering of orgone and wondered if it were not a subjective impression; he acknowledged that an inexplicable temperature difference Reich had discovered above his accumulators was a potential "bombshell." Reich then brought him a small accumulator. Soon afterwards Einstein reported that an assistant had discovered the critical anomaly was a result of simple heat convection from the ceiling. But Reich had also recorded the temperature difference outdoors, and he reminded Einstein of that. Einstein never answered his letter and never discussed the matter again. It was perhaps at this point Reich understood that he would be a pariah for the rest of his life. If the radical and open-minded author of relativity could not hear him, no one could.

It was as an "astrophysicist" and cosmic doctor that Reich came to his grand synthesis: eros, matter, plants and animals, starstuff were all formed within the same universal wave. Nature could not be an empty vacuum speckled with occasional stars and dust. This would deny its functional unity and integrity. Nature was a whorl of dynamic relationships, a cohesive field of primordial orgone. The universe we inherit from Reich is interpenetrated at all points with energetic streaming, differentiated in each zone by the interaction of shapes arising from this flow. We are autonomic self-healing "stars." According to Reich:

"What is important is that a functional relationship has been found between the movements of primordial orgone energy and matter that, for the first time in the history of astrophysics, makes comprehensible the fact that heavenly bodies move in a spinning manner. Furthermore, it makes comprehensible the fact that our sun and our planets move in the same plane and in the same direction, held together in space as a cohesive group of spinning bodies."[28]

Now Reich had an origin and definition for the charge in sexual intercourse and human procreation: it is a concurrence of the macrocosmic and microcosmic orgone streams. The living membrane traps the free energy of nature, historically and contemporaneously, and forces it to cohere. "The orgone, pressing forward and concentrated in the genital organ, cannot escape from the membrane. *There is only ONE possibility of flowing out in the intended direction — fusion with a second organism, in such a way that the direction of the excitation of the second organism becomes identical with the direction of the orgone waves in the first.* . . . With the superimposition of the two orgonomes and with the interpenetration of the genitals, the pressed and therefore 'frustrated' tail end can allow its orgonotic waves of excitation to flow in the natural direction, without having to force them back sharply. . . ."[29]

Two structureless orgone streams approach, penetrate each other, and superimpose their "tissue," translating their excess energy into a unified galactic system. Spiral nebulae arise, their limbs flung out in an embrace which lasts for an eternity (at least of our time). Within their "arms" the microcosm forms (our sun with its planets was generated from two enormous streams of orgone energy which marked their center by the star and spewed out the planets like an animal birthing its young). Our own love-making repeats this rhythm, even as the cells within us fuse, exchange, and divide. The functional unity of the cosmos is the orgasm cycle: tension, charge, discharge, relaxation. Human beings are individuations in a cosmic orgone ocean.

This is either psychoanalysis writ large or nature itself viewed as a psychic entity.

From Freud's intuition of the dreamworld and the cavernous unconscious, through the frozen smiles and sunken chests of Reich's patients, to the worms and jellyfish of northern Europe, the ocean-charged sands of Maine containing a blue life force, dissolving armor before his eyes, the gnostic "Reich" represents the whole universe as a qabbalistic or anthroposophic drama. The galaxies themselves are huge "beasts," engaging in copulations billions of years long, extended through the very fabric of time and space, separated from us by a mere peristaltic membrane, that also connects us to them.

The social and political objections to sexual freedom now become not only ludicrous but blasphemous. Sexuality is not an "invention" of human biology, eroticized in the "mind" of the instincts. It is the driving force of the sun and other stars, a gravitational import trillions and trillions of time the size of any one organism; nature itself is sustained from end to end by its attraction. Eros is the abundant visible starstuff we call "light" or "gravity."

Humanity imagines itself locked in contactless empty space on an isolated planet, but Reich sees this "old" science (and religion) as a symptom of the contactlessness felt by neurotic scientists (and clergy) and distorted into a theory of nature. Scientific man has denied the objective fact of the universe; religious man has slandered divine energy in the name of God. Reich writes:

"On the human stage, it is forbidden by law under punishment of fine or imprisonment 'or both' to show or even discuss the embrace between two children of the opposite sex at the age of three or five. Somewhere in the audience sits a human being, broken in his emotional security, full of perverse longings and hatred against what he has lost or never known, who is ready to run to the district attorney with the accusation that children are being misused sexually and that public morals are being undermined. Outside, on the meadow, however, the genital embrace of two children is a source of beauty and wonder. What drives two organisms together with such force? No procreation is involved as yet, and no regard for the family. Somehow this drive to unite with another organism comes with the newborn when it passes from the meadow onto the stage. There it is immediately squelched and smolders under cover, developing smoke and fog.

"Inside, on the stage, the embrace between two children or two adolescents or two grownups would appear dirty, something totally unbearable to look upon.

"Outside, under the glimmering stars, no such reaction to the sight of the embrace of two organisms would ever occur in sane minds. We do not shudder at the sight of two toads or fish or animals of other kinds in embrace. We may be awed by it, shaken emotionally, but we do not have any dirty or moralistic sentiments. This is how nature works, and somehow the embrace fits the scene of silent nights and broad meadows with infinity above. . . .

"Outside, a child is a child, an infant is an infant, and a mother is a mother, no matter whether in the form of a deer, or a bear, or a human being. . . . Outside, to know the stars is to know God, and to meditate about God is to meditate about the heavens. Inside, somehow, if you believe in God, you do not understand or you refuse to understand the stars."[30]

During his career as an orgonomist Reich moved further and further from conventional forms of psychoanalysis. He feared that mankind had become so diseased the very protoplasm was deadened. The best he could do was to heal with orgone itself, drawing on sublimated life energy from the ocean and sky to treat physical and mental disorders—cancer and schizophrenia alike (a modern philosopher's stone). Using different methods of orgone vitalization, he was initially able to prolong the lives of cancer patients; however, after reductions in their tumors, the draining of systemic "poisons" and emotional disturbances apparently led to their reappearances (even as they were their economic cause initially). This confirmed Reich's pessimism.

In 1949, as he began to test orgone as an antidote to radiation, his experiments led to a powerful "radioactive-like" cloud being released, a contamination which permeated the laboratory and surrounding buildings. Many collaborators abandoned Reich out of fear they had encountered a force they were not equipped to handle. However, after extensive investigation, he concluded that only the initial "response" of orgone to radiation is a kind of anger (not unlike the reaction of a neurotic to a penetration of his resistance). After this pathological excitation the radiation is successfully antidoted. Ultimately Reich named three basic forms of orgone energy—orgone, oranur, and dor. According to his co-worker Lois Wyvell:

"Clean, sparkling, soft orgone energy is free-flowing, beneficent and life-positive. When it is irritated by nuclear radiation (as Reich found in the Oranur Experiment and as has been evident from the effects of nuclear bomb tests), orgone is aroused, "angered" as Reich put it, and turns into a highly excited, hard pushing energy he called "oranur." This over-charge, over-expansion, of the atmospheric orgone leads to a contraction of the energy (just as over-expansion does in the biological realm), and the energy becomes "stuck," stagnant, and definitely life-negative (again, as in the biological realm). This condition Reich called "dor" for *deadly orgone* energy. The effect of over-charge is more difficult to assess, but it upsets the beneficent natural life-energy rhythms and can be deadly.

"To repeat: Oranur is an energy expansion that can't be discharged in the normal way and thus becomes immobilized and turns into dor.

Our own natural orgone energy is free-flowing and clean, but when it can't be discharged fully and naturally (in the sexual embrace, for instance), it may become dammed up, "stuck," and we become despondent, dull, depressed, and bored. The biological energy stagnates just as does the atmospheric energy, and when it does, it tends to become putrid, like a stagnant pond that has no outlet.

"The difference between dor and oranur is distinct in most respects, since they are in fact diametrically opposite; one being the stagnant energy synonymous with death by aging, by undercharge and loss of movement, and the other by over-charge, pushing movement and hyped-up emotions and actions. It seems to me, however, that there is still considerable confusion in some orgonomic writings. Some authors lump the evidence of both under 'dor,' and others lump them under 'oranur.' Reich called his experiment that brought nuclear energy and concentrated orgone into contact the 'Oranur Experiment,' not the 'Dor Experiment,' perhaps because he tended always to emphasize the positive, but most probably because the initial reaction of orgone to nuclear radiation was irritation and swelling anger.

"Dor and oranur are opposite in color, too. Dor is a dirty yellowish grey or brownish yellow, while oranur is usually purplish — complementary colors. Oranur can be reddish, too, but the red combines with the orgone blue to give it a purplish cast. Orgone, of course, is blue, the blue of the clean sky and the clear horizon. Most typically, it is indigo. On sunny orgone days, shadows and horizons are indigo blue.

"On sunny dor days, the shadows and distances are devoid of blue and the air looks dirty, while the horizons are a dirty yellowish brown or yellowish grey. Have you observed the day through a very dirty window? That is the way dor looks. It smudges the sky. On dor days, when you look at the dancing points of light in the sky, you will also see what looks like pepper sprinkled throughout the sparkles. Reich found that dor is not sheer, unalloyed radiation, but a transition between pure energy and matter. . . .

"The glaring white haze that covers the sky after an atomic test . . . is another indication of oranur."[31]

Reich perceived that deadly orgone in the atmosphere was a cause of droughts and ultimately, deserts, so he devised a "machine," called a cloudbuster, for drawing dor out of clouds and dissipating it in the healthy orgone from running water. The device consisted of several twelve-foot-long metal tubes concentrically mounted on a sort of tripod and connected with hollow coaxial cable to a source of running water. Stagnant dor is drawn from the atmosphere through the tubes into the flowing water. The effect is to stimulate the atmosphere in much the same way as an acupuncture needle stimulates the body. On several documented occasions Reich brought sudden showers to drought-stricken areas. In one instance, two blueberry farmers invited him to the Bangor area to help save their crops, and after the cloudbuster was employed, a fine drizzle began, followed by a strong steady rain. This recalls the ancient profession of the shaman who was both healer and rainmaker because these were the same.

Like all of Reich's experiments the "rain-making" lies outside of orthodox science. Few have tested his cloudbuster because the concept is so outrageous. Any institutional scientist would jeopardize his reputation by requesting funding for such research. Reich himself wondered why, with so many people looking through microscopes no one saw the bions — with so many telescopes and astronomers no one reported the sparkling of orgone among the stars; he could only conclude: "Because no one is looking for such a thing."

Now, after a lull of about two decades, there has been a surge of new interest in Reich's work. Robert Harman, M.D., has recently replicated Reich's discovery of the bions. Using sterile solutions, he has been able to "create" entities showing the lifelike characteristics of movement and pulsation. Courtney Baker, M.D., et al., have performed a classic study using mice in which they have demonstrated over several years how orgone energy can be used to facilitate the healing of wounds. Erecting their own cloudbuster, James DeMeo et al. have achieved some rather dramatic results in alleviating droughts, notably in the southeastern United States during 1986. Jutta Espanca, in a series of experiments spanning a decade, has exposed both seeds and seedling plants to concentrated fields of orgone energy and measured their growth against untreated plants. She has achieved an improvement in the number of tomatoes and in the weight and size of individual tomatoes grown from seeds that were kept for a period of time in an orgone accumulator. Jesse Schwartz, using an orgone seed sprouter, has demonstrated similar differences in the growth of corn and soy bean sprouts. [See Footnote 32 for references.]

During the years in Maine Reich was under repeated attack. The old innuendos about sex machines, orgies, and the mad scientist creating life in the test-tube joined new ones about cancer-quackery machines, rainmakers, and mail-order miracle cures. Reich's fiery personality and lack of patience with anything outside his research con-

tributed to a popular caricature. After a series of scurrilous and inaccurate articles, he became the victim of a protracted Food and Drug
Administration investigation.

Since both the FDA and the scientists it hired shared an assumption that Reich's propositions were ridiculous, the conclusions of their
tests were preordained (any positive reports or results were of course
ignored). The idea that such a simple "box" could trap a "cosmic
energy" seemed the height of chicanery. Reich had again presented
the scientific and medical bureaucracy with an epistemological riddle they were in no position to resolve.

As FDA agents continued to visit his lab and interview doctors
and patients who had contact with him, Reich became more bitter,
isolated, and paranoid, and, at the same time more fanatic about the
cruciality of his work. He saw himself as an important contributor
in the battle against the Russian inheritors of Stalinism. He fantasized
President Eisenhower as a secret ally; he wrote to the Atomic Energy
Commission offering to lend his assistance in countering the pathological effects of radiation. He interpreted jets flying over his laboratory alternately as government protectors and as enemy spies. He
perceived that UFOs were some sort of alien craft either intentionally
or unintentionally polluting our atmosphere with dor. In curious resemblance to G. I. Gurdjieff and Immanuel Velikovsky, he came to
blame the human scourge, the planetary plague, on an external space
disaster. Now alone awakened to the threat, he sought to repel the
invader. It is a strange scenery as his son Peter describes it from
memory of when he was eleven years old:

"When I got back upstairs, Daddy was looking through the telescope. 'Here, look through. See if you can see. I can make out a thin
cigar shape with little windows.'

"I looked through the telescope and focused it. It was bright, bright
blue and glowing, but I couldn't see the windows.

"'Do you see it?'

"'Yeah, but I can't see the windows.'

"'Well, they are there. Run to the cloudbuster and make ready.
Unplug all the pipes and pull them out to full length. I'll be right
there.'

"My boots pounded against the dry dirt. My jacket was open, and
each time my arms went back the sides of the jacket flapped against
me and the fringes sounded like rain. As soon as I got to the cloudbuster I jumped on the platform and started unplugging. The pipes
were like an old-fashioned telescope and had two more sections in-

side that pulled out. Bill and Eva [Reich's son-in-law and daughter] drove up just as I pulled out the last pipe. They parked near the truck.

"Bill pulled his binoculars out of the case and put the strap over his neck. 'Where is it?' he asked.

"I pointed to it and Bill raised the glasses. He whistled.

"'Boy, it sure is something,' he said, handing the glasses to Eva.

"She looked for a while and said, 'I knew it would come. I felt bad all day and said to Bill that I thought there was something in the atmosphere.'"

Later, after Peter himself succeeds in driving off the invaders when the others have failed, his father puts his arm around his shoulder and says:

"'Yes, we are really engaged in a cosmic war. Peeps, you must be very brave and very proud, for we are the first human beings to engage in a battle to the death with spaceships. We know now that they are destroying our atmosphere, perhaps by drawing off Orgone Energy as fuel, or by emitting DOR as exhaust. Either way, we are the only ones who understand what they are doing to the atmosphere and we can fight them on their own ground. The Air Force can only issue misleading reports about the flying saucers and chase after them helplessly, while we are dealing with them functionally, with Orgone Energy. . . . We are dealing with the knowledge of the future. . . And you, Peeps, may be the first of that generation of children of the future. Here at the age of eleven you have already disabled a flying saucer using cosmic Orgone Energy. Quite a feat.'"[33]

Reich had now reached the top of the mountain. There was no place to go. He was an avatar and magus who had changed the face of the Earth forever. To such a one the FDA investigation was ludicrous. Here was a millennial scientist being challenged as a perpetrator of petty fraud. He ignored an injunction to appear in court on the grounds that the legal system was in no position to judge his work, to decide whether or not the universe was full of orgone. When the court, in the absence of a defense, found in favor of the FDA, Reich was in essence enjoined from further accumulator sales. However, associates continued to deliver the devices across state lines. Reich subsequently was summoned, appeared, and was found guilty — not of medical fraud but failure to obey the original order. He was imprisoned in 1956 and died in the Federal Penitentiary at Lewisburg, Pennsylvania, in 1957.

Even today the FDA's behavior seems shocking and extreme. Their representative mocked Reich in court and pushed not only for conviction but the harshest sentence possible. After the ruling, Reich and his associates returned to Rangeley to destroy their laboratory and its equipment as ordered. They carried out the task in brutal masque, using axes, as FDA agents looked on to assure compliance. Reich's books — not only those dealing with orgone but all of them — were burned en masse in a public incinerator.

How can we explain such a violent reaction? Reich believed that the human suppression of biological energy was so deeply ingrained that the authorities, in the name of the masses, would turn against anyone who revealed its true nature and the extent of our sickness. Late in his life he wrote *The Murder of Christ* in which he presented Jesus as a biologically free, unarmored person crucified by those who could not bear the force of his love. Christ's murderers were now the Stalinists, the fascists, and the Higs (Hoodlums in Government as he called the FDA and other officials).

The extremity of the FDA reaction suggests that Reich had indeed released an unknown energy, had unlocked the power of rain and the sun, had neutralized radiation, had found the one universal medicine. We need not imagine a conspiracy to steal this discovery from him to suspect an unconscious impulse to drive the jinni back into the bottle.

But what was that jinni: The vital force? Alien cosmic energy? Love itself?

Pure Reichian science still cannot be practiced or defined. Even now we do not have a name for it. And so Reich's life stands as an allegory against our time.

"Your honor:

"We have lost, *technically only*, to an incomprehensible procedure treadmill. I and my fellow workers, have, however, won our case in the true historical sense. We may be physically destroyed tomorrow; we shall live in human memory as long as this planet is afloat in the endless Cosmic Energy Ocean, as the Fathers of the cosmic, technological age."[34]

Models and Meanings

XVII

Bodywork

Therapeutic bodywork is an ancient tradition. We have seen it in Pacific Island systems of massage, Bali dances, and the craft of bone-adjusting, which Daniel David Palmer and Andrew Taylor Still remade, as if from scratch, into "guilds" in The New World. Later postural realignment systems, like Rolfing, kinesiology, and Feldenkrais, owe at least as much to this lineage as to Reich. In fact, there was a pre-Freudian psychological tradition involved in somatic work with patients, best exemplified by Georg Groddeck (1866–1934). Groddeck dismissed the possibility of reaching most of his patients on a conscious or linguistic level, believing that disease lay deeper than language or consciousness. So he regularly bathed, massaged, and adjusted his patients and prescribed exercises for them to do. These methods, he thought, would speak to the "It" of the patients rather than to their persons. Obviously, this is as much a pre-Freudian view of the unconscious as a pre-Reichian view of deep character analysis, and, in fact, it is from Groddeck's It, the thing which could not express itself through language, that Freud borrowed his term "id."[1]

Reich was influenced indirectly by Groddeck, though he rejected him on the basis of his mysticism. Freud's work, in a sense, had drawn attention away from the use of massage and bone adjustment in treatment of mental illness and toward unconscious dynamics. The unconscious was such an important insight that the earlier physical methods were forgotten. When they were picked up again by Reich, they were already being reorganized in terms of those new Freudian dynamics, so it is almost as though they were being discovered again as something else.

The curative aspect of simple contact between doctor and patient has been acknowledged and cultivated since the beginning of our species. What Reich did was to rediscover therapeutic bodywork and systematize it according to the psychoanalytic definition of the unconscious. Most somatic therapists today either make deliberate use of his model or inherit it anyway unaware. The different "cures" achieved by each style of treatment and its interpretation of motility and resistance may have unique meanings to their practitioners, but they are probably not differentially less functional, and even if they are we could only know that in terms of larger archetypal systems and lifelong processes of individuation.

Sheer human activity is curative: the organism breathes, the bones and flesh pulsate; the pulse is integrated into more complex neuromuscular and emotional events. We have a profound liquidity in our chest, eyes, forehead, guts. Self-healing precedes any theory and extends beyond any definition. Therapeutic bodywork is a channel for self-healing transmitted from one organism to another. It also makes the energy basis of the neuromusculature conscious.

Between any two people—*any* two people—there is a quality, whether it interests them or not. It can be anger or repulsion; it can be attraction or warmth. It is the basis for the common arrangements people have, including marriage, community, and healing. Although Freud focused on the symbolic interpretation of psychological data, he understood the importance of transference. It might well be that the transference, in the context of mutual insight, is what cured people in psychotherapy—not the interpretation but the behavior. In the discussion of a dream, it does not matter what symbolism doctor and patient agree on as long as in the process they establish a curative relationship between themselves, as long as the collaborative interpretation evokes appropriate behavior in the future. Likewise, when communities and cultures actually work, it is not because of their beliefs or ideologies but because the people within them respond to each other in satisfying ways. Just as no ideology can force this, a community which has this will generate appropriate institutions from its feelings and sense of connection. This is the political basis of the holistic health philosophy, and it is meant to be an epitaph on the shallow idealism of 1960s' political organizations.

Bodywork, in all of its versions, tries to grab the disease by the tail and follow it in—the tail being anything it wags at the moment of interaction. Insight followed by transcendence is a favorite Western mode. But bodywork maintains a more Oriental equanimity: the pursuit of internal sources of distortion is never subordinated to a sudden flash of meaning, no matter how brilliant, no matter how suggestive of the great artistic and philosophical traditions. This is also the difference between symptomatic art, which allows the artist only to deepen the pathology, and curative art, which transforms the pathology into new activity.

The penetration of attitude is a medicine, and one that shares more with the bone cracker and acupuncturist than the psychologist. The shock of inner recognition is crucial. The personality develops around the issues of its own survival, and though its intellect can recognize the value of retraining (it can read books about it, for one), the self acts only on the basis of what it knows for certain about life. The intellect, no matter how sweet and convincing, cannot tell it otherwise. In fact, the self already knows all the tricks the intellect has for convincing it, so it cannot be convinced. That is the role of the healer. He reaches the animal inside the person, the animal on whose needs everything is based and who can die and take the body with him, without the mind ever suspecting the disease began in human conflict and symbolic distortion rather than germs.

So tricky is the personality that it will take any lesson it learns from the self and exaggerate it in order not to have to learn anymore. The difficulty of realignment is how not to replace one exaggerated gesture with another.

As Buddhists have long noted, people often mistake their desires for intimations of their inner beings. Sexual titillation is not the aim of bodywork, and this is never clearer than when the doctor and patient are of different sexes. For the patient, the intimacy of the situation may spark desire, but beneath that desire is a more fundamental holding back. If the doctor is lucid, the desire comes out, without seduction, and then exhausts itself until the patient tires of it. Farther beneath is a deeper sexuality that is slow and serious and has no compulsive quality; it is the fundamental arrangement the self makes with its male or female personality, and from it deep sexual feelings can emerge.

This is particularly significant in light of the evidence that the problem of psychiatrists' having sexual intercourse with patients has reached alarming proportions, discussed as an ethics issue at the 1976 meeting of the American Psychiatric Association.[2] Although the speakers tried to blame it on the failings of specific doctors, it is more clearly part of a breakdown of the mode of therapy. The desperation is not only the inability of the psychiatrists to produce positive change in their patients but their lack of self-esteem and clarity that results from that failure. There *are* therapies of sexual relations practiced in the world, but they do not arise improvisationally from insight analysis.

Part of the physical basis of bodywork begins in the language basis because speech occurs on two levels; one as words, shaped by the mind into meaning, and the other as sound, shaped by the breath and mouth into expression. Chanting is clearly somatic, but talk is also. How a person talks is part of how he moves and how he breathes, how his body talks to him and how he talks to his body.

Health is closely related to breath and body rhythm. Violations in the coherence of the organism, including shallow breath, nervous speech rhythm, disorganized posture, tight control of diction, are symptoms not just of emotional disturbances but also of skeletal, muscular, and visceral diseases. These are waves locked in a single pattern. There is no other way we could expect the heart and the liver to express themselves. Language comes out of the body and speaks its mind, and, as the bioenergetic therapist Stanley Keleman tells us in the very title of one of his books, the "body [also] speaks *its* mind." The teaching of the mind is philosophy, but the teaching of the body is not athletics. It is the body's version of philosophy and is just as difficult, subtle, and multileveled. In fact, they are the same, reflected at different levels of being.

In chiropractic, for instance, social and psychological health is maintained by the organs' correct positions in relationship to one another. If behavior is aberrant, then the organs must also be out of position. It cannot matter which came first, which initiated the drift; it is functionally the same. The chiropractor believes that by adjusting bones he adjusts muscles; by adjusting muscles, he changes tissue qualities; the changing tissue qualities cause the body to reorganize itself; and as the body reorganizes itself, the intellect instantaneously begins to reorganize its life.

The philosophy of the body is usually enacted in body and voice exercises. Not all of them are strenuous. Some are as simple as tightening and loosening the throat or trying to experience breath in a certain organ. For most people simply to stand symmetrically at their natural height is a major undertaking. The strain from the exercises is not caused because they are punishing; it is caused because the patient is organized away from them as normal functions, usually out of fear. He is avoiding the feelings that go with them. As feelings rush up, a rhythm from the system tries to impose itself, and since the rhythm is more fluent, more coherent than the person, it will run into personality blocks. The person will tighten and resist, and this will be felt both as pain and the wish not to continue the exercise. Although the discomfort is immediate, it is primarily historical. It hurts now because something else hurt back then, and the body organized itself away from that in protection.

Since the feelings are perceived as pain, there is often the fear that to persist in the exercises will cause injury or disease. The irony is that the disease feared, such as heart trouble, is caused more directly by the lack of than by the exercise, by the decades of stiffness, shallow breathing, and withholding. Fear of disease, in this case, is fear of self; and from fear of self, disease arises. Reich left little doubt that he considered cancer and heart disease literally diseases of the personality, the heart, and the genitals. If such is the case, character exercises are a viable preventive medicine.

Some of these issues are presented in a story the Chinese *t'ai chi* teacher Benjamin Lo tells about his contact with American doctors:

"'The doctors in Palo Alto asked me to come and teach them how to have their patients relax. I thought that this was a good thing. Patients should relax. They wanted me to teach them *t'ai chi*. They wanted to teach it to their patients to help them relax. I came there, and they were so tense. How can those doctors cure anyone, tense like that? I show them the first moves, and they are unable to do them, they have too much tension. I say, 'You can't go on, you must first learn to make the body soft, have less tension. Then you can teach your patients and be better doctors.' But they say, 'We don't have tension. You give us hard postures, straining, awkward; they are not natural.' But what did I ask them to do? Did I ask them to lift heavy weights? No. Did I ask them to lift even a piece of paper? No. I asked them to hold up the weight of their own bodies. And they cannot do it. How can a doctor like that help his patients? If the old Chinese doctors are like that, no one goes to them.'"[3]

The complaint that these kinds of exercises are merely calis-

thenics is more a confirmation than a criticism. They *are* merely
calisthenics, but not calisthenics in which one pushes himself past
the point of feeling or numbs himself to pain in order to achieve
some victory or heroism. There are no Olympics or competitions,
only the self. The work causes feelings to bubble up and surge. The
athlete may sometimes be able to use these feelings to spur performance; other times they are overcome as distractions. In bodywork,
one must understand the feelings aroused by the use of the body exactly as they come up and in the way in which they come up—first in
the exercise, then in life itself. There is no extraneous meaning or
revelation, no goal; the meaning is simply: this is what's happening—
no place to go.

Deep into an exercise, the patient may become the animal he is,
wailing and shouting animal sounds, doing animal movements; the
inner being is brought into alignment with the surface personality
and shares an expression of coherence with it. This coherence is so
sweet and medicinal that its obviously unattractive traits are a price
worth paying.

The voice speaks for the "It" also. A physiological change takes
place—muscles are stretched, the skin changes color and temperature, liquids move through the system—all in the context of feeling.
In experiencing these things, the personality understands that there
is another life it has not been living. There is a point, past exhaustion and past the driven expression of the emotion, where the self begins to express its own being only. This pours through the flesh of
the person like an elixir, but also as a familiarity, a recognition. Suddenly anger or passion no longer needs a situation; it is one of the
things in the body.

Fake psychodrama perhaps, but then no one protests that a pill or
an operation isn't real because it is given or performed by a doctor in
a clinical setting. As mind and body work together and realize their
nondifference, the tension momentarily lightens. The sky outside the
window seems as blue as Reich, in his vision of orgone bliss, would
have us believe it is. The blossoms on the trees hang as globes of
fuzzy light, expanding eternally without weight and made of tenderness more than of matter. Memories flood the body and mind,
memories that seemed to have been lost forever. Life becomes so
large and expanded in them that it is itself sufficient and ample;
there is enough to drink forever, but there is not so much that one
would drown. One's size changes, the sense of being cramped in a

body softens; the torso expands to hold a figure which is at once more muscular and firm and more angelic and graceful. For the duration of the feeling, lost functions are recovered, but no one such experience changes the life or treats deep internal illness. It is the gradual accretion of such moments and perceptions that ultimately penetrates character at its base.

The inside experience is important and not generally discussed. For instance, *Lomi* breathing work, and other massage-breath forms, have a moment in them where one feels one simply cannot go on breathing fully. This is exactly the point at which one must go on, for it is fear, not physical pressure, that holds one back, though there is a weariness and a sense of not being able to push on or maintain concentration. Once one gets past this point, the breathing begins to be freer. The body is transformed into a hidden unity of muscles, emotions, organs, and breath (for which breath is the catalyst and universal agent). Instead of resisting, the flesh tingles, concentration becomes easier; attention hangs in a suspended state. There is a joyous, paralyzed feeling. One is paralyzed by one's own flood. From that point it is possible for the person to use his own breathing as a healing agent.

Bone adjustment can be like standing on a very high mountain, looking at everything far away. That's how bones are. They create the sense of space the body encloses. If a bone is damaged, the disorientation is vast, and a person becomes shapeless. At the moment the adjustment takes place—the famous bone cracking—there is not so much pain as immense surprise. The shape within changes, and the muscles momentarily hang on nothing. The viscera respond immediately. The stomach expands and fills the shape of its own hollowness and sadness. The lungs and chest fill with air as if it were magnetically drawn into them. They expand and contract easily and fully, and the air rushes into them as into deep, sucking cavities. Fundamental disorientation may lead to fear, but a very faraway fear, as seen from a mountain. At the moment when the bones crack and right afterward, one possibility is: the person is standing above a river, a river which rushes between his legs, limitless in both directions. Suddenly he is lifted above the river and dropped on both sides of it at the same time. He struggles to his feet, but he is on both sides, he is on opposite sides, he is on the wrong side from himself and must somehow cross it in order to get back together, but as each half tries to cross it, so does the other half. There is the momentary fear that he has ended up on the wrong side and he can never get back to the right one.

In the end, it does not matter what side of the river one is on or what happens when the tingling stops. Life continues from there, as whatever life is.

It is a mistake to think that this process is not universal. In ancient Africa, Amerindia, and Australia, health was maintained by functions like these. In its present form, bodywork has certain promise and power that the original planetary therapies did not have, even as it lacks other olden skills and powers. Although they are not documented as such, we can find hundreds of cases of ceremonies which obviously have a character-emotional import in the ethnographic literature. For instance, take the following two ceremonies from Australia and Bali, respectively. We do not know the inside of them, but it is clear that they have physiological as well as mythological impact on the recipients, and, furthermore, that even their mythology, i.e., their inner voice and drama, has physiological impacts.

The first is a physician initiation in Australia:

". . . a very old doctor threw some of his crystalline stones and killed the novice. Some of the stones went through the latter's head from ear to ear. He then cut out all his insides, intestines, lungs, liver, heart, in fact, everything, and left him till next morning, when he placed more of these stones in his body, arms and legs, and covered his face with leaves. After 'singing' over him until the body was swollen up, he put more stones in him. He then patted him on the head, causing him to 'jump up alive,' and made him drink water and eat meat containing magic stones. When he awoke, he had forgotten who he was, and all the past."[4]

The second describes part of a public healing ceremony in Bali:

"By the spell, the krisses in the hands of the men turned against them, but the magic of the Barong hardened their flesh so that, although they pushed the sharp points of the daggers with all their might against their naked chests, they were not even hurt. . . . Some leaped wildly or rolled in the dust, pressing the krisses against their breasts and crying like children, tears streaming from their eyes. Most showed dark marks where the point of the dagger bruised the skin without cutting it, but blood began to flow from the breast of one, the signal for the watchmen to disarm him by force."[5]

Reich redefined therapeutic activity in libidinal terms, making dissolution of the body armor and release of the orgastic response the universal goal of somatic rituals, whatever their original intention. In that sense he sustained the ethnocentricism of Freud, who also submitted non-Western cultures to analysis by Western symbolic processes. But that doesn't mean Reich was wrong; it just means that he objectified the libidinal aspect of all healing, so any somatic system derived from him adopts a sex-economic priority at some level (likewise, any bodywork system practiced by a Hopi shaman will be taken under Hopi mythology).

Although there remains an orthodox Reichian hierarchy, most post-Reichian bodywork now spreads in its own popular folk movements, incorporating elements of zen, yoga, chiropractic, Alexander technique, Feldenkrais work, etc., electing to blend European science with other traditions. Thus Reichian therapy has been synthesized with skeletal adjustments, massages, herbal remedies, yoga, aikido, and karate, respectively.

Pure Reichians may lament dilution and bastardization, but contemporary bodywork traditions have enlarged the framework of function and motility, allowing varied experiences of somatic freedom and self-awareness. After all, meditation and the martial arts incorporate thousands of years of empirical testing, and though they do not diagnose in a psychoanalytic manner, they still address our paradoxical condition from a tradition of wisdom and subtlety. Interestingly, many bodyworkers have rejected Reichian dogma on the same basis that Reich first criticized Freud: the system doesn't have the clinical effect its ideology implies — it doesn't work. Karate and zen *do* work (so does Reichian therapy of course, but within a less ambitious framework than Reich required: it does not have a universal application).

Reich came to the same pessimistic conclusion as Freud did, late in his life — people are too sick to be healed. By adopting orgone — a vitalistic current that transcended psychoanalysis — Reich implicitly abandoned character analysis. Yes, he still recognized the need to work somatically with patients after orgone treatment, but he made orgone a requirement of healing in a malefic civilization (in that gesture he embraced the esoteric Hahnemann of miasm theory). Today orgone therapists and character therapists are usually different individuals, often practicing in the same community without any awareness of each other.

Reich left behind a variety of therapeutic tools, but in the end he became methodologically fixed. Instead of remaining an intuitive healer, he came to require a specific sequence of removing segments of armor (from the eyes down) and ignored contraindications. In fact, he even mentioned to Ola Rakness, his Norwegian disciple, that he left certain cases out of his writings because they seemed to improve without conforming to the rules.[6]

Although it was not his intention, Reich set a standard of absolute orgastic potency against which men and women have had to measure their own shortcomings. Reich said, in effect: Most people are ruined from early childhood and will never feel "the real thing." This was a quintessential power play, and its consequence is a legacy of "feeling" elitists and promiscuous orgasm-seekers, all looking for the perfect wave and claiming to be his children.

The followers of Reich do not condone this simplification, but they do emphasize orgasm. The basic difference, for instance, between the Reichian orthodoxy and the bioenergetic tradition associated with Alexander Lowen and his disciples is that the emphasis on performance is replaced, in bioenergetics, by an attention to feeling. Orgastic potency becomes less crucial in a world of varied hopes and relationships. Reich had adopted an idealist position, so his system has difficulty preparing individuals for the bioenergetic "middle ground," that is, for sustaining a charge without erupting or exploding — and for tolerating the wide, often-uncomfortable range of ambiguous emotions.

As a doctor, Reich was a prophet; he wanted to transform humanity: without a planetary revolution, individual cure was meaningless. Nowadays, absolutist post-Reichian models of cure, like Arthur Janov's "primal scream," ostensibly produce "healthy" individuals who can make no peace with the "unhealthy" world around them. They must be vigilant, guarding against relapse, and there is nothing for them to do in this scenario of unreal people and fake goals.

The feeling model avoids ideological postures and follows Buddhist method: experience arising from situations and situations being changed by the nature of experience. There is no singular solution, no negative prognosis for humanity. One simply lives out the individualized fact of his or her life.

It is a testimony to Reich's accuracy and also his blindness that so much of his methodology replicates yin-yang medicine without his having been aware of it. His general view of mysticism was tainted by his contempt for the German theosophists and anthroposophists who took a mythological rather than empirical view of nature. Denying life as the final reality, they sought meaning in spirit, outside of psychology and biology. Reich considered this so-called philosophy mere mystification and armoring, but his own revelation of blue divine energy, living streams of starstuff, and UFOs strafing the atmosphere with deadly orgone has delighted mystics ever since. Reich gave us an illuminated Darwinian/Freudian version of Gnostic and Zoroastrian hermeneutics.

Looking back from our perspective, we can say that it is not orgasm which Reich most significantly defined, but objective soma, i.e., the organs, nerves, and muscles, of which we are not aware except collectively and kinesthetically. By dealing directly with our resistance to knowing our own habitual patterns and somatic blocks, Reich made possible a discovery of and connection to our core selves. The empiricism of his character analysis and somatic work suggest a twentieth-century zen.

In Hindu mind/body science, *prana* is the energy which travels in channels through the body, is activated by the nerves and fanned by deep, regular breathing, and is finally dispersed through the skin and pores. When these channels become knotted, disease develops, but disease can be cured by restoring the flow of *prana* through yoga and meditation.

The *chakras* are the reservoirs and activating centers of this energy. They are located at the base of the spine, in the sexual organ, beneath the solar plexus, within the heart, beneath the larynx, at the third eye spot in the center of the forehead, and in the brain. Another has been suggested at the large toe, which happens to be the point at which bodily sensation is said to awaken embryologically and join to the central fissure of the brain. Mythologically, this *chakra* is represented as the river Ganges sprouting from the large toe of God.[7] How much the *chakras* are actual physiological points and how much they are versions of something else, experienced as parts of the body in the cerebral cortex, is a riddle suspended between systems. In Hindu psychology, if something happens, it's real. The issue of brain or body, spine or skin, thoughts or sensations— which mirroring which—is never raised because it is taken as a level of artificial objectivity.

A particularly potent form of *prana* is the *kundalini*, a power represented as a serpent because of its violent uncoiling from the base of the spine where it is grounded. Modern parapsychology offers a version of this in which the spine itself is grounded in the planet, and the pulse, passing up the spine, is pitched to the Earth's resonant cavity which is formed by the solar wind with its magnetosphere and plasma envelope. The Hindus say that *kundalini* connects man to the universe.[8] Reich's "cosmic superimposition" is no stranger to this business. The cerebrospinal-planetary connection has very deep embryological implications, with the *kundalini* maturing as another component of the nervous system through the amphibian, reptile, and primate phases of the fetus. Dormant at birth, it contains a map of biospheric history and the cosmos.

If not integrated, the *kundalini* is very dangerous. The flesh tingles and vibrates, and extreme heat builds up in the body, often at the extremities, reminding us that radiating physiological heat is an attribute of healers. There are colored lights and flashes, blue pearls and red curtains dance, and the inner hearing whistles, roars, chirps, hisses, and plays the flute. This is the serpent rushing upward along the spine to its destiny in the brain. Some trainings demand that the student learn to receive him in the brain or he will turn back on the body as disease and insanity.[9]

In Gurdjieff's system, which is a mixture of Oriental and Islamic doctrines, the "unconditioned side of creation" was called "*Trogoautoegocrat*," built up from Greek roots meaning "I eat and so keep myself." The hydrogen and nitrogen cycles are science's recognition of spiritual law: the disintegration of stars and the decay of organic materials, from which all higher substances are made. There is an upward cosmic transformation of energies; matter is transformed into cells and life, and life is transformed into thought. Thought passes out of the hydrogen and nitrogen cycles into the creative force that lies outside the world of light and dimensions, into the realm of the absolute.[10]

Man's goal is to transform the food he eats and the air he breathes into higher and imperishable substances. He does this through conscious labor and suffering. Gurdjieff used the most basic sort of bodywork: endless repetitive exercises, exhausting and boring, to break down the false habitual sense people have of how the world is supposed to be. The Moon feeds off us, he warned; it eats the unfinished souls of men. Other humans are turned into light—"the souls of the damned," he called them—by whom the present living see the creation. It may sound like mythology, but Gurdjieff meant it as frightening, physical law. He trained his disciples to spend their lives working against habit to evade the hungers of heavenly bodies millions of times their size.

Of course, each culture and mythology gives its own meaning to the process it transmits, and what remains, as in the Australian and Balinese cases, is the exercise itself. The Bushmen of the !Kung bands of northwest Botswana obviously do not know the Hindu serpent by name, nor do they have a context for therapeutic bodywork or the relation between their spines and the universe. Yet they describe a fact:

"You dance, dance, dance, dance. Then n/um lifts you in your belly and lifts you in your back, and then you start to shiver. N/um makes you tremble; it's hot. Your eyes are open but you don't look around; you hold your eyes still and look straight ahead. But when you go into !kia, you're looking around because you see everything, because you see what's troubling everybody. . . . Rapid shallow breathing, that's what draws n/um up . . . then n/um enters every part of your body, right to the tip of your feet and even your hair.

"In your backbone you feel a pointed something, and it works its way up. Then the base of your spine is tingling, tingling, tingling, tingling, tingling, tingling, tingling . . . and then it makes your thoughts nothing in your head."[11]

Each system has its own way to set the healing energy flowing. Reich's apprehension was that sexuality would be softened because the public would be terrified of it. But how much more terrifying could it be than the hungry Moon and the *kundalini* and the "tingling, tingling, tingling"? If there is a dispute, it is not with orgasm, even as it is not with *prana*. The possibility of pure and fundamental energy remains, but the decision that we fully understand it or have located it must be postponed.

Before the healing takes place, at any point during the process or afterward, there is only the individual. Healing occurs because there is unity, because there is a parallel between the doctor and the patient. A message is sent to the wholeness of the body, either emotionally, by meridians, by muscles and nerves, structurally, or by language and other codes; the basic integrity of the system resonates in the message and organizes around it anew.

Healing cannot sustain fragments or parts of cures. It is a wave, with an amplitude and a periodicity. Elements may change, but the wave reasserts itself. Even a healing experience which is a shock or jolt expresses itself finally as a wave. The cure may be a crack or a ping, but the ripples from there are perfect wholes.

The healing wave lies at the frequency present in the patient at the beginning and is tuned to the healer or healers. The fact that the wave exists prior does not make the healing less authentic. The patient experiences the wave, *is* the wave, but in a fragmentary sense. He does not feel his living being as a unity. Thoughts are scattered, purposes are at counterpurposes, physical movement is uncoordinated, and responsiveness is uncommitted and interrupted. The wave is broken, or experienced intermittently; the signal is still uniform, but the body does not perceive it singly nor take its own existence as a serious event—"Tired of livin' an' skeered of dyin'," as the black dockworker Joe sang in *Ol' Man River*. The resiliency of life is not there, but one also shuns the ultimate singleness imposed by death. If the organism cannot express its whole nature, it seems to need all of time in which to accumulate and express its partial natures. Life and death both are violations of its hoard of fragments. Phenomena in nature, like rivers, are also driven by springs, and when the springs snap, their properties dissipate; their single existence ends.

A good healer does not try to do too many things. He tries to do the one necessary thing. The person who is being healed cannot truly judge the experience from one symptomatic relief or proposition. It is up to both to assert the wave and not become distracted.

Bone cracking is "silly," but the bones that are cracked do not laugh. Their pulse rides into the body like a horse throwing back its head in midflight. They snap or cast an arc of essential nature. Spasm may interrupt unity, but eventually it completes itself because it is already there. In native situations, indigenous mythology is necessary to complete the link. We have our own mythology.

Single therapeutic gestures may fail if they rip open a blockage or a tightness but do not communicate a unity. Disease also has a singleness of expression, and it will reimpose itself if there is no event to sustain the insight.

Usually it does not matter if the patient and doctor work together often. Once the cure is correctly begun, their relationship is a connection. Changing the frequency or the stimulus does the same thing it does to a wave; it changes its quantity without changing its quality. Its shape may be different, but its congruence remains.

A wholeness comes on gradually. A person first feels better, has fewer chronic symptoms, is less depressed. Then he feels more coordinated. Relapses may be resting periods before greater movement. Later on, the person feels springy and responsive. He mocks himself less in interactions with people. He takes himself and his life seriously. If he laughs, that is also coordinated and part of his expression as a living being. Eventually the wave will express itself in life decisions; he will make better decisions, have more coherent thoughts, experience more poignant and relevant ideas. The unity becomes unavoidable.

He may have the feeling of dying or being about to die. His death is now a single thing too, and he must face it, as part of the wave, with deep feeling but no longer anxious nostalgia. If the life itself is made up too much of nostalgia, and feeling is always in the past as sweetness of memory, then the experience of the wave will be, temporarily at least, the experience of a dying, for the moments in the past are no longer necessary to having the feeling in the present.

It is important to see that this process is called "bodywork" not because it is physical rather than mental but because it takes our incarnation in a physical universe as an irrevocable condition of therapeutics. It little matters whether we believe that spirit has arisen in matter or matter itself is possessed of remarkable attributes: the cure requires an acceptance of the body's exact terms. We cannot out-think our anatomical destiny; we must think in it; we must find mind through it. In this sense, bodywork is a restatement of the condition of birth. We come into being through the body of another who came into being likewise, back to the beginning of a universe. The therapist must repeat, in some sense, the act of birth. It is not that he has to be a maternal force, but his cure cannot evade the seriousness of biology and genetic continuity. He must impose himself into the biological message with the same seriousness with which the mother *is* the biological message.

When doctor and patient begin to work together, a breathing together is established, and everything in both individuals will be represented in that breathing somewhere.[12] The two bodies re-open the ancient message—or, as Johnny Cash sings: "Flesh and blood needs flesh and blood, and you are what I need."

He means loving not healing, but the meaning could not be clearer.

XVIII

Healing, Language, and Sexuality

Healing has a dynamic all its own. It defies any science which turns out doctors by a standard procedure from its medical schools. It proposes to accomplish the same cures without any of the tools. Although a healer may be skilled in medical mechanics and knowledgeable about physiology, he practices, in whole or in part, by intuition and charisma, and this challenges the basic mechanics.

Orthodox medicine trains doctors, not healers. Healers gain their power elsewhere: either they are "born" with it (however one takes that), or they develop it through personal discipline, prayer, and/or initiation. The resulting ability transcends any individual system. A healer seems to be able to use any particular system he is trained in to get to the core of the matter. Quesalid, the Kwaikiutl shaman, discovered he was such a healer when he became proficient in the very system he had proven was a fraud (see Chapter VI).[1] We need to go back centuries in our own tradition to get to the time when medicine was the weavings of the gods into the texture of the physician's mind, but this is not so unlikely a premise even now. The Greek gods, who are still the demonic intelligences in the West, are the closest affinity our medicine has, at this already late date, with the supernatural sources of the shaman. Our own healing and faith healing is an extension of exactly that element of pre-Socratic thought which is also proto-Christian. But many of our doctors come upon their technique as mysteriously as Quesalid did.

Herbert Barker, the early twentieth-century British bonesetter, discovered his skill when he treated the dislocated elbow of a fellow passenger on a sea voyage to Canada. He had had no training at the time, but a cousin later taught him the rudimentary bonesetting methods. He proceeded to realign bones, joints, and ligaments spontaneously and was so successful that the British War Office employed him *sub rosa* during World War I (much as the United States Army used dowsers fifty years later in Vietnam).

Barker, in a way, failed his supporters, for he could not defend himself against the onslaught of medical criticism, and he could not describe his own method. He said he was not even sure how he did it. He was unable to train any successors, so he died like an artist, leaving his masterpieces but no system behind.[2]

Oral Roberts, the American TV evangelist, describes hearing an inner voice when he was young that told him to "be like Jesus." Several months earlier he had been healed by a preacher who laid his hands on him (he had had tuberculosis for many years). His own first healing success was spontaneous, during a test he set up for himself before twelve hundred people, when, during his sermon, an old woman's withered hand spontaneously came alive. With that sign, he began healing others in the room.[3]

Harry Edwards, the great contemporary British spiritualist healer, like Quesalid, practiced at first as a skeptic. He had been told by several mediums, on their own, that he had a gift of healing, so he began to test it on people who were seriously ill. The first time he put his hands on a sick person, he felt an amazing energy in them, as though the cure were passing through him.[4]

Years later, his mind caught up to the wonder, and, in an interview, Edwards says: "Spiritual healing is a *science*. It does not depend on a person's faith. To overcome a given condition does require specialized treatment to induce change that is needed and to overcome the affliction. Therefore it is a *planned* effort. To carry out a plan needs an intelligence. To a healer the curable is only the so-called 'incurable.' It indicates that an intelligence superior to man's is operating. Therefore, it also implies that the spirit intelligence who carries out the healing has a knowledge far superior to human science. It also means that it has a much more extensive knowledge of the laws that govern physical science, energies, and things like that."[5]

Mind entering matter and redirecting it is an ancient theosophical tenet. Whether this is what happens or not, it is what seems to happen; as with the bloody down that Quesalid produced, the patient proclaims himself cured after the treatment. John Lee Baughman, a contemporary American healer, describes four spiritualists and a doctor praying together to rid the doctor's wife of cancer:

"We saw these cells under the influence of God, and the action stemming from the subconscious to the cells, wherever they were, and they were being fed their proper direction again, and their form, and their movement."[6]

Baughman also claims no knowledge of the physiology, attributing the cure to the precision and efficacy of prayer. Thomas Johanson, another contemporary British healer, was "chosen" by a Roman Catholic monk in trance as a man with healing ability. He was placed, despite his own protests, in a Catholic clinic and took to putting his hands on patients and praying. *He* was aware of nothing, but the people he treated reported a strange heat emanating from his hands. At present he heals between eight hundred and a thousand people a year.[7]

Healers come from all over the Earth and use a variety of methods, some of them startling and absolutely inexplicable, as the psychic surgery of Tony Agpaoa of the Philippines and José Arigo of Brazil; these "doctors" cut open the flesh with their hands or a small penknife, do something quickly to the tissue, and close the wound without a scar. At least this is what is reported by hundreds of professional observers and what has been recorded on film. John G. Fuller's description of Arigo includes an account of the first time Andrija Puharich, the American physician who also worked with the Israeli psychic Uri Geller, and his friend Henry Belk observed the Brazilian's surgery:

"Puharich and Belk watched incredulously as the people moved up in line to the table, rich and poor, of all ages. Arigo would barely glance at them. For most, his hand began almost automatically scribbling a prescription at incredible speed, as if his pen were slipping across a sheet of ice. Occasionally he would rise, place a patient against the wall, wipe the paring knife on his shirt again, drive it brutally into a tumor or cyst or another eye or ear, and remove whatever the offending tissue was, in a matter of seconds.

"There was no anesthesia, no hypnotic suggestion, no antisepsis—and practically no bleeding beyond a trickle."[8]

At one point Arigo suddenly asks Puharich to perform the operation on a patient's eye. He is terrified to hold the knife, certain he will slash the eyeball. He hesitates, but Arigo says, "Do it like a man!," so he plunges the knife against the eye.[9] He expects the worst, but instead experiences a repelling force coming back from the tissue. He operates, but he never actually penetrates or damages it. Mechanically, physiologically, it makes no sense. But what about the Navaho patient who rises from the sand painting chant cured? What about the revival meeting when the lame throw down their crutches and walk away?

The only thing that stands *for* these events is that they happen. They vanish like snowflakes, for no general case or science can be made from them. The idea itself of a healer is too hypothetical, too subjective, and too idiosyncratic for the medical tradition to handle. It is even an uncomfortable matter in holistic health circles, where the general belief is that the unorthodox techniques are themselves the causes of cure, not the doctors. The cured person takes his health home with him, and his immediate associates and family explain it by his faith; the local doctor may question whether he was sick in the first place, or whether each next test will correct the previous error and reveal the still-present disease.

All medicine which works inexplicable cures runs into the same dilemma: there is no way of establishing a relationship between the medicine and the cure. If a patient treated by acupuncture or homoeopathy improves, what can the improvement be attributed to? How can fine needles stuck in the arm correct a stomach ulcer? How can pills with no chemical material remaining in them relieve diarrhea? How can an adjustment of the spine help a nervous ailment? The practitioners of these medicines all have theoretical explanations of energies and vital properties; this is their post-scientific bias, even as the shaman's certainty of spirits and supernatural forces is a pre-scientific bias. But any cure could equally well be explained by the ubiquitous placebo effect, by the curative benefit of the experience itself or, in parapsychological circles, by the telepathic intercession of the doctor in the disease, no matter what his trick or technique.

One lay homoeopath told me the story of his sister, who had stomach pains for ten years and had been to a number of doctors without any cause being found. She was a total disbeliever in homoeopathy, but she saw no harm in taking pills from her brother. When he didn't hear from her for several months, he assumed that the medicine had not worked. But eventually he saw her and asked about the pains.

"Oh, the pains," she said. "They just went away."

"Was it when you took the medicine?" he asked.

She thought about it, and then agreed it was right after taking the medicine, but she considered that a coincidence.

In telling me the story, the practitioner added, "That's the way it is. The cure is so profound that the disease just slips away. The body knows something profound has happened; it changes. But the person doesn't have to know anything in their mind."

In fact, many faith healers recall praying over "atheists" at the request of worried family members and healing them of life-threatening diseases.

We can use three models to deal with miraculous and charismatic healing. Although the models are different, each may be valid at a different level or as an expression of a different partial truth. In fact, we will deal with them collectively as well as singly.

First, we have the dialogue between the healer and the sick person. Some quality of compassion, recognition, or curative potential is transmitted from one to the other. This dialogue exists not only apart from but *despite* the express methodology of the healer. Chiropractor, shaman, and surgeon are all human beings, part of a life chain, and, despite their differences, they work most fundamentally and unconsciously from this "prejudice." They also have its biological power.

Orthodox medicine may rely on mechanical intercession, but it also includes an unacknowledged dialogue. Diagnosis involves communication as well as information gathering, and surgery itself conveys personal meanings that go beyond the act. A good surgeon may well be one who can communicate the essence of healing while making the appropriate organic adjustments in the patient. The faith healer communicates the same essence, but in a different language, without the physical manipulation.

The "worst" doctors, in a sense, are the ones who simply cannot be spoken to and who say nothing. They continue to talk in the deceptively neutral language of technology. They insist on abstracting the patient and in being abstracted. They may be "nice" to a fault, but that niceness is impenetrable. Furthermore, they cannot help but communicate the persona of robot they aloofly mime. This robs them of a valuable tool.

In this kind of work, there can be no promises and no outlaws. If a psychosurgeon or preacher can get through where a trained physician cannot, this does not cheapen the cure. The cure, in fact, cannot be cheapened. The explanation, even the need for an explanation from outside the experience of change, is a residual issue for our intellect to resolve.

The language itself of the cure gives us a second model. Somehow, somewhere, either in the nervous system, the various auras hypothesized around the body, and/or the cells themselves, a meaning conveniently called "cure" is transposed from the medicine and treatment onto the living flesh. It does not require contact or pills, for many medicines involve language, movement, or the acting out of gestures. Yet there is something in the cure that makes it sudden and effective, that causes it to stand out from the rest of life.

About such a message we finally guess at its terms from what we know of different medicines. It is not in American, of course, because it is not in language, though language, including those of music, art, body code, etc., affects people to the quick, and is part of a larger message. We would like to think, along with the optimistic homoeopath, that matter can be spiritualized and then communicated to the intelligence of the soma. But we are also stuck with this: that the *idea* of the mentalization of matter is not the same as the fact of it. Likewise, the science fiction stories of mind over matter in other galaxies and dimensions are projections of our own isolation in just such a condition. When parapsychologists tell us that healers communicate directly to the etheric and astral levels and that this message is then enacted on a physical plane through the embryogenesis of new cells, we can understand that this is only what *must* happen, given not only that we are on the outside looking in but also that it is in our minds and bodies themselves—the only way by which we know existence at all—that the experiment occurs.

The dialogue between the parties in an act of healing and the language of the cure are virtually indistinguishable in the holistic medicines. Current alternative medicines share this feature with faith healing and many of the tribal methodologies. If they "cure," they do not do so by demonstrable pharmaceutical and surgical techniques. Instead, they place an implicit emphasis on the body's powers, and they seek methods of communicating with and inciting those powers. For this reason, each medicine develops its own method of reading "character," both of people and illnesses, and sometimes also of medicines. In psychiatric medicine, character is defined in terms of personality, but in many other medicines character is defined mythologically. Likewise, the medicinal "meaning" is not its pharmaceutical drug action, but its functional relationship to a chain of medicinal symbols.

From this perspective, we can look back at Wilhelm Reich. His *Character Analysis* is a basic text for reading character. It would serve for the chiropractor, the homoeopath, or the psychiatrist. Freud gave the first prescription in reading character: Pay exact attention to what the patient says. Reich went a notch further: It is not what he says but how he says it—his mode of description, his breathing and movement while he talks, the eye contact he makes or fails to make, his choice of words and underlying speech bias and rhythm, the general sense he has of who is doing the talking. This character knows much more than the doctor or patient about the source and nature of the ailment.

An M.D. does this as a matter of course. His job is to see behind the description, to pay attention to the actual physical events *in* the patient rather than what the patient says. But from Reich's point of view, the doctor has to read the patient absolutely; he cannot use diagnosis as an excuse to single out those things that are heavily stated. He has to "see" the disease.

Most native medicines are also based on reading character. In their case, though, character is manifested in unique cultural circumstances and may appear as a toad or killer whale, a stone or a spirit. The language may include larger ceremonial and mythological reference fields, and the bodywork is often an acting out of demons and supernatural beings or a community dance. African, American Indian, and Aboriginal Australian character exists always with respect to gods, supernatural forces, and a system of totemism, even as our character appears in respect to our own cultural system. A poor doctor, in any culture, fails to grasp the relationship of the many levels of psyche and soma and drives the patient around in a repetitive mythological, symbolic, and, hence behavioral circle. An unwilling patient simply does not "see."

Primitive and alternative medicines share this other feature: The diagnosis seeks to grasp the basic coherence of the person, his or her *essential nature,* even if the healer knows nothing of the disease, the history, or the idiosyncrasies of the person.

The healer has already established that he will not be working in parts, so he does not need different remedies for different aspects of the disease or strong medicines to penetrate the stubborn physiological mass of the body. Older magical law prevails: If a thing is a one, it can be altered by altering, even to an infinitesimal degree, the nature of that one. Where holistic practitioners fail, by their own definition, is when they miss the whole. It is one thing to *seek* to grasp essence; it is another to grasp it actually. No partial solution can correct this; the healer is committed to the whole he discovers. If it is the wrong whole, he has missed the case. But unity still holds him to a solution. His error becomes part of future interpretation: he may well come to the whole by successive instructive errors. Homoeopaths do this all the time; a wrong remedy can throw everything into perspective and show why something masquerading convincingly as the whole is not the whole. A present stomach inflammation may be less important than a speech impediment or slight lameness, if these go back further historically and join more tightly to the roots. The body itself is precise and acute: a limp or stutter might throw the organism many degrees from center, with flaring up in the stomach one symptom of the tilt. A terrific headache, with much weeping, might seem psychiatrically to have its origin in a personal event, whereas a chiropractor could find it at the fifth vertebra, making the psychological origin secondary and superficial.

The regular physician, remember, follows Ariadne's thread through the labyrinth of his diagnosis: he can stop at any point, effect a partial adjustment, pick up, and follow his thread on, to further partial adjustments. The holistic practitioner has no territory in which to follow such a thread. He can never be proven right or wrong except by the spontaneous response of the patient. Thus, he must go from whole picture to whole picture, even if they both are erroneous, and whole pictures are never connected by a thread.

It is here we must look again at the so-called dubious armamentarium of the alternative practitioner. He lacks the standard surgical tools and antibiotics; if he has access to X-rays and laboratory data, it is on a different basis. In their place, he has needles, potencies, exercises, and his picture of a whole and the angle of tilt of the organism. But neither the remedy nor the diagnosis works in terms of a gross material adjustment even when there are obvious physiological elements in his method, such as manipulation. However little we really know about it, the remedy must communicate one tiny thing to the essential nature of the organism. All medicine rests on the promise of such a message, even medicine which avoids it as an issue.

At the same time, the various healing systems are not bound in a universal somatic language. Breathing, pulse, and bones are in the same body but they use different linguistics. What binds them is that all the doctors, in reading the "character" of their patients according to the systems in which they work, stand as mirrors in which the sick persons see themselves. The mirrors are there before any medicine is administered. They are part of the diagnosis, but they cannot be separated from the cures. If a reading is accurate, the effect of that on a patient may rival, as a message, the effect of the remedy itself.

It is on this level, of being the mirrors, that preachers, shamans, homoeopaths, psychologists, and surgeons come together. Oral Roberts or Quesalid may be a more successful healer than a trained doctor. Cure is an unquantifiable and indefinable event. We still do not know what medicine is, or what the real meaning of even our present orthodoxy is, i.e., what those treatments say to the system all the time they are doing their chemical and surgical number called "cure."

The ancients did not distinguish between the herbal message of a plant as tincture and its vital message as deific force; they did not distinguish between the messages passing within nature and the phenomena of nature as messages themselves. The pure spirit of the plant could be identical to the vital energy of the plant and the plant's position in an over-all matrix of stars, seeds, and affinities. It is our obsession with the single chemical voice that has made "divine" cure difficult to explain.

It is no great surprise if we come to believe, after all that medicine has done for us, that the cure is obscure; after all (and we have not forgotten this), our own lives are obscure. A system of healing must reach *actually* within them, and touch their imperatives, as the Yellow Emperor reached within the lives of his patients. It simply doesn't work to give all up to science and technology and to the verdict of Western history and ask them to solve it, and then only when it is manifested as disease and discomfort. We are more in the battle than this.

And it is no wonder that we come back to language as the key because we are obsessed with it and have been since it drove us from pure animal being into the villages that became the cities of our lives as humankind. Freud hoped to return language to the nervous system, to prove its origin there and read the literal event of character disorder in physiology, but that is only a small part of the hieroglyphic. It is doubtful we will ever find it comprehensively there. The later French psychoanalysts, Jacques Lacan among them, read from their "Freud" that it is all language, that there is no true moment in it, no literal disease formation. Language is the common denominator of the obscurity we have reached in our history and culture, meaning that our claims to a historic location are diagnostic not historical. We are located in the "languages" of embryology, cell growth, mythology, technology, and so on, and so on, all the languages we have known as well as the languages we have spoken with our lips. Even the way of phrasing past and present or mind and symptom is a contemporary convention. Behind known language is unconscious language—not only the associative codes of psyche, but the dense and buried structures written by ancient trails through the jungle and fractures in stone knives and smoke from forests and factories, and untold even unremembered dreams. The writing of the world on its own body, which they call "grammatology," must approach us as intimately as the disease.[10] In orthodox medicine we try to argue this language away literally because we believe it must be true. We use those things which are presently literal. In the other medicine, we believe it too, but we call it objective psyche and soma, not because it is true in any local sense but because we *are* it regardless.

Then, from entirely different sources, most of them vernacular compared to the French academies, we hear that great masters cure by addressing the disease (as language), by speaking through its condition, making words and chants into instruments of power. The sages speak in "divine" rather than "social" voices. Born in Oklahoma, Oral Roberts can stay there; he doesn't have to go to school. If a school is needed, he can start his own. It is not that anything *else* he expresses is "eccentric" except the fundamental bias, which is "Sooner." The school can have the usual subject matters, libraries, and basketball team; we can overlook the Christian bias of the curriculum, which is after the fact. The fact is that the patients he heals are also Sooners (or "Okies") in some fundamental way; he must touch that part of them, which can recognize him as the true other.

Babiji, the mysterious Hindu master, was bothered repeatedly by a yogi who could not practice because of a pain in his knee. Finally, he paid him some attention, saying, rather lightly, "You have a sick knee; I'll fix it." Then he spat on his hand and threw his spit at the knee with a gesture of disinterest. But it was healed.[11] Some might claim, as the teller of the story, that the holiness of the spit is what worked the cure. But it could also have been the gesture, "spoken" so precisely it cut into the obscurity of the other's life. It spoke to the deep tilt, of which the knee was only a warning.

Sticking to this model of unity, character, and message, we can see the relationship between different holistic medicines. For instance, the chiropractor reads character from the functional shape of the body. It is not simply a matter of something out of alignment, but where the subtle tilts and inhibitions occur and what they indicate about the life and responsiveness of the organism. "Signaling errors" are transmitted from within the viscera and occur in the skeleton and the personality. The chiropractor must read the signaling error from a character point of view, not taking the body's awkwardness or asymmetry per se as completed functional statements of illness. The chiropractic formula for adjusting is: the minimum force, in the correct direction, with the maximum speed. The movement must be done confidently and with a meaning that transcends its initial physical effect.

Likewise, the homoeopathic materia medica is a compendium of character statements. The doctor must match the image of an individual with the image of a medicine; it is not sufficient simply to find parallel symptoms in either. For instance, *Nux vomica*, the poison-nut remedy, is used for a diverse range of ailments, but always on the basis of underlying traits of the medicine which are more character than pathology. The *Nux* person is supposed to be husky, strong, ambitious, hard-working, but also distinctly overambitious to the point of being driven to work all night and day. He is self-destructively competitive, fastidious, and lacks perspective, preferring to drive himself. He is also prone to stimulants and kinky sex. We must emphasize, first that these are the character traits beneath the visible pathology, and second that they are derived from the potentized substance itself in provings and prescribed only on the basis of the Law of Similars.

Acupuncture would seem to rest primarily on the subcutaneous transmission of energy from the needle, opening internal channels for the circulation of *chi* energy. The acupuncturist, however, diagnoses by the patient's pulse. Each wrist has three pulses, and each pulse can be taken at two different levels; in each of these twelve pulses there are twenty-eight common readings, every one a distinct "character." The pulse may be empty, disappearing on pressure. It can be too urgent, too sunken; it can float on the surface of the skin from the Wind Evil. It can slip and slide; it can overflow from Fire floating and Water dried up. It can bounce like a fiddle string; it can be larger but leathery from the cold; it can be blurred; it can be shaped like an onion stem, hollow from great loss of blood. It can be overquick and halting or soft and fine; it can be shaped like a bean from fright.[12]

According to *The Yellow Emperor:*

"The feeling of the pulse should be done according to method: for when it is slow and quiet it acts as protector and guardian. In the days of Spring the pulse is superficial, like wood floating on water or like a fish that glides through the waves. In Summer days the pulse within the skin is drifting and light, and everywhere there is an excess of creation. In Fall days the torpid insects underneath the skin are about to come out. In Winter the torpid insects are all around the bone, quiet and delicate like the nobleman residing in his mansion."[13]

The application of the needles can come only after the disease is diagnosed. The doctor must read the person's character in terms of the system and then put the needles in with correspondence to seasons, hours, whether the point tonifies or sedates, color, sense of element, and relation of organ to other organs by elements.

Mythology and psychiatry *are* dynamically similar systems of character analysis, but we must learn to read myth as an expression of character before we can see the relationship. The Yellow Emperor was the psychoanalyst of his time:

"Beginning and creation come from the East. Fish and salt are the products of water and ocean and of the shores near the water. The people of the regions of the East eat fish and crave salt; their living is tranquil and their food delicious. Fish causes people to burn within (thirst), and the eating of salt injures (defeats) the blood. Therefore the people of these regions are all of dark complexion and careless and lax in their principles. Their diseases are ulcers, which are most properly treated with acupuncture by means of a needle of flint. . . .

"Precious metals and jade come from the regions of the West. The dwellings in the West are built of pebbles and sandstone. Nature (Heaven and Earth) exerts itself to bring a good harvest. The people of these regions live on hills, and, because of the great amount of wind, water, and soil, become robust and energetic. The people of these regions wear no clothes other than those of coarse woolen stuff or coarse matting. They eat good and variegated food and therefore they are flourishing and fertile. Hence evil cannot injure their external bodies, and if they get diseases they strike at the inner body. These diseases are most successfully cured with poison medicines. . . .

"In the North is the region of storing and laying by. The country is hilly and mountainous, there are biting cold winds, frost and ice. The people of these regions find pleasure in living in this wilderness, and they live on milk products. The extreme cold causes many diseases . . ."[14]

This is absolutely literal stuff, but only when we have penetrated its other, surface literality. It is beyond us to know exactly what it means, but it is a closed system of diagnosis and maintenance of health, and it is a system which works, prior to the application of needles, on aspects of being and images that conduct the underlying qualities. The unknown originators have not chosen forms because they are picturesque and suggest Oriental painting. They have chosen them because they are already imbedded in their world, hence in their personality. These images describe the pulse of their life. We talk about "living waves" and a "literal pulse," its quantity rather than its quality, but, in the over-all run of things, this difference is a difference between symbolic systems.

The methodology which, perhaps, best demonstrates the relation between cure and language is the "Curative Eurhythmy" that arises from Rudolf Steiner's anthroposophy. Eurhythmy is simultaneously a paralinguistic code and a rhythmic interchange. The medicine is "taught" to the patient as a motion made up of the letters of a "word" the therapist has chosen. He demonstrates the word over and over, and the patient imitates it until he picks it up. The correction process *is* the healing process. Each imperfect spelling communicates to the inner self, and, as the spelling becomes truer and truer, the whole cure is transmitted. As in many of the medicines, the inner self, as it improves, also imposes a truer and truer rhythm on the body.

The Steiner language system is made up of the Germanic vowels and consonants acted out as body postures and movements. Each sound has a gesture. The gesture itself is simple and can be placed on a number of different planes or scales by the different organs. A "U" for instance can be written close to the ground or high in the air. It can be suspended vertically or extended horizontally. It can be made with the toes or fingers or with the whole body.[15]

Steiner took language as basic to being. The vowels and consonants are our psychic and somatic seeds; they precede us, since we discover them in our own emerging consciousness. Although words seem to be semiarbitrary semantic codes of sounds, Steiner considered their phonetics a fixed aspect of the meaning. While the semantic "meaning" is communicated to the conscious self, the inner self "hears" the discrete quality of the sound. In fact, regional dialects indicate the nature of civilizations—so that the emergence of English or German civilization *is* the English and German languages writ large.

The curative power comes from the potentization of the alphabet, which translates the seed forms of these sounds into sequences which have meaning for the human personality and anatomy.

The relationship of the sounds to actual words is not arbitrary, so the sound "M," wherever it appears, from "mother" to "hum" to "rhythm," is the same eurhythmic seed, set off by its relationship to other seeds in the cluster. "S" in "sun" and "sleep" and "asthma" is the same "S," so a remedy with many "S's" might be given to someone with asthma, although this is not the only diagnostic procedure, and those "S's" might well be mixed with other seeds (note the "S's" here too) in making up other qualities of the disorder. For instance, a person with heart disease might well be given "H's" and "R's," but only to the degree they were specifically relevant. He must also be fed "L's," which would not be surprising, since "L" is "love" and "light" and "life."

T'ai chi, like eurhythmy, emerges from seed forms, but while the seed forms of eurhythmy are basic notes of human speech, the seed forms of *t'ai chi* are movements of animals—snakes, birds, fish, monkeys. In the former case, the body is spoken to in terms of the origin of human language, on the possible assumption that the etiology of disease and the etiology of words share a connection in human phylogeny. But *t'ai chi* takes mind and language as a hindrance. Man must imitate not his own forms of speech but those movements ani-

mals make, because animals exist in the pure expression of their bodies, *as* language but prior to language. There is no hedging in the escape of the fish or deer, the attack of the snake or tiger. These are
objective expressions of their total being, and it is the sense of self as
objective being that man learns from them.

T'ai chi has its own self-corrective message. The form of the "single moves" is done over and over again, from day to day and year to
year, with the general alignment of the body and organs improving
infinitesimally but constantly. In Benjamin Lo's description: "First
you do it incorrectly and don't know it. Then you know there's an
error but not what. Then you know what is the error, but you cannot
correct it. Then you correct it."[16]

T'ai chi also raises the important issue of medicine as martial art.
After all, protection against sickness and poisoning is incomplete
without protection against physical attack. If a person moves correctly, the organs in his inner body line up and he throws off disease,
but also his outer body is so soft that an attacker cannot injure or kill
him and will actually harm himself trying to do so.

The connection goes even deeper. The martial movements of *t'ai
chi*, done with a different focus, are the movements of massage (as in
the Japanese form of *shiatsu*). The points of the opponent's body are
the same ones on the patient's body. The formula is rigorous: too
much energy harms, maims, or kills; less energy stimulates and heals.
"Shoot Tiger," for instance, is a move for immobilizing an opponent
by twisting his arm upward and back and delivering a blow to his
shoulder blade. The same motion, with gradual pressure applied instead, is used to heal tensions at that point as well as diseases forming along that meridian. If the movements are done even more softly
and with slightly different intent, they become lovemaking, seduction. Even while the connection is erotic, it retains its healing aspects for both parties (as in the Reichian embrace).

The particular series, from martial to curative to sexual, clarifies an
important aspect of healing. It is always in a continuum. It becomes
healing through a very special focus and intention. Though we do not
understand the relationship between fighting and lovemaking in a
Taoist sense, we still find it in our culture. Lovemaking verges on violence unless the implicit violence of the people is understood and integrated. Where sex becomes violence, as in some urban street cultures, something else, such as dancing, sports, or tenderness within

gangs, must take on the healing function usually expressed in lovemaking.

In our culture, men and women are often made uncomfortable by the healing implications of lovemaking, and they resist it almost electrically. They make sex into any number of other things: cool, chic, ferocious, power seeking. If someone should challenge the tough sensuousness of the playboy image of sex, those who hold the image rebel. Call what they are doing anything but the charge and the conquest—or, most provocatively of all, call it healing—and they will deny it. The closest they will come, in countercultural circles, is an agreement to "exchange energies." This verges on healing, but becomes so only when the energies are processed through personality, where the healer and healing potion are identified with each other and understood as one. Just as there is no healing machine, there is no lovemaking machine. For the same reason, rhesus monkeys reject the cloth mothers that experimenters saddle them with.

Opening a day-long class on Chinese medicine in Berkeley, Paul Pitchford commented on the fact that the class was made up almost entirely of women: "Women are already into healing. They are natural healers. Men have to learn how to become healers."[17]

This statement has both a biological and a cultural meaning. Women are natural healers in bringing life into the world and nurturing it, and then they continue to develop the part of their being that is receptive to healing. Men seek sex so much more ardently often because they lack (i.e., have not developed) their own natural healing function. They are dependent on others (women) to supply this necessity because their personality and cultural role prevents them from developing it in themselves. In another culture, men may develop what seem like feminine aspects of their personality but which are actually healing aspects originating in a receptivity to the natural rhythms of creation.

The third model of healing is one of external intervention. Previously, we had only the mind, body, and history of both the doctor and patient. Now we must consider the possibility of a force from outside this dialogue or emerging within it from alien sources. In the simplest sense, it is like a housecall to a UFO, and it is no accident that extraterrestrial beings are called on in Western science fiction cycles to intercede and save a sick and erring humanity. Long before, there were gods, angels, and splendid demons.

Once we consider outside entities, there is no end to what is possi-

ble. Disincarnate intelligence or energy can be summoned by the
healer in behalf of the cure. Beings from other worlds and dimensions can contribute tools of a technology still removed from us by
billions of billions of years. By such a time, argue the advocates, anything will be possible, including intervention in our present world.
At the same time, these external powers behave identically to the
postulated hidden intelligences of the cells and auras of the body, so
they may always be another way of explaining the same thing. The
extraterrestrial beings become like gods, or ancient astronauts. Even if
they never visited the Earth, they could communicate the same images to us telepathically across galaxies, intrabiologically through
plants, or even as messages in a nucleic acid with which they seeded
the Earth from afar, which then spawned not only our bodies but
our collective unconscious mind. At such a point, the occult rituals
of the Egyptians, reenacted by Aleister Crowley in the cult of the
Golden Dawn, become etiologically synonymous with the wisdom of
the Jovians or the beings from the planet system of Sirius.

L. George Lawrence, in experiments conducted in 1971 in the
middle of the Mojave Desert, in Southern California, seemed to pick
up messages from living tissue on planets in Ursa Major, or rather he
picked them up as recorded in the sensitive tissue of terrestrial
plants.[18] If such signals can reach cacti and wild oak, they could also
enter some aspect of human intelligence.

Robert K. G. Temple, the British astronomer, proposed in a book
published in 1976 that the mythology of Africa and Egypt contains
such exact references to the solar system of the double star Sirius
that the Earth apparently was visited by beings from one of the
planets in this system around 4500 B.C.[19] He suggests that his own
book may be the "cosmic trigger," signaling these beings, who are
still monitoring the Earth, that our planet is now ready for direct
communication. From this book, Robert Anton Wilson takes the
title *Cosmic Trigger* for his book propounding his own conspiracy
theory, which links these events and the plant communication with
the prison martyrdom of both Wilhelm Reich and Timothy Leary,
and the discovery of the psychocosmic potential of LSD by Leary, a
conspiracy so vast and overwhelming as to encompass all of history
and to include the assassinations of John F. and Robert F. Kennedy
and Martin Luther King, Jr.[20] By such a point, almost anything is
possible, and Wilson proves this by suggesting that the development
of an immortality medicine is the key to the solution of these planet

mysteries. It is only by a longer life-span that man can hope to inhabit space and complete the galactic mission by traveling in body back to Sirius. Leary's LSD is the forerunner of such an immortality drug, and Leary himself is quoted as saying that he fully expects to be alive when our local Sun bursts into a supernova and burns to its icy core. The mystery is heightened by the possibility that human DNA comes from the system of Sirius and continues to receive or activate messages from there. If Leary and Wilson's contemporary America is key to this plot, then the political assassinations become intergalactic murders, perhaps connected to a government plot to squelch the immortality drug and the colonization of space.

Going to the extreme clarifies what we are up against, both in its manifested and potential complexity. External agency will always be an issue, in healing as it is in other science fiction and parapsychology. At the same time, all this is the expression of our state of being on the Earth. It occurs to us for a reason, perhaps different from the reason it prophesies. Alone or in cosmic company, etheric or physical, immortal clone or link in an eternal planet biology, we still must make our own world. We can think about external entities and await UFOs or spirits, but if they should appear in glorious science fiction terms, our response to them will come from within our lives, and our preparation, in fantasy or vision, may not be preparation at all. This is why one can welcome the remarkable energy and grasping at stars that these prophecies contain and use it, in itself, as an elixir and, at the same time, be unwilling to commit our great riddle to such flagrant and intimate aliens.

The research of the future will continue to be done by physicists and parapsychologists, and it will be, like the other hurried research of Western culture, for new energy sources, for intelligence in outer space. We will continue to hear about plants communicating, the terminally ill being healed, and enormous Russian machinery, sunk in the Earth, sending psychic waves through the planet. In the meantime, we can set aside the promise or danger of these experiments and deal with the reality we have, which has been the reality of mankind as we have known it and as it has made us human.

XIX

The New Medicine

Shamans and medicine men stand near the beginning of this book, as though at the beginning of time. The elemental doctors of the early Eurasian world were their unwitting followers and apprentices. By other names, their torch was passed through the European Renaissance, surviving the birth of industrialism, into the modern world.

In this context, professional medicine is a particular Western adaptation, begun with the occupational stratification of society and hastened by the scientific revolution. It has since spread globally, giving the impression that all less "scientific" forerunners bear merely a trial-and-error relationship to the corrected Western system.

Many other medical traditions have survived the turmoil of generations and continue to be practiced somewhere on the Earth. They represent the most grass-roots challenge to a standardized Western medicine, for they are far older than modern science and they are the background against which it arose. Collectively, they include our legacies of faith healing, herbalism, mineral cures, meditation, diet, exorcism, etc.

But the rise of scientific medicine against the background of ancient healing has also produced other hybrid systems, systems which reflect some of the profundity and empiricism of original medicine and which, yet, are the products of the tools and concepts of modern scientific thought. Homoeopathy and psychotherapy are the two most stunning offspring of this dialectic.

There is no single thread to this book. Even the linear historical structure is misleading. So before we identify the "new medicine," we should review the simultaneous understandings and misunderstandings we have come to.

By implication, we have romanticized native medicine. It would seem that much of the toughness and strength of both homoeopathy and psychotherapy comes from their retention and/or recovery of primitive features. But that is only one face of their genesis. Their radical innovations and their potential for incorporating the subtleties and complexities of modern life are equally significant. A fleshy primitivity is not enough, and a parapsychic futurism is not enough either. The virtue of all medicines of the middle ground (between healing and science) is the process they describe and embody, whatever their origin or philosophy.

Our romanticization of the native and his technologically primitive society is both true and false to the theme of this book. On the one hand, it is essential that we see the vacuity behind modern arrogance and chauvinism, that we understand the rightness as well as the profundity of non-Western and even prehistoric cultures. On the other hand, as scholars and historians, we speak only for ourselves and our culture; our glorification of primitive peoples is an attempt to say something about ourselves and, by proxy, to enlarge our real scope and wisdom. The humanitarian justification for this monocultural dominion of the Earth is that man is one, and our salvation lies eventually in a mutual sharing of all knowledge. But this, again, is our idealism, and, though representatives of other peoples have come to share it and have participated in our globalism, we still do not speak for objective humanity first; we speak for science, modernism, and our own utopian fantasies. The difficulty many Marxists had handling a non-Western revolution in Iran is one clue to the potential shallowness of our most fabled universalisms.

We exist in the present. Our knowledge of other cultures and other periods of history is, as we have said before, a state of our contemporary culture. We do not have these other things at hand either to reenact or deny. What we have is our image of them, our reflection of our own bias. We may also have something of an intimation of the truth, but it sparkles and then it fades, it goes in and out of clouds, it is dazzling and then it is nonexistent; it is certainly not a clarity or consistent form.

In that sense, it is false to think that primitive and ancient medicines are the sole origin of this book (despite the fact that they *are*, in some ways). It is a convention of structure that places native medicine at the beginning of a sequence concluding now with contemporary holistic medicines. The real origin of this book is in the spiritual and material crisis of modern civilization and in our own quest for a voice, for a moral and rationale in our time. The ancients help us in this. But we come to know our ancestors only long after we have internalized our own system of thought.

This book begins in the place that primitive medicine has in our contemporary mythology. It works from there to the place that alternative medicine has in the same myths. These are not separated by millions of years, or thousands of years; they are parallel designs, aspects within the same design. The book could as easily begin with the contemporary revolution in healing and medicine and then work back, through the image of holism, to the forerunners we discover and our messianic images of them. Let us neither overestimate nor underestimate the relationship of primitive medicine to holistic health. They are connected in two ways—first, by the fact of an actual lineage (much of it unconscious), and second, by the ideological affinity we have given them in our search for new meanings.

The alternative medicine movement in the United States deceptively appears to have arisen in the 1960s. There *was* a revival and even a revolution in the 1960s, but there have always been "other" medicines in America, many of them involving much higher percentages of the population than the present publicized group does.

North America is a melting pot of world medicine, as of so many other things, and, despite the dominance of a universal scientific medicine, "street healing" and sectarian medicines have flourished, some of them regionally, some of them nationally. The multiplicity of different healing styles rather than a commonality of theme has distinguished the sectarian medical movement. By contrast, holistic health is a synthesis by which many individual medicines have been made more similar and integrated into a loose system of methodologies and ethics.

A brief survey gives the flavor and variety of sectarian medicine in the nineteenth century. Indian pharmacy, of course, was discovered in place, but it gave rise to numerous different naturopathic schools, including the Thomsonians whose wide popularity we described in Chapter XIV. Other pharmacies and systems of healing were imported with immigrants or slaves and continued to be practiced intact. Faith Mitchell, the Berkeley medical anthropologist, describes a system of African herbal and "hoodoo" (hex) medicine practiced in virtually its aboriginal form in South Carolina as a result of the importation of slaves directly to the Sea Islands.[1] Homoeopathy itself, of course, was imported from Germany and established its own American schools.

There are also many "new" American medicines prior to the twentieth century, medicines that may not have been absolutely new but which had a distinct New World quality separating them from any Eurasian forerunner. The Christian Science of Phineas Quimby and Mary Baker Eddy is an American original, native to Maine and New Hampshire. Edgar Cayce's life readings and metaphysical cures read "Illinois" as clearly as Rosicrucian Europe. Andrew Taylor Still (1828–1917) was a country doctor in Virginia when he "invented" osteopathy in the nineteenth century, proposing health as the full arterial circulation of the blood. Daniel David Palmer (1845–1913) was a grocer and lay spiritualist in eastern Iowa when he translated osteopathy into chiropractic, with his emphasis on an intuition of animal magnetism. The twentieth century saw a translation of these into new models of spinal integration and over-all nerve-muscle coordination; by the 1960s, kinesiologists were presenting a version of chiropractic synthesized with Asian interpretations of anatomy and a healing method based on "ensalivating" herbal and nutritional materials.

Many of the so-called alternative medicines were invented or flourished in nineteenth century America. Forms like chiropractic, homoeopathy, and osteopathy now have both conservative schools and schools formed by the current revolution. And it is impossible to say which is closer to the original visions, in any of the cases, for it is impossible to say which are the original visions, or even if the ostensible founders are themselves original or derivative of some older form.

The present syncretism of holistic health has made an unlikely but dynamic alliance among such diverse treatments as those of native American Indian medicine, Christian faith healers, chiropractors, Reichian therapists, homoeopaths, *t'ai chi* masters, vegetarians,

masters of yoga and breathing, and general spiritualists. It has re-
formed and redefined these things in terms of each other, so that the
traditionalists have either been converted, along with a version of
their tradition or have been abandoned. The systems themselves
have converged on certain features which they did not all have in the
original. It is safe to say that each individual system has contributed
at least one belief or practice to the holistic collective and has also
adopted at least one totally untraditional aspect. Some of the synthesis has been intentional, reflecting a developing ideology; some of it
emerges naïvely from the over-all cultural matrix in which the revival
is occurring. To understand these forms in their present use, whether
North American, Eurasian, or of other heritage, it does not help us
to know the old medicines, their forerunners, as they were. The new
"holistic" meanings of traditional treatments are contained in the
deep structures and meanings that underlie the holistic theme. And
this theme itself is the product of a number of different philosophical and political movements that collided creatively during the
mid-1960s and early 1970s.

Of all the forerunners of alternative medicine, the one that provided it with the largest ready-made niche within the professional
mainstream was psychoanalysis; it is the "holistic godfather" in that
sense. By "psychoanalysis" we mean a particular tradition arising
from Freud, not necessarily the one he sanctioned but the radical
cutting edge he set in motion. Freud himself passed on his scepter to
a mainstream orthodoxy, and its farthest extension is in a series of
behaviorist and related psychotropic schools that pay no homage to
the founder. They have reinterpreted what were already derivative
Freudian insights in terms of reductionist biochemical research, and
have, unwittingly, gone back to before Freud, when mental illnesses
(and the mental life in general) were treated as potential disrupters
that had to be manipulated and controlled. Radical psychotherapy
might have been just as unappealing to the conscious Freud, but all
masters have had their unintended offspring, and few would be as
prone to such instructive mischief as the very doctor who revealed
the workings of unconsciousness.
     In general, practitioners of radical forms of psychotherapy have ac-
cepted Freud's basic energetic dynamics of the mind and body but
rejected his clinical methodology and his explanations of resistance
as an expression of thanatos (death instinct). Despite their dif-

ferences from one another, they have emphasized the regenerative capability of the human being as the basis for the restoration of health and function. Like advocates of all holistic disciplines, they locate the dynamics of the illness in actual personal behavior. Many are somatic, but this does not exclude a strong verbal component. In gestalt therapy, for instance, language is used, but as a psychodramatic expression of the present situation rather than a historical consequence. The gestalt therapist does not deny the existence of traumatic events, but he wants to know their contemporary form. He wants to see them in action, and it cannot be a matter of mood or chance. In fact, the laws of holism demand that everything be present at every moment in some form. So he attempts to locate the current form, however submerged and resisted, and he puts aside, methodologically, the proof of an original traumatic charge.

Inevitably, these somatic and gestalt forms of psychoanalysis merged with other pre-Reichian bodywork traditions like chiropractic, osteopathy, acupuncture, and massage, with each giving the other a slightly different meaning. The physical tradition supplied new tools for diagnosing body states and abnormalities, and the psychological tradition supplied an emotional-affective basis for interpreting and working with these states. For instance, the traditional chiropractic, which was marked by its intuitive jarring of bones and its general uneducatedness about anything else including the meaning of diseases, becomes far less thin when it combines with somatic therapy and "understands" the dislocations and subluxations as psychosomatic traumas. It also gains a new credibility for its claims of being able to cure serious organic and emotional diseases, if these in fact are psychosomatic and reachable by manipulation. Likewise, somatic psychoanalysis gains decades of actual practice and training in working with patients and modes of physical alignment. It literally becomes the "hand" of the chiropractor and the "mind" of the psychiatrist working together to reach a space that is neither and both. This synthetic mode is so active today that we can have a treatment like kinesiology, which is a mixture of chiropractic, acupuncture, and some form of psychic healing. Acupuncture imposes its map of the meridians on the chiropractic skeleton, but the doctor works by hand rather than needle, and he intuits a range of "sensitivities" and "aversions" to a variety of substances that is part of neither system.

Somatic therapy also merges with schools of dance and body align-

ment, so that its range extends to the entire human tradition of
teaching movement and posture. Traditional dance already includes
forms of improvisation and movement therapy, forms which deal
with somatic structures not only in a clinical context but also as a
repertoire of individual gestures and creative movements. Nowadays,
though, there are dance forms directly intended as medicines, which
evoke the "feeling" body. Besides these, there are many other dances
which are experimental and radical only in terms of the movements
they propose. They are aesthetically inventive, but not necessarily
therapeutic. They are more involved with choreographing and expressing a shape than with the somatics and quanta of individual
moving bodies.

One of the results of holism is that all activities are reevaluated in
terms of each other and in terms of mind/body unity, so it is no
wonder that dance as art and movement as therapy should be unable
to escape each other. But not all movement therapies are technically
dance, even if they arise from dance traditions; equally, though, not
all creative and avant-garde dance styles are healing or healthy, no
matter how "new age" their movements seem or how evocative they
are of healing imagery and human change. This does not mean that
in order to be curative, movement must be aesthetically sterile. The
combination, however, is rare.

Posture has never been as confused with technical issues of artistic
perfection as dance has, but it suffers from a parallel history. Individual postures and body stances have come to reflect rules of etiquette
and professional or martial discipline more than underlying somatic
requirements. Thus, people *become* their niche in society or their job
rather than themselves. The disciplines of postural reintegration assume that these rigidities lead to organic and psychological as well as
structural diseases. Polarity, Alexander technique, Feldenkrais work,
and Rolfing are all forms of realignment and body balancing that are
intended to affect the entire personality and state of the organism.
Psychoanalysis has provided a new bioemotional depth to this kind
of work, even as it has added a layer to movement, dance, and bone
manipulation.

The revision of Freud's work has not led only to somaticization.
Carl Jung proposed his own regenerative healing energy, and he developed it in the opposite direction, or, at least, what is considered the
opposite direction by current mythology.

Jung took the Freudian unconscious, an obvious storehouse of primal creative as well as destructive energy, and invested it with additional dimensions. It now contained the collective racial, planetary, and cosmic memory of man—in some form or other everything he had been, as matter, as mind, as animal, as prehistoric tribesman, as bearer of civilization. Synchronistically, anachronistically, all these things were one and were collectively shared as the archetypes. Their contents could not be known as fact, but they were expressed in human enterprise, in all the shapes and numbers and structures created by mankind. The archetypes contained the most powerful healing energies imaginable, or, stated otherwise, healing itself and the doctors that practice it are archetypes; that is the only way healers discover treatments and the only way we are able to recognize their healing and allow it.

The archetypes contain, in part, geometric and crystal forms, plant and animal remnants, ancient wisdom from past civilizations, and intelligence of an order beyond humanity. How these merge with the individual psyche is uncertain, for Jung found them already there; their origin itself must lie beyond space and time and consciousness and thus not be at issue. But it is the destiny of every living being to discover this cosmic network within himself and learn how to assimilate it and to grow and change from it. An unexplored psyche is a potential disease. Dark images spawned there attack their unwilling carrier in nightmare and waking anxiety. The unconscious only appears evil and rapacious when it is ignored or suppressed and that is because it is urging the personality to regain its life harmony in the only way it can.

Jungian spiritual dynamics are startlingly similar to Reichian biological dynamics. The objective psyche is no more or less mystical than the objective soma. Both come mysteriously from chrysalis of seed and egg, merging with the personality of childhood, growing with the organism into its mature form. In Reich's reading, we are the remnants of vaster physical systems: galaxies and planets and orgone. In Jung's version, we are the remnants of vaster psychic systems: equally galactic and originary. Reich spells out the consequences of ignoring soma, in pathology and distorted function. Jung reminds us that psyche continues to exist and will merge with us as sickness if we will not open a way to it as health. In modern therapeutics, psychic and somatic healing tend to oscillate as different versions of the same image. There is nothing optional about either one.

Jungian therapy seems mythological in orientation because it tries to put a person in touch with his psychosomatic sources through hidden images rather than bodily integrations. These are seen to contain the meanings of individual existence. They might come from anywhere, most obviously from one's own culture and religion, but also, conceivably, from the myths, gods, and symbols of remote cultures or from accidental ancient material stirred up by dreams and experiences. For example, an acquaintance looks like a Greek god. One dreams of a hunched-over woman who suggests the Navaho creation goddess by her appearance. These associations were not arbitrary to Jung. "Synchronous" is what he called them. Meaning itself abides in nature and forces connections that have in them potential for further meaning, like an endless, unfolding system of divination. It is from this largest field of connection that individuals are enlightened and healed.

Every disease, in that sense, exists in the archetypes, has an archetypal counterpart; if cured, it is cured archetypally. The personality and ego bind one to a disease—they alone. In therapy, the patient becomes aware of a larger sphere around his personality; he begins to allow cosmic and archetypal images through, and, by kinship of psyche and personality, they are integrated.

Physical and mental disease converge in the archetypal sphere. If the symbols go that deep, then having them transformed into flesh is no larger matter. The actual life occurs in the remnant vibrations of the universe and is flesh only at one level of mind, one level of body. Images and symbols strike to the core of matter, as Hindus, Buddhists, and theosophists propose, and as Seth has recently reformulated from his seeming space between a world of mind and a world of matter through his medium Jane Roberts.[2]

Jung tended to emphasize the heroic integrations of artists, alchemists, and other exceptional people. James Hillman, a contemporary Jungian, has called the process "soul-making," at the same time making it a part of ordinary life and making ordinary life itself epic. The very formation of a human being with the potential for "making himself" is heroic and mythic. "Even without artistic talent, even without the ego strength of great will, even without good fortune," Hillman writes, "at least one form of the creative is continuously open for each of us: psychological creativity. Soul-making: we can engender soul. 'If you have nothing at all to create,' " he adds, quoting Jung, " 'then perhaps you create your soul.' "[3]

The proposition that self-knowledge and self-deepening are curative is axiomatic to most of the new medicines. It is, in part, an acceptance of the Jungian connection of healing with symbolic and artistic processes. This is the key to the manifold Jungian contribution to holistic health. For instance, today bodywork may be done according to Reichian principles but with Jungian associations and meanings. Feeling one's self as a rich-leafed tree, wind blowing in its branches, could emerge suddenly upon the freeing of deep breathing. It is the archetypal tree of the nervous system, with nerves and axons for branches and buds, and skin and ducts for wind, but, at the same time, it can be Yggdrasill, the great Norse ash that connects Heaven, Earth, and the Underworld by its roots and branches; it can be the sacred Druid yew and the Qabbalistic Tree of Life.

We may change physically in an exact moment of body and mind, space and time. We also change archetypally, and that is also instantaneous and real, also body as well as mind—but it places the moment of flesh and vision in an eternal continuum of time and space. Thus, we might fairly say that synchronicity and instantaneousness are the respective Jungian and Reichian properties of the same healing event within the nonsectarian holism.

The most dominant nonmedical forces in the new medicine are the Oriental spiritual disciplines. In the last two decades, psychoanalysis (particularly Reichian and Jungian) has provided the language in which Eastern thought could be translated into Western terms. So, in many ways, the psychoanalytic contribution and the Oriental one are the same thing.

Oriental teaching is *like* psychoanalysis. The doctor-patient transference in the latter resembles the master-disciple transmission of the former. Conventional medicine and religion are also alike. They both involve faith in authority (priest or doctor), passivity on the part of the congregation, and a relatively superficial investigation of subsurface mysteries.

Pure psychology, like pure meditation, seeks to get to the actual bottom of things, at least insofar as there can be one. Neither thought nor health have any absolute meaning or value; they are the result of the organism working through its existence. Almost parallel with Reich's "character analysis," Chögyam Trungpa, the Tibetan Buddhist master now in Colorado, writes:

"In the practice of meditation all thoughts are the same: pious thoughts, very beautiful thoughts, religious thoughts, calm thoughts

—they are all still thoughts. You do not try to cultivate calm thoughts and suppress so-called neurotic thoughts."[4]

The paradigm of "working on one's self" as a life goal is the aspect of Eastern science most generally adopted by the holistic medicines. Of course, Buddhist as well as Hindu teachers have traveled throughout the United States and Europe, and many have set up schools. Inevitably, their teachings have been synthesized with somatic, gestalt, and Jungian therapies. In becoming Americanized, they have given their own depth and experience to the systems in which they have been translated. Freud may have opened the conscious West to a vision of its own unconscious, but psychology has since discovered that Asia had been developing, over millennia, a language for unconscious process and a methodology for integrating unconscious materials. Earlier we suggested that the system might be as old as the vision quest carried across the Pacific by Australians and American Indians. If ancient Asia began by testing her warriors and priests, civilized Asia has inherited from aeons of initiation an exquisite inquiry into the nature of mind and body, of a philosophical depth touched in the West only perhaps by advanced physics and abstract mathematics. Even if Reich and the chiropractors had not established a tradition of bodywork in the West, it would have arrived, eventually, from Asia.

The key point on which the Oriental and psychoanalytic systems agree, providing the ethos behind holistic health, is the requirement of working on one's exact mind and body impulses, of dealing with resistances, distortions, and distractions exactly and only as they come up in a life-style or a delegated practice. They are situational not prescriptive. As circumstances occur, they suggest their own solutions; but they must occur—they cannot be posited hypothetically. At any moment that something "important" does not occur, something else is happening, and this "something else" is the basis of the work. A preference for another situation, one not occurring, would only rigidify and delay the process. Trungpa says: "Situations are the voice of my guru."[5]

In Buddhist tradition, mind/body is very simply our most precise tool of knowledge. In seeing who we are, we see what everything else is. These are parallel processes. There are no facts outside of our existence as such, though certain externalities may distract us as if they were objective.

In standard Western terms, by contrast, the limitations and disorders of the mind/body are neither interesting nor a source of knowledge; they constitute an inconvenience and a burden. In that sense, we are in the way of our own experiment. The Buddhists would have it differently: we *are* the experiment. If we get distracted, we produce a temporary sideshow. The orthodox East, where it still exists, considers the entirety of technology and global civilization one such sideshow, a machinery that will be destroyed, inevitably, by the passage of worlds. It remains a trivial event beside the forces that control the universe, and it is not worth the attention of a liberated man.

Western medicine is a technological distraction, from the point of view of the yogi or the Buddhist healer. In their view, it is a message of the most trustworthy and elite lineage. Ancient Chinese tradition opposed surgery as violating the sacredness of the body, but this is no doubt a partial translation, for surgery also violates the sacredness of the mind. The blame or incidental cause for illness is irrelevant. Disease is an opportunity, not a condemnation. To get better superficially, without learning the accompanying lesson, is to be doomed to repeat the disease. Such improvement has no dignity and is never profound or complete.

We might say that the Oriental doctor trains his pupil to heal himself, but that is misleading, for, in many cases, he is not even a doctor. He trains him to tune his body to its finest degree of awareness and insight, as fine as cultural conditions allow. In the ideal situation, the disease is seen, through the clearness of mind/body, and the right adjustment is made; if necessary, herbs and needles may be used.

Self-healing requires pain, hence disease, as a focus. It sharpens the message and gives the system something exactly descriptive of itself to be conscious of. If the Oriental doctor is not a doctor, it is because he is almost an "antidoctor." Where there is no palpable disease, he creates the likeness of one. Tension is generated by forcing the body's limits. Where pain comes is where the difficulty prior to disease and unclarity resides. But the antidoctor does not seek suffering in and of itself; even though he may make his patients sick unto death, he is still a healer (we have all seen pictures of the emaciated but bright-eyed ascetics). Yoga is a preventative medicine, though the natives do not think of it this way. The patient is experiencing the difficulty of his own meaning beforehand so that it will be clear as it emerges. In the Gurdjieffian sense, he is the victim of "con-scions" suffering. *The Tibetan Book of the Dead* itself is a script, after all, of lifelong preparation for death.

A very sick person may suffer "needlessly" or even die before his time. But since these spiritual systems accept karma and reincarnation, the information learned will be invaluable in future lifetimes. It will protect the reborn personality against future disease, for the lesson of the fatal illness will be imprinted on the deathless part of the self. The mind that survives has nothing to do with conscious mind, or even unconscious mind, and certainly does not carry secular memory. Whatever this attitude says about life after death, in the meantime it directly affects the health of the person living it.

To believe in a purely East/West dichotomy is naïve and antiseptic. Distraction exists in the Eastern part of the Earth as much as in the West, and few in the East practice this extremely refined science (even as few Americans practice physics). It is not the issue here to figure out what populations practice this healing or if it is a significant demographic event. The ideas themselves have a profound planetary impact.

It is also important to see that Eastern mind/body work and psychotherapy diverge on at least one extremely important issue—not on spirit and body, which would find Reich and Jung on opposite sides and both with supporters in the East, but on the relationship of both spirit and body to emotion.

Reich gives his basic formula as the arousing of feeling, the full experience and integration of that feeling, the passage of it into neuromuscular rhythm, and the expression of that rhythm in orgasm, which then relieves blockages simultaneously in the organs and the character. Not all Asian systems agree on a formula, nor do they all reject the importance of orgasm. To them, it is simply one more event. Buddhism in particular teaches nonidentification with the emotions—not their unimportance but the greater value of transcending them and translating them into something objective, lasting, and sublime. Orgasm is not the major curative or culminative experience. But this does not mean evasion of the physical or that a nonphysical component of orgasm takes priority over its biological ramifications. It simply means that the sexual experience is translated into a different mind/body system and interpreted according to other rules. There are Taoist yoga and Hindu tantra practices that explicitly prescribe withholding sperm during intercourse so that "it" (i.e., the internal visualization and *chi* of it) can be driven back through the body as medicine and power. Both Reich and the Asians agree on the amount of energy contained in genitality and even on its usefulness in breaking down mental-corporeal stagnation. They disagree on the role of the emotions in translating that energy into medicine.

Trungpa gives the Eastern version: "If one actually feels the living quality, the texture of the emotions as they are in their naked state, then this experience . . . contains ultimate truth. And automatically one begins to see the simultaneously ironical and profound aspects of the emotions, as they are. Then the process of transmutation, that is, transmuting the emotions into wisdom, takes place automatically."[6]

For Reich, yoga and meditation were "diseases," not medicines. They were grotesque exaggerations of body armor. "The breathing technique taught by Yogas," he wrote, "is the exact opposite of the breathing technique we use to reactivate the vegetative emotional excitations in our patients. The aim of the Yoga breathing exercise is to combat affective impulses; its aim is to obtain peace." He went on to compare yoga to compulsive neurosis and to blame its spread to Europe and America on the fact that people "seek a means of gaining control over their natural vegetative impulses and at the same time of eliminating conditions of anxiety."[7]

Present-day holistic practitioners have integrated Reichian exercises with yoga, meditation, and Oriental martial arts to create new therapies for the balancing of mind, body, breath, and emotions. But Reich saw only the rigid outer face of yoga from across the Eurasian divide, and the pure lineage that follows from him allows no such rapprochement or synthesis.

The next element we shall consider is perhaps most important as the catalyst and glue of the new medicine: it is the political-ecological union which emerged from the 1960s, in part battered and in search of new goals, in part refined and toughened by its struggle and deepening its common denominators.

The radical ecology movement inevitably translated its concern for the biosphere to a reconsideration of the human body. Not only was man part of the biosphere, the part that perceived it ecologically; he was also the chief disrupter. Possibly, then, pollution and disruption were his own malignancy projected outward in a vicious circle which continued to make both him and the planet sicker. Sanity, an unpolluted body, a community in balance with the living world, and healthy people not only require each other, but also new foods, new understanding of natural cycles, and new medicines.

Bodywork merges with farming or farming gives rise to bodywork anew, a refined exercise which makes a better farmer and also a better organism to farm. Building homes and inhabiting bodies are parallel modes. Alternative sources of energy and alternatives to drugs suggest each other on every level. In fact, in many ways the oil industry, the drug industry, and agribusiness are the same conglomerate. Radical ecology proclaimed the importance of people being stewards of nature, and left-wing politics demanded a brotherhood of mankind based on economic and judicial equality. But all of these—the steward, the politico, and the warrior—require the "healthy mind in a healthy body".

These are not just mythic images. Radicals separate themselves from the prevailing culture so that they can move freely and create their own institutions. Inevitably, this leads to self-sufficient medicine, which contains within it a critique of the medical establishment. Furthermore, the health of people doing creative and revolutionary work is generally better than the health of people locked into society.

It would be a mistake, for instance, to see the homoeopathic revival in the Bay Area of Northern California as primarily the result of an interest in homoeopathic medicine and its principles. It represents at least as much a rebellion of younger radical doctors against the medical establishment. They may emphasize the failure of industrial medicine to deal with chronic disease, but they are equally concerned with its use for social control and for making enormous profits for the whole establishment, including the construction companies building the hospitals, the insurance companies, the drug monopoly, the medical bureaucracy, the schools, and the doctors themselves. Antibiotics, tranquilizers, hormones, and pain pills are not only superficial remedies, but they serve the interests of the prescribers more than the patients. They generate huge profits for the ruling and professional class, and they are also used to reduce the pain and anger of, and hence the danger from, the socially deprived, to palliate diseases arising from social ills, and to "jail" their victims.

These issues are so historically seminal to Bay Area homoeopathy that it is clear that homoeopathy itself was adopted as a means of furthering a revolution. Many of the doctors have less education in homoeopathy than in politics, and they trust this difficult and controversial system almost to the degree to which they distrust the establishment. As graduates of medical schools, they admit they don't have the slightest idea how the potencies work, but then, they claim, no one has the slightest idea how regular pharmacy works either.

This does not mean they are not credible homoeopaths also or that there are not many less political members of their group. It simply means that understanding the politics of the new homoeopathy is essential to an understanding of its revival as a holistic medicine.

This is what distinguishes the homoeopaths from liberal doctors who bring health care to the poor. The latter may find the new health maintenance systems, such as the Kaiser Foundation Health Plan, radical and progressive; they may also favor national health care. The former see such systems as assembly-line medicine, absurdly unequipped to deal with deep chronic disease, and in fact productive of new chronic disease. Their alienation is deeper, hence their solution more radical.

In general, new medicine spawns a life-style which stands against the luxuries and palliatives of modern materialism. This made it attractive to the veterans of sixties' left-wing politics, who then radicalized the new medicine. As it became clear that it was impossible to overthrow the system and that the system had gotten into one's guts and cells, the important thing became to change one's self, to make one's self into a new person, an actual revolutionary who purges the somatic-psychic fact of having been born and raised in the belly of the giant. Unless we change, they thought, we are doomed to repeat the thing *they* have made, for we are their children and their successors and have no knowledge or training otherwise. The failure of so many of the sixties' communes and cadres is exactly their failure to practice a healing discipline. Ultimately, the ancient and famous unconscious and the internal poisons expressed themselves. No matter how strong their communal ideology, it was transformed from within into something either alienating or deadly.

Very early on, emerging from a twenty-day fast, the comedian Dick Gregory said: "They control us by the food we eat. We must stop."

The new medicine has developed its own political base in the 1970s, having found the perfect mirror of the Vietnam-era Pentagon and military-industrial complex in the medical establishment. Other politicos have gone into radical agriculture as their own transition from political ideology to seminal action. The New Alchemy Institutc scientists were political radicals before they were agricultural radicals. They changed from being scientists protesting against corporate America to scientists living out a different possibility. Of course, not all activists became farmers and healers, but much of the essential idealist and utopian thrust of that movement and that epoch has been captured in the momentum of this one. If the 1960s provided some of the images, in mythological form, of a new world, then the 1970s, in a sense, have provided many of the tools and disciplines for realizing a small part of that. The sixties bit off the whole nation and then the whole cosmos, which was more than it could handle; obviously the United States would not reverse world history or the history of consciousness. But it provided forms and images, and they have not been lost. The models have been criticized, found wanting, etc., and some of them have ended in dismal failure, as the holocaust at Jonestown showed. It was certainly the first and most devastating statement on the largeness of failure in the sixties, for we learned that ungrounded rhetoric can lead to anything, even the opposite of its stated goals, that pacificism can lead to brutality and murder as long as it is only a word and the American body remains.

But healing and farming have tended to take on the small piece of that cosmic vision that can work, and for many involved in the transition, it seems natural and smooth enough. It does not seem as though a great era was necessarily lost in its own shadows and hallucinogens.

In Western as well as Eastern tradition, healing has a long occult lineage. Ritual magic provides the form in which ceremonial healing occurs. In a sense, the Western occult is a continuation of the visualization of inner meaning and forces from the preliterate world of shamanism and spirits. Alchemy and homoeopathy are themselves one in Paracelsus, and astrology and herbalism join in the astrological botany of ancient and mediaeval times. Today astrology has merged with several psychoanalytic methodologies of character reading to produce new modes of interpretation. Sufi and Christian mysticisms are also healing sciences, a fact which shows up strongly in the Rosicrucian churches from the seventeenth century on as well as in the more vernacular faith healing of Mary Baker Eddy, or, currently, Oral Roberts and Rex Humbard.

But occult medicine is also dangerously authoritarian. It requires faith and discipline and will often worship any leader who seems to have contact with the spirits or gods. This is why so many are led to satanic cults or their own destruction. Once they are committed to an individual as a link, they must follow, and this is true equally in tribal Africa, South America, and the theosophical churches of Los Angeles and Detroit. All charismatic healers are susceptible to the fact that healing has been the tool of hierarchical, nonhumanist, and nonprogressive traditions; at the moment the healer loses interest in his patients, they merely serve to aggrandize him and increase his power. "Brainwashing" is a catchword for this process nowadays, and it is employed by faith healers, psychiatrists, and cult leaders, even as it has been by secret police, military, or by Hitler before and during .World War II. The possible corruptions of healing are limitless, and we must live with them as long as we require this radical insight into our lives, as long as we maintain this willingness to internalize unknown materials and change who we are. This is the present risk.

Occult medicine, it should not be forgotten, has a strong mainstream tradition quite different from its uses in holistic health. Faith healing has some of the same Christian sources as alchemy and homoeopathy. As old as mankind, it is an incredibly dominant Mid-American tradition. Far more people are affected by just one Billy Graham crusade than perhaps are involved in somatic therapy and holistic health. The latter remain essentially upper-class practices in America, with strong regional concentrations among educated people in urban areas in California and the Northeast. Faith healing literally awakens the mute masses and calls out something deep and silent in them. It is shamanism on a mass scale. But it would be wrong to think that the healing done in the name of Jesus is competing with the new-age medicine and its own communal gatherings and festivals. These are different faces of the same mystery. We have called it "planet medicine" in this book. It is reassuring, perhaps, that Ruth Carter Stapleton can visit the Berkeley Holistic Health Center and perform her Christian faith healing there in absolute harmony with a celestial rainbow healing evening and a *t'ai chi* class. Likewise, along another long dormant line of contact (Georgia to Africa), her brother Jimmy Carter, President of the United States, can appeal to the Black African continent on the basis of the atheism of the Soviets. At the bottom line, this means the spirit church, the voodoo church, the Church of Africa and the Mississippi, which is also the Rosicrucian Church of Bohemia and California, or the joined traditions of Rudolf Steiner, Wilhelm Reich, and Carl Jung. There is an optimism in this, even if it is presently no more than a mythic allusion to a legendary time. It *is* the healing tradition of a planet whose military tradition is all too well known.

What we are finally face to face with is a movement made powerful by the fundamental ideological divergence of its separate tributary streams. As incredible as it might have seemed once upon a time, the political activists and the spiritualists have joined on a common path: the radical ecology movement gave them a joint platform. Preservation of the environment has the same spiritual as political meaning. Health is the basis of the new Marxist man or the new Buddhist-Christian man—health and sanity. But, at the same time, this movement includes the most Fundamentalist traditions of Bible-reading America, the revivalist and millenarian churches of the urban ghettos, and the echoes of the shamans and medicine men of dying cultures. This is potentially a powerful alliance. But it still must come down out of the clouds.

It can also be the road to death, as the Reverend James Jones showed a disbelieving world. He showed that there is a road from the urban slums of Indiana to the communes of Northern California to the joint Marxist-Jesus revival church to the jungles of South America, a road which cannot be taken straight from Indianapolis to Guyana. His journey was overcome by the death forces of the sixties: paranoia, drugs, righteousness, and apocalypticism. But he showed the road.

The merging of these worlds—spiritual and political, native and Western, mute and wise—is tribal and incipiently Third World at its core. No wonder New Left people were willing to abandon their own rhetoric for the revival language of those dispossessed people with whom they most identified. It happens in the reggae music and jazz, which has become part of the New Left, but also the New Medicine underground. Here the shaman and voodoo master are not far from the doctor and politician, not far at all. The revolutionary spirit might still have more of the jungle and the Snake Dance in it than Russian and Chinese bureaucracies will allow. Is this the America that Jimmy Carter unknowingly wooed Africa with?

When people notice the new medicine movement now and are surprised at its swift rise and sudden popularity, they must not overlook that it is the fruition of much that was going on for a long time. It is a single common rallying point now. But its potential is barely yet realized. It *is* dynamite, for it challenges the principles of government and the principles of science too, and it holds the seeds of new values that might actually not be the old values in new clothing. It is not simply another tyrant awaiting the convenient overthrow of the present regime.

XX

The Political and Spiritual Basis of Medicine

Medicine has no meaning. That is, medicine cannot supply the missing meaning or direction to a life. Cure more defines the system to which it is being applied than it does its own content. It can increase freedom, awareness, motility, feeling, but it cannot replace the life; it cannot live the life for the person.

Many people involved in the new medicine look to it for answers it cannot provide. They assume that something has become wrong in them or was always wrong and that a radical treatment will correct it. They will get "better" always. They will become the correction instead of who they were or are. There are holistic health junkies who go from treatment to treatment, looking for the one that has the special insight and power to recognize them and to intercede in their behalf. But this very activity is alienating and off-center. The search for a cure becomes the symptom of another illness, and the longer the quest goes on, the less chance there is the person will regain his own necessity. Even the best healers and gurus run the risk of habituating their disciples to the cure and themselves to the system. Failure to recognize this then becomes part of the disease.

Especially in California, enlightened M.D.'s who feel stale and alienated try to get in touch with the new music without a sense of the real difficulty. Some adapt versions of acupuncture, chiropractic, homoeopathy, and macrobiotics into their general practices. Some regularly attend holistic health meetings as authorities and give papers on "wellness," biofeedback, biodynamic nutrition, life after death, and the cosmic healing energy of swamis and gurus. The worst of them are as enamored with the language and imagery as they would with being physicians to famous athletic teams or rock groups. They are trapped by the compulsion of hipness and fashion.

There is a holistic health elite whose main and unfortunate contribution has been the promotion of "superhealth"—the all-feeling, self-healing, responsive human being. These doctors preach a mixture of religion, life-style, health, exercise, and charisma. They discuss powerful natural healing agents and oneness with the cosmos, and these are alluring products to have presented by those with scientific background and training.

Not all holistic health practitioners fall into this stereotype; in fact, it is fully realized in only rare cases. But the ghost of this person hides behind many people, representing the guise that exploitation takes on in the new medicine, even as it takes on a different guise in the traditional AMA. We can paint the caricature—he is compact, California brown, with leather pants, sometimes suggesting Charles Atlas in the presentation of his build, but with an occult (astrological or Tibetan) medallion hanging in his chest hair and the classic holistic health smile. He jogs, does *aikido*, enjoys teaching women how to improve their orgasms. He looks as though ancient wisdom has come through all of history to visit him, which is a common "born yesterday" New Age fantasy. In battle with mainstream colleagues, he will go quickly to his training in physiology and the "hard" sciences if pressed. There is also an exaggerated feminine expression of cosmic ripeness.

Another danger is the professional who adopts some version of holistic health as his own solution to a mid-life crisis; he begins practicing homoeopathy, kinesiology, or visualization with no more training in them than an average educated person would have in surgery from reading a few books and attending public lectures. He is legally entitled to practice, whereas the person whose lecture inspired him may well lack the necessary credentials. Bad homoeopathy and kinesiology from an M.D. is as risky as any street medicine.

Patients develop equal inflations. In seeking their own holism, they can become solipsistic and righteous, unconsciously. While maintaining a surface image of holism, they break with their own culture and thus distort unity on another level. Losing a sense of appropriateness and interaction with other people, they begin acting like a medicine, which is really like a disease.

The victim of disease is blamed and even taunted for it. After all, holism says that the fiber and quality of the life is reflected in the body and the mind. Nowadays cancer is spoken of as retribution in some circles, as archetypal disease, the cells themselves picking up the nihilism of the person, rebelling and going crazy, punishing the failure of faith or belief with disease. Once again, this is the authoritarian face showing through.

It is not so simple a matter as that. Whereas the Jungian tradition rightly indicates that disease is destiny and is not arbitrary or meaningless in terms of the life of the organism, it is also true that much of this happens on such a deep and unconscious level that no one but the most enlightened saint or yogi could possibly control his absolute health and destiny, and these can only for a period of time before they too submit to natural law and decay.

The trouble with all this new insight and holistic cure is that it is too good to be true, and terribly misleading. It has nothing to do with the lives most people lead, so many end up chasing the impossible promotional image itself and get very far from what it is to experience themselves. They end up preferring the imported decorative images of enlightenment to their own souls. Carl Jung diagnosed this in 1929:

"One cannot be too cautious in these matters, for what with the imitative urge and a positively morbid avidity to possess themselves of outlandish feathers and deck themselves out in this exotic plumage, far too many people are misled into snatching at such 'magical' ideas and applying them externally, like an ointment. People will do anything, no matter how absurd, in order to avoid facing their own souls. They will practise Indian yoga and all its exercises, observe a strict regimen of diet, learn theosophy by heart, or mechanically repeat mystic texts from the literature of the whole world—all because they cannot get on with themselves and have not the slightest faith that anything useful could ever come out of *their* souls. Thus the soul has gradually been turned into a Nazareth from which nothing good can come. Therefore let us fetch it from the four corners of the earth—the more far-fetched and bizarre it is the better! . . . Were it so, then God had made a sorry job of creation, and it were high time for us to go over to Marcion the Gnostic and depose the incompetent demiurge. . . . But man is worth the pains he takes with himself, and he has something in his own soul that can grow."[1]

Something new *has* been emerging, from within our individual and collective souls—but it is different from entire holistic health movement. It is both more and less—potentially more but presently less. There are two movements—the true political medicinal revolution and the one in flight from it which borrows its symbols and tries to masquerade as the same thing. The true one comes from within our historic process, and *is* our historical realization. The other seeks to enlist every passing stranger and foreign official, in hopes of postponing any real change. So close together are these two that for a moment now they seem to merge and unfold together.

One radical therapist tells the story of leading a breathing exercise during which a man suddenly crawled onto a young woman who had recently given birth and tried to suckle her. When she pushed him off and struck him, he shouted, "Bitch!" as if *she* had violated the terms of the exercise. Then he added, as if in explanation, "I'm expressing myself."

And the therapist suddenly wondered, "What are we teaching these people? What kind of a world are we telling them this is?"[2]

That moment, made up collectively of hundreds of such moments, now hangs over the whole Western world, like a wave—the idea that there is no planet, no history, no context, only the elusive search by individuals for their inner psychic power and lost lives. Among the masses it becomes the unabated (and unabatable) appetite for materials and goods that will somehow confirm their own flimsy existence. One does not have to accept the whole message of the Russian exiles to understand they are telling the truth when they say: "There is a world out there, and it's got teeth." The historical situation in which we find ourselves is real and cannot be replaced by an imaginary asylum, or even by a distracting greed.

One gets nowhere simply lying on the floor pounding and breathing more freely or escaping on a science fiction journey through the silver needles of the Yellow Emperor. Each episode comes to an end, and the same issues in the world prevail. Otherwise, we have lost the meaning of being born.

After the healing, deep-sea divers return to the sea; musicians return to their music; philosophers go back to language and reality. As Werner Erhard, L. Ron Hubbard, and other "human potential" business people have proven, money-makers continue to make money—more money. A medicine can be proposed around any process and play into a variety of possible meanings. The same skeletal adjustment can lead to quiescence in one person and aggression in another. Healing can also be martial, as *t'ai chi* and *aikido*. Assertiveness training, looking out for *Numero Uno*, etc., are merely some of the present-day cut-rate versions. The equivalent of such training has gone on for decades—in fact, for millennia—in the corporate academies and the "schools" that preceded them. Only it was not called "medicine." Business success has always been an episode of shamanism and self-cure.

At exactly that point where bodywork, yoga, and medicine come together, the human being cannot be understood only as an abstract physical system to which a corrective measure is applied. What is at stake is the life, the quality of life lived—a point easily missed when "cure" is emphasized. What good is the cure if the person cannot use it and the life ends in darkness and obscurity anyway?

It is a subtle, even evasive point at which the healer works both toward curing the disease and giving the patient the lesson *from* the disease. Native healing, as we have seen, cultivated this at the expense of high percentage first aid. We have lost and are forced to regain that meaning in our own medicine complex because in our time society has become mechanical and nihilistic, and there is no meaning as such which sustains the exact tilt of any one disease.

The writing of this book is a small act of coming to awareness, like turning within sleep to an unvisited level of dream. When the roads are flooded, the citizens call a town meeting and discuss the problem. The discussion itself will repair nothing; still, it is necessary.

We now require such a discussion in our culture at large. We cannot skip this stage of awareness or we will cure the wrong things. In this century, in our haste, we have cured many wrong things. And it has left us with a science establishment and a government that are out of touch with both history and disease.

The arguments in our culture about what constitutes actual death and when to stop trying to save someone when they do not want to be saved are telling indications of the dilemma. When we don't know why we are alive and have bodies, nor how to inhabit them harmoniously, we put the issue to every desperate test. At the same time, we stand stupefied before legalistic and problematic definitions of things we must ultimately know from the inside if we are to know them at all.

It is as though people try only partially to be healed, only partially to be alive. The dichotomy becomes: now I do this/now I am me. When they are being cured of something, they withhold their more sophisticated part, making the experience as if a cure of someone else to whom they have special access. The ultimate hope, though, is that knowledge from being, from the flesh and bones, the nerves and meridians, can enter into our science and philosophy and change them, and society with it. This cannot happen as long as we talk about "therapy" and "holistic health" and "alternative medicine" rather than the thing they are: a revolution of those who lie deeper and more oppressed than the workers or the peasants—those actual beings whom previous decades got away with naming "peasants" and "workers," selling them to themselves that way and thus consigning them to the revolution—to *that* revolution, which now swaggers toward the hinter edge of its century, as Russia and Cambodia, just as unaligned, the dispossessed just as exploited as before.

In his discussions of alienation and economic structures, Marx raised real medical issues. Reich and Marx form a possible unity: hygiene and revolution require and nurture each other. Politics *is* medicine, but medicine is also politics—a thing many of the new healers have still to learn. The claims by some doctors that their patients do not want to go back into society because society is sick and they are now well is a miscarriage of historical process. It may sell out currently in California, and, for all we know, the children of the oil-producing nations may buy it next, but it means nothing in terms of Blake, or Whitehead, or Marx, or Mao. And these are finally where we are too, if we are anywhere.

In the words of one therapist: "Having a sixty-year-old man run around in diapers crying may have therapeutic significance, but as a statement on the human condition, it's fucked."[3]

In our emphasis on hidden process and the unconscious mind, we have forgotten consciousness, where our lives and selves as we know them occur. It is at least partially in the conscious mind that systems of medicine form and the doctors do their diagnoses. It is in the conscious mind that will is sparked and a decision to get better is initiated. The discipline required by the most powerful societies of ritual magic and healing should suggest to us that the conscious mind has a required role in this affair.

As a long-term healing method, *t'ai chi* realigns and softens the body so that *chi* energy can flow through its pathways. The exercises, by necessity, begin at whatever point the person beginning them is. They are repeated thousands of times, tens of thousands of times, day after day, for years, and finally for a lifetime. The new student is told, in effect, to practice. There is nothing the teacher can do to help since he cannot do *t'ai chi for* another person any more than he can eat or sleep for him. All he can do is demonstrate and correct, demonstrate and correct. At some quite early point, the student runs into extreme difficulty; he finds it painful to move through the positions in the correct manner, so he adjusts to take strain off his weaker areas. The teacher corrects this, and ultimately the student is asked to correct it himself, to learn to observe when one part of his body tightens to allow another part to carry out a movement. The corrections are painful and exhausting, but the goal is to move as a whole, according to principle, despite the pain. This can happen only if the student is willing to keep his attention on the correctness of the moves.

There is a relationship between conscious will and internal intelligence. One must suffer in the end, either in directing his attention under difficult circumstances or in having his life changed by the redirection of attention out of altered unconsciousness after being healed passively. Systems which involve direct suffering allow a person to participate consciously in his life changes and to learn things about the nature of himself in the world. Such bringing to consciousness is one of the clearest things life *is.* In his spiritual school in France, Gurdjieff hung aphorisms on the walls of the Study House, including:

"The worse the conditions of life, the more productive the work—always provided you remember the work."[4]

"Only conscious suffering has any sense."[5]

We are reminded of the moment in Jean Cocteau's *Orphée*, where Death and her helper Heurtebise struggle to force time backward in order to undo their damage. Heurtebise screams that it is impossible, as the invisible wind ripples his hair and every muscle strains. They lean back against the events and force the film to unravel to its beginning. Death continues to shout at him, urging him to use his will, reminding him, "Without our wills, we are cripples."

Medicine has long known that the organism must want to get well in order to get well; it must want to live in order to live. The wanting goes to the core of one's existential being and has little to do with surficial greed for life. It also does not mean that all diseases are finally curable if the patient wants to live. It means that the medicine itself is not the final court; the individual is. The medicine sets into action the healing force and reminds the body of its implicit desire to be well (the same desire that originally led it to *be* at all). As we have seen, this must be a single message and not a mixed message; it must be a specific unignorable shot. The body core knows how to resist mixed messages.

An irritation can be more compassionate than a salve when it is more definite and communicative. It is brief, swift, and precise, like the ideal homoeopathic remedy. Acupuncture uses a needle, and it is no accident the needle is as sharp and fine as a filament. The bioenergetic therapist seizes the patient's compulsion and fear and exacerbates, recognizes it. Nurturing is necessary too, but in the context of a hard truth. After all, an organism can be irritated into exhaustion or terror unless there is something in the irritation to which it can respond positively.

A change in bodily attention is then communicated back to the will to express itself in the life of the person. It may not be recognized as coming from the medicine, but the mind—sweeping back and forth across its accustomed territory—seems to come up with new ideas.

Discussions about whether a person wants to get well are doomed to go around in circles, for wanting and not wanting can be indistinguishable ploys of the self. Not wanting to get well is itself part of the disease, and it is also the irritant behind the cure.

During his seminar in Vermont in 1977, Theodore Enslin was questioned along these lines when someone raised the issue of the relative importance of symptoms in homoeopathy, implying that the wish not to get well *must* be a more significant symptom than calluses on an elbow.[6] Enslin objected:

"If you're really going to get into homoeopathic thinking, you have to erase those artificial boundaries—that thought is different from a hangnail. It's not. It's a manifestation of you. I've always loved that story about the guy who went to [Charles Godlove] Raue, who was one of the Philadelphia school, a really very eminent homoeopath. And he was an old man. He had many many things wrong with him. He had gout. He had prostatitis. And he had loose teeth. And he had all these things. So Raue gave him a pill. He said,

'Well, now, is this for my gout?, or is it for my loose teeth?' and so
on. And Raue finally said, 'Your name is Miller, isn't it?' If you were
really going to be a good homoeopathic patient, there wouldn't have
to be any more discussion. You simply realize *it's all one thing*. You
cannot consider one ailment or another. You have a burn on your
arm which doesn't heal. The aim of usual medicine is to clear that
one spot. Cure it. Fight it. Homoeopathically, we don't think that
way; we think about the whole organism. Because there is that one
disease manifestation, there is an indication that the entire organism
is diseased and you've got to treat it that way."

"But still," the questioner persisted, "isn't not really wanting to
get better such a basic and serious symptom that one won't even
seek out a doctor in the first place? How do you overcome *that?*"

"Well, that is a personal decision," Enslin replied. "There *are* certain medicines that can bring you to the place where you *do* want to.
But sometimes not. Some so-called failures of treatment can simply
be traced to a personal resistance."

"But then isn't a personal resistance just another symptom?"

"Yes it is. Yes it is. Of course we're always looking for the miracle
that will cure us of everything. I don't think that homoeopathy or
very much of anything else will ever do that for us. And when people
weren't talking about psychosomatic disease, Hahnemann himself
was the first one, by saying, yes, the mental symptoms are equally
important. But they are sometimes hard to deal with. You get to the
point of Kent and the mental symptoms are more important than
anything else. I think he got to the place where perhaps he *overem-
phasized* them. He did because there was absolutely no support for
them anywhere. I mean there *is* a balance. The thing that we really
need to do, the thing that more than anything else can get over that
kind of resistance, is simply the admission that there is no difference
between any kind of symptom and any other. The old division of
mind and body—with all our philosophizing about it—means we still
think we are superior to the animals, we still think that somehow our
thinking brain is going to bail us out."

He paused for a moment and then continued:

"You asked in our earlier talk: 'Would you say we are, as a race,
diseased?' I would say, 'Yes, we certainly are.' Because we place an
emphasis on something which has nothing to do with what makes us
move. We think—we *think*—this is the problem."

The questioner proceeded: "Whose chances of cure are greater:

the person who wants to get better but doesn't take a homoeopathic medicine or the person who doesn't want to get better but has the right medicine prescribed for him?"

"Well, the chances of cure without a homoeopathic medicine are far greater than without a feeling that one wants to be cured. I mean there are many instances of the whole placebo thing. A person is convinced that this *will* do it, and he *really* wants to be cured: therefore he *is* cured! That, in a sense, is a homoeopathic high potency. It is a strong enough wish in the person to outrage the system to the point where it will cure itself, which is the principle behind all of this."

"But where does the resistance to being well come from in the first place? How do we get to the bottom of it?"

"There is a direction to your repeated question. You're hammering at this one particular thing. But you see, in doing that, you're actually doing what we all do when we depend upon our thinking processes. It's a very difficult thing, because somehow we're going to have to do it in reverse if we're ever going to get to the place where all of these things are in balance. But there are places where probably this is the wrong direction to take—if you really want to know. If you really want to know, don't want to know! I mean, enlightenment never comes if someone wants to be enlightened."

This recalls a curious moment in the history of medicine and philosophy. The wish to be cured *does* locate in the will, but it is not the conscious self-expressed will we understand in language; it is the real inner will of the body, the It. The conscious will must, at some point, work counter to literal intention, to itself, in order to incorporate the "meaning" of the deeper will. The way a person expresses to himself that he wants to get well may in fact be the way to stay sick. One thing is clear: the ambition is not the desire; the ambition is the disease. So the person must suddenly discover how *not* to want to be well (which is certainly not the same as wanting not to be well).

Enslin continued:

"I think the only real problem and the only real resistance to this whole way of thinking is this refusal to admit that there are no divisions. You can sit and talk philosophically about it, and it's very popular to do that. You can talk about a holistic universe and so forth and so on, but we don't *think* that way. If we started to do that, probably there would be far less disease. And homoeopathy or any other specialty would fade away. You wouldn't need this particular way of looking at things because everything was looked at in the same way."

"What would our lives be like if we did think in that way?"

"I have no idea. It would seem to me, from every indication that I've had personally, simply looking at animals, trees, or anything else, that it would be far easier to do things that we really want to do, or say we want to do. We have simply forgotten. We think. We think we are the masters. We forget that we aren't any more important than a raccoon. We think of *our* lives, the preciousness of *our* life. Even a man like Schweitzer: he is a humanitarian, but he is not a totalitarian—the reverence for life; but there is always the feeling, 'human life—this is more important.' If we could just drop this, maybe we wouldn't have to go through this backward trip through the labyrinth to get to where we could really function."

"Well, we can say we're going to do that. We can theorize it—"

"Don't theorize it. Do it! Of course it's impossible: therefore do it."

Once we drop the idea of medicine and think instead of wanting to be well, wanting to live, it becomes clear that everything is a medicine, a realization we have come to at many points of this book.

People say: "That woman is my medicine." "My work is my medicine." "Dancing is a medicine." "Rock and roll is a medicine."

Interviewed on TV, the rock singer Bruce Springsteen said: "When I was a kid, rock and roll was the only thing that always came through. It was the only thing that never let me down. Now I can't let those kids out there down. I let them down and I let myself down."

It is the same for the Cherokee chanter. He grew up hearing the voices. They were his medicine. They delivered him into life. Now he is their voice.

Not a medicine? Watch how the audience responds rhythmically, expressing an inner pulse and emerging feeling. Not a doctor? Watch how the wave emanates from him and how he leads them through the exegesis, the riff.

When people live for something, that thing becomes engaged with their psychic and physical process. The will to live may not be expressed as that directly, but it is expressed through love or an art form. When disease is encountered, it is transmuted through the event. The more complex and true to the heart a dance or painting or religious ceremony, the more access it gives the artist to the depths of his or her own being. But we must not have the illusion that these visions are imposed on people, like visitors from the beyond. Rock and roll and abstract expressionism arise from the very fact of human life in the biosphere. They express the direction and the yearning of that life, the satisfaction of its biological and spiritual core. That is why they are so effective in melting and transforming the difficulties people bring to them.

The artist, whether he knows it or not, works side by side with his health. The development of a style and work, initially in youth, becomes part of his maintenance system. It works on a level prior to division, hence prior to medicine. The inspirational moments in an artist's work, as well as the great plunges into the depths, are entanglements with the roots, where the seeds of being are. Inspiration is literally breath.

Sometimes these plunges stir up material that the artist cannot deal with; many have lost their health in their work, too—Vincent van Gogh and William Faulkner are examples. But if they can learn to transform those seeds in their raw primary form, they can enact a cure prior to the disease. The language of poetry is so valuable exactly because it is the language of the self. The dance, if done authentically, is the dance of the self. This is the real burden of authenticity in art.

Moby Dick was Melville's cure, given how sick he was writing it and the calm that came upon his life afterward. *Pierre*, his next novel, reads as the sweating off of a profound disease in its last vestiges. Laura Dean's dance of spirals, performed in 1978 in New York, shares features with the complicated color and positional code of the Navaho sand-painting ritual; they are both attempts at psychosomatic objectification. Why shouldn't they contain the same sort of incipient healing possibility? It is the dancers as organisms that matter, not the publicity of the forms. Cecil Taylor's music is an old African medicine, a theme Pharaoh Saunders makes explicit by naming one whole tune *Healing Song*. Art and politics are as old as medicine—why not as primary? Why are not all three overseers and handmaidens of our creation?

Occasionally, art as medicine is admitted explicitly. Stan Brakhage, the experimental film maker, spoke of his early films as medicines for his asthma because of the way in which they taught him to breathe in visual rhythms and put breath into the visualized landscape.[7] The

poet Robert Kelly has long considered the breathing in poetic syntax
a means of bringing hormonal and metabolic rhythms into the self-
curative urgency of the organism.[8] Art, through being a way to live,
enters the primary dialogue between the self and its underlying intelligence. Dr. William Carlos Williams writes:

> My heart rouses
>   thinking to bring you news
>   of something
> that concerns you
>   and concerns many men. Look at
>   what passes for the new.
> You will not find it there but in
>   despised poems.
>   It is difficult
> to get the news from poems
>   yet men die miserably every day
>   for lack
> of what is found there.[9]

It is, literally, "my *heart* rouses," not the mind and not the voice,
which later give it shape.

In that sense, art is our natural folk medicine. Young street artists
each pick up a tradition and a style. In tracing origins through learning the skills, the trade, they are taken more deeply into their own
origins. It need not be highly literate art; in fact, it rarely is. "Satur-
day Night Fever" is both the medicine and the disease for which it is
the cure. Nothing but disco can carry these dancers into a sense of
their desires, unshaped personalities, and potential for absolute freedom. In the dance, they are alive. Outside of it, they are inert,
trapped.

Native society invites this spirit regularly to its ceremonies, but it
has been taken away in the transition to civilization. So we are in a
position of having to recover the performance which is also a ceremony and a medicine. Current forms of experimental theater are
working toward this original authenticity. Some dancers use the
dance to recover lost and unconscious forms of human movement.
Their patterns are far more fragmentary than those in conventional
dance, but they also reach a different level of mind/body consciousness. Joanne Kelly, Carolee Schneeman, and Yvonne Rainer do
healing dances, each in her own way. Meredith Monk has integrated

shaman voices of the American Indian Southwest into her perform-
ances; these may not invoke the same things in her audience that
they do in the native circumstance, but they could be the beginning
of a different curative mode. It is through improvisation and "crazy
wisdom," to use the Tibetan-Americans' translation of their own ancient name for it, that we change as a culture, that suffocating modes
are replaced by dangerous new styles of being, breathing, and
moving.

It is no accident then that the new medicine is so closely associated with the arts; its public fairs include music, dancing, poetry,
and ceremony, and many of its practitioners are also artists.

As the boundaries between medicine, healing, artistic expression,
political action, praying, and teaching break down, new forms and
institutions begin to emerge to replace old ones that have failed us.
At a time like this, healing and medicine become the forerunners of
other changes, for they call our attention to the flesh and spirit we
are living out. They give us the simultaneous cue of "cure" and
"change."

This book is timely not because medicine has become such a hotly
discussed topic. It is timely because, through the new approaches to
healing, we have begun to see where we fall on a planetary scale and
where the current epoch comes in world history. The book ends,
rightly, at the moment when medicine returns us to our own inevitability.

The Present State of Holistic Health:
How to Choose a Healer

In this book we have come to see medicine as a flux of practical techniques, remedy provings, scientific experiments, and ancient symbols. It is a cul de sac but also an infinitude, for there is nothing in the cosmos that is not an aspect of a disease, that is not potentially a medicine too. Only our clarities and distortions determine what each thing will become.

The dynamic interplay of primal energies does not respect categorical boundaries. How we behave and how we treat the other entities on this world affect relative disease and health. Peasant ailments run banshee from the village doctor into the hills, and they return armed as revolutionaries. If they were deeply sick, the illness is transformed by a new possession; but it is not cured, for history presents merely a succession of diseases. They sit behind corporate desks, dealing out lives and deaths more mundanely than any surgeon. Their medicines also abound on any city street—images, colors, vibrations, people, feelings, unknown substances that are part of every impression and breath.

It is certainly true that until all living things are healthy, no living thing can be healthy. That is the inevitable proviso of a Freudian-Marxist dialectic. Now communist and capitalist nations prove that pure ideology is bankrupt and that labor cannot be abstracted from the hidden desires and violence of mankind. The law of yin and yang assures that alcoholism, whale slaughter, and global industrialism are shades of the same materiality, rhythms within a single current. Poisonous urban sprawls and military machines mark the absence of vitality. Like the capacity to kill without compassion, these are symptoms of powers suppressed and distorted, not powers achieved. Gangs of juveniles preying on the old in the cities and derelicts lying on the pavement are specific eruptions of collective diseases. But within the planet's homeostasis they are also statements of relative health, for as long as there is a vital force left, we will not see the disease, we will see only our desperate stands against its ravages. This is what punk ritualized decadence must also reflect: our natural resistance (so close is the malady now to the heart). To become the disease is, esoterically, to attack the disease. This remedy may well not cure the single junkie or gang-member, but its vibration will fan out to the society at large.

Our dilemma is that all of these processes are latent, interwoven, interdependent, while other forces that do not share our consciousness or its goals weave about us. The parapsychologist Jule Eisenbud has mentioned on a number of occasions the possibility that thought can injure and kill—but nowhere as dramatically and eloquently as in his recent book *Paranormal Foreknowledge*.[1] Given the violence we carry out routinely toward one another and with "mere" external tools, and given our unadmitted psychokinetic power, is it any wonder, asks Eisenbud, that our death wishes may be collectively more pathogenic than all the germs on the Earth? Our responsibility for this ongoing murder, erupting in plane crashes and heart attacks, may be the primal guilt which Freud displaced onto the Oedipal event because he could not acknowledge the full impact of mind on matter. We may still doubt the evidence and the interpretation, but Eisenbud is speaking from fifty years of research and against his own likings (". . . . a vital part of me rejects the whole as pure nonsense.").[2]

There is clearly something there—dangerous and unfathomable— whether it is this factor or another. Eisenbud's paradigm at least alerts us that there is an intruder in the house. The creative energies assigned to *chakras*, auras, meridians, and thought-waves throughout history may have their negative counterparts in curses and "evil eyes." We cannot begin to diagnose a plague that the primitive shamans were thousands of times closer to than we, and it is a joke to think we can cure such disease without returning to the origin. We cannot even tell when our own headaches begin: at the moment the first symptoms are perceptible the condition is already irreversible. When the poisons start to eke out, the poisons have also already been made. To "banish" them with distractions is to waste our time and delude ourselves. Imagine—those who cite "a clear and present danger" think that by arming ourselves with nuclear weapons aimed at the Russians we could become safer! Not when the elemental forces of voodoo still rule this world.

"It may be one of the most tragic paradoxes of history," writes Eisenbud, "that throughout the tortuous course of what is somewhat charitably referred to as 'the ascent of man,' the repudiation of such an aim (the 'destruction of the enemy,' to use the utterly emotionless military abstraction) in the ordinary transactions of everyday life has led to a never-ending assault on an omnipresent and protean enemy-by-proxy on a scale that would have been unimaginable to the primitive."[3]

In one of our imagined ideal medicines of the future, doctors will treat how the nation is ruled as well as its rulers, and how goods are transferred as well as the buyers and sellers, but they will not be called doctors, and there will also be no politicians or police in the present sense. "Polis" will stand as a synthesis of justice, production, and healing. Doctors may be artists and inventors, but this work will not be distinguished from medicine. They may also be senators and corporate directors, but they will still be philosopher-scientists. Confucians and present-day disciples of the Yellow Emperor may insist that such a "polis" has already been, in Atlantis or Old China, and we have destroyed it, and continue to destroy its fragments today;[4] but this must not be true or we would not be in such disharmony; we would not have inherited millennia of war. In any case, we have only the present Earth to work from. And perhaps our idea is only a sentimental expression of the miasm of this age, and such a society will never come.

The "mean streets" and warfare in Central American villages may be one current of the contemporary toxin, but the future doctor is also slowly being born. He calls our attention now to the potential epidemic of nuclear war. Even if this is only a statement of his inability to treat the concrete medical consequences or to deal with human life in the aftermath of collective suicide (and not at all a critical review of the contribution of his profession to mankind's need for such weaponry), the mere fact of his recognizing the "larger medicine," the healing that transcends political categories, is a seed of the new medicine.

Doctors like yogis must begin to treat the nuclear weapons within us, the internalized war from which the external armaments come. It does not mean abandoning science, as critics of the spiritual disciplines fear; it does not portend a return to magic. It would be no more or less than an enlargement of science to include all its faces, inward and out. The mindfulness and bare attention of the Buddhist monk and the receptivity to archetypal symbols of the analytical psychologist are not irrelevant to the medical effort necessary to focus the tremendous energy now on the loose, to return it to its causes which alone can detoxify it. This cannot be done without facing the auto workers in Detroit and Hokkaido and the shipbuilders in Gdansk. This is the implicit message of holism, and it has the kind of teeth our newborn holistic health has still to earn.

If we face great disease now, we also face great power and wonder. The first people on the Earth knew that exactly because they were first. Our own proto-historic ancestors dimly recalled the dawn. And now we, the ones who are mesmerized by the externalization, must learn it again in the apparition of its shadow.

Even though there is every reason to be pessimistic in the midst of so much pathology, there is equal reason to be optimistic because we are alive in the unbroken flow of breath and insight. Even as we struggle against this decay of culture and contamination of nature, we are individuating and internalizing. The very process of life that brings us into being and sets our uniqueness against the vastness of nature leads to healing. We have untapped powers (if we cultivate them and permit them), and some of the changes we effect can heal not only ourselves but aspects of the world.

In our own lives we have the responsibility to find a correct "level of treatment," but the complexity of factors confuses us and casts a mood of hopelessness. There is always another system of medicine claiming that the real disease lies deeper, that cure of symptoms is not holistic and merely displaces the pathologizing force. The esoteric interpretation in both homoeopathy and Reichian psychology (and elsewhere) is that society is diseased, so even an ostensibly cured person immediately absorbs a new imbalance. As long as one is in mind and flesh it seems impossible to be healed.

There is, however, a gut sense of wellness whose "symptoms" are a clarity and the freedom to act, an ability to move without internal resistance. We may never be totally cured, but we can have intimations of what it would be like to be healthy in a healthy world, and we can set ourselves on that path by the guideposts that are intuitively most true. If this book has a practical purpose it is to sharpen people's senses of how to recognize those guideposts and how to keep their options open when medical rhetoric seems to cloud the already cloudy world of their existence.

We dwell within a polarity: on the one hand, everything is incurable and the world is submerged in millennial miasm; on the other, we are permeated with a universal medicine, and with the slightest impulse in the right direction our beings are capable of curing themselves of anything. At each moment we see both sides of the polarity, so one should not fear the darkness and woe. It will be there even at the best moments, rejoicing in our freedom and song, warning us in our high. For being one of us, it requires integration too.

We face another practical difficulty too. Our favorite healers and superstar holistic medicines are at war with one another. We hear one say that medicine is vital and energy-oriented, as disease is. Another tells us that the world is physical and muscular. One system requires mentalization; another says: "Physical bodywork or you are wasting your time." The planet pharmacy now offers us a choice of infusions of substance, potentizations, and images and archetypes of the same sorts of substances. Does one ingest the herbal remedy, distill it in Bach flower waters, seek the minimum nonphysical dose, or translate it into elemental psi and archetypal forerunners? If mixed, do remedies negate each other? Should the bones or the meridians be adjusted to heal the organs? Is rolfing the only bodywork "tough enough to face up to the facts?"

When the Greek homoeopath George Vithoulkas spoke in San Francisco, I overheard the Reichians outside the auditorium discussing how deeply armored he was—this present paragon of a homoeopathic physician. From a different part of the room a local homoeopath pointed to the circle of Reichians and told his colleagues: "There you see the pure sycotic miasm on the hoof."[5]

It is more than a lack of generosity; it is a failure of holism, for on some deeper level these dichotomies must disappear. True systems all heal, even if they begin at different points and work through different levels. In truth, we rarely know the level of being a medicine speaks to even if we have its cover story. Remember Eisenbud's caution: how can we be sure that the active elements of homoeopathy, acupuncture, chiropractic, or even allopathy are not simply psychokinesis guided by a therapeutic mythology?

This book does not tell the reader how to massage the zones of his feet or how to diagnose pathology from the irises of his eyes. It works toward increasing consciousness around diseases and medicines. Holistic health resource guides can become an exotic supermarket at which one chooses from varieties of wonderful ethnic medicines, each with its native paraphernalia. The sick person finally does not have this leisure; he wants to pick the right medicine, for he is going to have to live it. Attraction to the images can mislead. It would be difficult to cure most Euro-Americans by Navaho sandpainting and chanting because they would not be attuned to the levels of mythology internalized in the ceremony: they would absorb the exoticism rather than the dynamics. But this does not mean it is impossible. In a well-known healing paradox an American who does not know a word of Navaho is cured during such a ceremony, but another Westerner who has studied Navaho for years is unaffected. This is not only because we do not know the active properties of the medicine and the forces involved, but because we do not begin to understand the nature and source of our own resistances to treatment and cure or what attracts us to the pathology in the first place. We do not know on a biochemical level, and we certainly do not know on a psychological or parapsychological level. And this shadow play extends well beyond medicine. The rock concert or political rally that "heals" one person may well make another sick. The individuality of lives outweighs the commonality of the species. The modern allergist practices a pale replica of this protean medicine. The polarity therapist, reaching into the thousands of years of Ayurvedic provings, touches a deeper chord.

Medicine is a desperate act, and all cures are miracles. Healing works against the deep-seated and inevitable fact of disease and decay. But disease embraces life and is its close ally from the beginning when the fertilizing sperm is little more than a virus to which the egg accedes. Throughout the wondrous transformation that follows, disease is the basis of all the defense mechanisms and immunities that keep this creature alive. The final disease is the *nigrcdo* of the original infection. The point is not to evade disease but to keep it integrated with the living. "Of course it's impossible," Enslin told us. "Therefore do it."[6]

Shopping for medicines is like shopping for diseases. The very existence of a system of medicine is the consequence of a distortion, an illness which it reflects internally. Navaho medicine, like Yoruba medicine, Ayurvedic medicine, and the medicine of Galen's Rome, all arise from cultural and natural conditions in an integrated simultaneity with local diseases. By combining mind and nature, medicinal symbols mediate the disease process. In Navaho ceremony we see the overall mind of the culture and the reifications of the landscape joining in a *metadrama* through which pollution, infection, guilt, grief, excitation, and mortality are purged. The same is true in contemporary hospitals: Western medicine exists in its technological mode because Western society as a whole is in a technological phase and individuals respond to a medicine that embodies their cultural myth.

Medicines are always to some extent homoeopathic, since remedies repeat aspects of disease. Even surgery attempts to "outdo" the disease on its own plane, imposing its precise disfigurement and adding its didactic wound to the damage. Chiropractic adjusts skeletal tissue to restore health, but the original adjustment was carried out by the disease or injury which set the biomechanical potential for such alignment. When the healing shaman calls out the illness, he *is*, in that moment, the illness externalized. "I am the crocodile," he chants. "I am lightning. I am the flood of water, the lion. And I am the shooting star." Of course he only externalizes the illness to the degree that his patient internalizes him. As the translation of the force of power and destruction into their native language, he has become the aspect of that force which can heal.

Watch the players on the field in a sporting event. Despite all else that is happening (the millions of dollars, the heavy equipment, the attention of masses of people), they too are involved in a struggle to rectify some condition, the same condition that makes their activity possible. When they are done, it will end. They are not doing it for themselves, and what they are drawing out and shaping may not become visible in their lifetimes. Science and war are surface events too despite the concern of physicists and politicians for their professions. The activities are symptomatic, a visible arrangement of inner facts. They too will be cured in time. This activity is called medicine only when it is acted out within a paradigm of curing, but the true medicine is the life force moving from the interior outward, driving and driven by the disease.

The curative eurythmist has the patient twist out odd shapes and angles, letters to "unspell" a distortion. The student of *t'ai chi ch'uan* tries to hold himself up with a stiff torso and arms rigidly propped on the air; what is sinking is the *chi*, which is supposed to sink; but, against a history of damming, the pain is unbearable—for the disciples of Ida Rolfe and Frederick Alexander too. Gravity is a dread opponent. And images can be phobias, nightmares. Long ago the letters were articulate and wise, and the organs and bones floated. The Tlingit shaman in his chanting sounds positively demonic, even to his followers around him, but he is talking to demons who are already here and whom he can no longer keep away. How could he possibly address a world to which they have not come, and still hope to disperse them?

"One creates devils when one acts badly," says Eduardo Calderon, the Peruvian curandero. ". . . We should not confuse ourselves that the spirit, that the evil shadows, frighten us, kill us. One frightens oneself; it is not the shadow that frightens one."[7]

Healing is painful because so much has become unconscious in us; the cure is a journey to the Underworld to reclaim our freedom and lucidity. We are always working against time to save what is left and transform what is active—as are even the crews putting up apartment buildings in cities. We worry now about whether there are resources just in the sense of minerals and fuels for another century of this, let alone an eternity. But even as the disease is not visible, the true energy is not within our present frame either. So we pretend, with our cities and automated clinics, to conserve time and restore matter.

The whole of Western technology is an attempt to make life safer and easier by progressive externalization of the gross properties of matter and refinement of that externalization to produce and control energy. Such an attempt had to be made, and we are now the products and the overseers of its experiment. We (but also the undeveloped world) buy into this circus, they sometimes more than we for not having lived it yet. Passing through this monstrous externalization is crucial to all, from the Yellow Emperor proposing harmony in a shattered world to the Eskimo shaman cursing the

cold he cannot cure while the children die around him. It is our
only answer to the deep and dark voodoo of nature. We requested
this relief collectively and perhaps even psychokinetically. Some of
our most spiritual healers have requested it too, for they go to
technological doctors for their tumors and infections, whenever the
poison is so strong only an antidote will do. Non-Western medicines
give a better sense of the actual location of disease and healing
because, for instance, they assume the complexity of multiple
disease arenas. Even the place of healing implies a notion of cure:
the sterile, efficient stage-set and rapid factory-like processing of a
doctor's office or a Western hospital give the illusion that diseases
can be located as discrete events.

In our guide to medicines and self-healing we will use two major
parameters: the degree to which a given remedy is vital or mechanical (spiritual or material), and the degree to which a remedy is
internalizing or externalizing (generating activity or passivity).

Most people assume that they do not know enough to make a
judgement, so they act only at the existential moment of commitment when the decision, like the remedy, is more a dream than a
waking. There is nothing wrong with meeting the healer with one's
heart, but individuals are more capable of analysis than they realize.*
There is also a tendency to assume that if doctors are socially
enlightened and humane they will be medically sound. There is no
reason to assume either this or its inverse for either holistic or
technological medicine.

THE SPECTRUM OF LIFE ENERGY

Most holistic systems have crucial vitalistic components, and some
are completely vitalistic; they are, in the contemporary jargon,
"energy medicines." As discussed earlier in this book (pp. 122–3),

* I have known people who were attracted to try homoeopathic medicine by
the first edition of this book, yet who read right through my description of
the homoeopathic "pills" as containing no substance. They tried homoeopathy
because the overall description charmed them, but they never actually made a
commitment to spiritual medicine, never realized that such a commitment was
fundamental to their decision. This may not matter at all in the long run, but
for those still seeking treatment, a closer exploration of this dichotomy might
be helpful, even if only to remind them that in the absence of a personal
orthodoxy, they still have beliefs about the nature of the world.

there are two versions of vitalism: biological vitalism in which the vibrant energy is an unknown force emerging from living tissue in its organization; and spiritual vitalism in which the energy exists on a totally nonmaterial plane and is thus permanently irreducible to the realm of science. Since these are usually the same "energies" defined by different traditions, it little matters how we treat this distinction except to note that the biological vitalists are regularly designing experiments to locate the source of the vital energy and offering models based on interpretations of the nervous system, circulatory system, or some other "electrical" or "magnetic" field of the body.

To the dilemma of proof in energy medicine (i.e., the missing causal evidence for the basis of cure even where there is ostensibly cure) the potential client can have two basic attitudes: either to base his valuation of the system on his personal confidence in the physicians and a rationale that complete explanation for any phenomenon is impossible (either forever or at present), or to attempt to develop an explanation for the mode of cure (this could be a personal theory or an actual line of scientific inquiry such as the research into the physics and biochemistry of microdoses that Harris L. Coulter recounts).[8]

It is also important not to misidentify and falsely concretize elements of models taken from physics and paraphysics. It is of potentially great importance for healing that contemporary physics suggests convertibility of matter and energy, holographic universal unity, and reversal of space-time; likewise that experiments in paraphysics show seeming psychokinetic influence over substances and events—but how these incipient models affect actual healing systems remains substantially unknown. Quantum physics is not yet proof for or against energy medicine.

Let us begin with a simple spectrum from spirit to matter:

Vitalistic Medicine: Energy medicine: faith-healing, Bach Flower Remedies, radiesthesia, shamanism
Elemental Medicine: Vital and Mechanical aspects intertwined: all traditional Oriental medicine, including acupuncture, *t'ai chi ch'uan*, Ayurvedic and Taoist medicine; also many systems of bodywork, including Reichian work, chiropractic, meditation, yoga; some herbal medicine

Mechanical Medicine: Ancient surgery, poultices; some herbal
medicine and bodywork; all Western technological medicine

Since healing occurs in the physical world, all medicines must
have some substance, if only the substance from which a potency is
derived or the bodies of the participants. The acupuncture needles
are not pure energy, and the herbs of the Ayurvedic or Basque
doctor grow from real soil; even the mind has the external properties of the brain. The San Pedro cactus of Peru which, according to
Eduardo Calderon, transfers its light and vibration to the patient
and locks with his aura to drive all physical and mental aspects of
alienation to the surface, originates in the physical properties of
the desert.[9]

Oriental medicines do not distinguish between material and
spiritual planes. The vital force carries out the creation of the organs through tissue (which is material) and the meridians (which
require physical loci). The world "knows" the vital force through
its substance, but substance would vanish without the primal elements to sustain it at every second.

VITALISTIC MEDICINE

A year after finishing *Planet Medicine*, I spoke at a conference at
the University of California at Berkeley entitled "Conceptualizing
Energy Medicine." My opening statement contained the following
lines:

"I have no idea myself what energy medicine is, or what this
conference means to discuss. But from the preliminary discussions
of the participants, I see that everyone's intuitions and doubts lie
in much the same territory. 'Energy medicine' is the name for an
ostensible basic property of the universe, a property integrated in
living systems, or in the living aspect of all systems, a property we
have either lost in our millennia-long materialization of the cosmos,
never known and thus seek in some future science, or have in our
midst and resist and do not know how to define. We may not, in
the end, choose to call it 'energy medicine,' but at this stage of
things, 'energy medicine' calls into action the cluster of computing
systems and advocacies we would want. . . ."[10]

In pure energy medicine no perceptible physical substance is
used; treatment is on a vital not a material plane. This is true

whether the remedy is words, the touch of a healer, homoeopathic potencies, or archetypal symbols. Their physical aspect is the barest possible under the circumstances. If a court case arose from ostensible murder with a homoeopathic remedy, the "suspect" could not be incriminated by a forensic pharmacist. There would be no substance present in the Western legal and scientific sense (even though homoeopaths have traditionally claimed their high potencies are very dangerous).* The same problem would exist in a murder by voodoo or any psychokinesis. The person who accepts only the material reality of his life should realize that homoeopathy and other vitalistic medicines are functionally nonmaterial. There is no way their thread can be picked up later by a mechanist physician. If he noted strange effects, he would attribute them to something else.

The Bach Flower Remedies are a particularly exotic vitalistic system from the 1930s. For all intent and purposes the medicines developed from flower blooms by the British physician Edward Bach are spiritual. They are not diluted to even a fraction the extent of most homoeopathic remedies, but they are diluted past the herbal phase. In the original system there are thirty-eight blooms. The blooms turn spring water into medicine by being floated on its surface in bright sunlight for three to four hours. Brandy is added to preserve the essence; later the mother tincture is diluted a few drops to an ounce of water.

The remedies are given only for the emotional planes of ailments, translating their action to the corresponding physical disturbance which is understood as present simultaneously and at the same vibration. Rock rose, mimulus, and aspen are given for precisely different kinds of fear, gentian and wild oat for qualities of uncertainty, honeysuckle for living in the past, mustard for susceptibility to gloom, heather for always seeking companionship and fear of being alone, chicory for being overcareful of children and relatives. In addition Bach developed a thirty-ninth remedy, a composite of five blooms: star of Bethlehem (for shock), rock rose (for terror and panic), impatiens (for mental stress), cherry plum (for desperation), and clematis (for being bemused, faraway, and out-of-the-

* In Chinese and Indian pharmacy, chemical analysis simply reveals the present material display of the underlying elemental energy.

body);* this he called the Rescue Remedy, and he describes using
it for near-drowned seamen washed ashore, for victims of automobile
accidents, for shock from injury, fright, dental work, and other
crises—always with miraculous results.[11] As with all vitalistic medicines, the limits are unclear. Bach devotees may use Rescue Remedy
several times a day, for minor pains (rubbed on the skin), close
calls in traffic, business disappointments, and other unpleasant in-
cidents—much as primal screams are used during the working day
to stop minor traumas before they settle in, or as a Muslim cleanses
himself anew with prayer at appointed hours. Where there are no
overdoses and the microdose is a dynamo of "nuclear" power the
patient himself must decide how he wishes to live and what arrangement to make with the vital force.

Current Bach practitioners distinguish between homoeopathy
and the flower remedies on the basis that homoeopathy touches the
astral and electromagnetic planes of the body whereas the Bach
"speaks" through the archetypal language of flower morphology to
the emotional conditions, which are the flowers on another plane
of being.

With only thirty-nine remedies and thumbnail character-sketches,
both ethnocentrically selected, the Bach runs the risk of being
simplistic. A group in California has developed their own system
of native essences, and one could imagine equivalent systems from
Australia, Madagascar, or Japan. There are thousands of California
flower essences, some of which seem to have no curative properties
in this system. But why, if they are made by the same forces in
nature? The answer of the purists is that the Bach is a "perfect
state of the art;" Bach found the system whole. Since it works as a
whole, to enlarge it is only to diminish it.[12]

The key to vitalistic medicine is never the unknown energy in
principle. Medicines may be posed in vitalistic terms, but their
viability and popularity will always rest on their rate of success and
their social roles. The traditional vitalistic medicines have been
"proven" by centuries and, in some cases, millennia of apparently
successful remedies. Their vitalism has not been proven, but the
practice of healing in its context has been. Mythological and ceremonial medicines were developed by tribes according to local tax-

---

* Bach remedies are regularly mixed for the different emotional aspects of
one patient.

onomies in an attempt to heal people, and they were maintained because people were healed through or synchronous with them. This is empirical medicine. Bach did not initially ascribe spirit to flower blooms in sun upon water; Hahnemann did not propose increased power in microdose. They, like the ancient shamans in practice, found that something healed, so they continued to work in that mode.

ELEMENTAL MEDICINE

Elemental philosophy describes an original field of psychosomatic potential through which bodies, substances, mind, and spirit pass and transform each other. Elemental medicines (especially the Oriental ones) are grounded in somatic work. Even if herbal remedies activate vital forces, even if massage and yoga quicken the energy in the *chakras*, the person must still integrate these processes on a physical plane. The elemental transformation must be reenacted in mind and body. In energy medicine, ironically as in mechanical medicine, the cure is often given for free.

In elemental systems remedies simultaneously affect the colloidal and dynamic properties of the tissues and cells and the transmutational qualities of the subtle body. Eastern practitioners do not deny the energy present in the meridians and in potentized substance, but they do not assume they can draw that energy simply and spontaneously onto the physical plane. If it fails to manifest without treatment, then the blocks are complex and deep-seated and must be dissolved by the same elemental principles that incarnated substance and form. Cure occurs on the physical-spiritual spectrum according to the actual development and relative health of people. Nothing is transcendent until something has been transcended. And that takes work, in one lifetime or another.

For thousands of years classical Indian medicine (Ayurveda) has practiced pharmacy, surgery, and psychology, and has developed sciences of embryology, anatomy, and nutrition. One of the oldest and most elaborate bodies of medicines on the Earth, Ayurveda has compiled a system of constitutional provings from accumulated cases going back to the dawn of Indo-European history. By comparison the homoeopathic repertory is an infant.

Classical Indian theory (called *tridosha*) postulates three *doshas* at the heart of every being. These *doshas* are both somatic and characterological and are formed of the five elemental, preorganic *bhutas*, the subtle material potencies which are never found unmixed in nature: *jala* (which is heavy, dense, flowing, moist, and cold, and associated with water) goes together with *prithivi* (which is bulky motionless, steady, and hard, and associated with earth) to generate *kapha-dosha* (which is called "earth," "water," or "mucus"). *Jala* goes with *agni* (which is light, hot, penetrative, digesting food through the organs, imparting a glow to the body, and associated with fire) to make up *pitta-dosha* (which is called "heat" or "bile"). *Vayu-dosha* ("wind" or "air"), an active element with more diseases ascribed to it than *pitta* and *kapha* together, is made up of *vayu* (which is light, transparent, cold, dry, and associated with air) and *akasha* (which is porous, soft, smooth, light, and transparent, rules the sound-matrix, and is associated with ether).[13]

If these are pictured as simple elements and humors, one tends to simplify their substantiating aspect and miss their existence as dynamic forces and psychosomatic vectors. Gerrit Lansing writes: "After learning to recognize them in one's own daily body experiences the conditions they signify become verifiable without necessity to reduce their range of application by translation."[14] They are not abstract phenomena but psychosomatic physicalizing forces.

The seven *dhatus* (body-components) are formed embryonically by the different vectors of the *bhutas* in the field of the body. The *srotas* may be translated as "channels," including capillaries, fatty ducts, semen ducts, and intestines, but they are the projections of space through the body from its seed potential. The substances they generate and which trickle and ooze through them give basic existence to the *dhatus*. *Srotas* that terminate at orifices (eyes, ears, breasts, genitals) are points of contact between the subtle roots of the physical body and the external world.[15]

There are 700 visible *siras* (veins) but countless minute ones; their continuous pulsing keeps the body irrigated and nourished. The *dhamanis* (arteries) are associated with circulation and rooted in the navel. When the elements become imbalanced or aggravated, the distortion appears in all the *siras, srotas,* and *dhamanis* simultaneously, for each of them carries all three *doshas.*[16]

The *doshas* have aspects which tend to be described by concrete Western anatomy: *bodhaka kapha* as saliva, *pachaka pitta* as gastric juice, *ranjaka pitta* as hemoglobin, *prana vayu* as oxygen, and so on, but this portrays only physical aspects of the vital flux. Each of the five aspects of vayu not only sustains the body but keeps the mind clear, generates speech, carries the senses, and activates the body to remove waste. If apana vayu is kept from moving downward, the passage of urine and faeces is stopped, so medicines which stimulate downward apana vayu are prescribed.[17]

Gerrit Lansing writes: "The three functional 'forces' in the human psychosomatic substance are considered to be ideally in an individual harmony or balance. Disease is finally an unbalance, not simply of two polar principles, but of three potentiating factors."[18]

Foods are digested by aspects of the *tridoshas* which are passed to the organs, such as mouth, intestines, and lymph. Each of the *doshas* in the character-soma reacts differently to individual tastes. For instance, *kapha* is aggravated by sweet but soothed by bitter.[19] The five tastes reflect underlying potentialities, so medicine relies not only on diet in the nutritional sense but elemental interaction on a psychosomatic plane. Diet and mind are parallel and simultaneous functions within the clarity of *vayu* and the bitter fire of *pitta* against the colloidal mud of *kapha*. We think of tastes in the coarse sense of surface qualities, but they go deep into substance where their elements meet the characters of the *doshas*. We and what we eat are the same potentiated field. Cooking, pharmacy, and herb science are one; chemical alchemy becomes alchemical yoga.

THE SPECTRUM OF HEALING

All medicines can be viewed in relation to one another on a spectrum from Internalizing/Active medicines to Externalizing/Passive medicines. Most holistic and non-Western medicines are based on the internalization (internal transformation) of events and substances. The images in the sand-painting; the darts, sigils, and swords of the shaman in his *mesa*; the letters fed to the patient in the eurythmic alphabet; the foci of meditation; and, on another level, the qualities of food and herbs—all of these are meant to be taken into the whole being—absorbed and assimilated, redefining one's self.

Just as the medicines of internalization involve external substances, so the medicines of externalization must internalize too, though often the external remedy has a different internal meaning from its external intent and even its external biophysical effect. The long-range consequence of an antibiotic in the latency and potentiality of the body/mind is often more profound and medicinal (even if pathologically so) than the original disease (even if the external activity is successful in reversing the external form of the disease). Initial iatrogenic pathology is severe enough; liver damage, change in blood chemistry, kidney dysfunction, neurosis, slurred speech, and fungal infestation are all regular by-products of popular antibiotics. The real problem is that since the medicine is not chosen according to any laws of cure* (Hahnemannian, Ayurvedic, Navaho) it can be internalized only pathologically. After surgery removing his spleen a patient may have no further physical symptoms, but the field of his meridians, his emotional balance and kinesthesia may be so altered that psychosis develops.

In general, a person should choose the most internalizing medicine of which he is capable and which the immediacy of the disease allows. At the same time, he should be developing other more internalizing methods as an aspect of overall personal development. Here is the spectrum:

Internalizing/Active Pole
First Level: Meditation, Prayer, Self-Reflection
Second Level: Activity (Dō-in, T'ai Chi Ch'uan, Chanting)
Third Level: Diet and Herbs
Fourth Level: Healing by the Senses (touch, vision, hearing, dreams)
Fifth Level: Bodywork (Massage, Adjustment)
Sixth Level: Acupuncture
Seventh Level: Surgery, Radiation, Drugs
Externalizing/Passive Pole

* I mean to reemphasize here the earlier distinction between "rational" and "empirical" schools of healing. The "laws" of modern orthodox medicine are rationalizations of cause and effect from models of biomechanical action. "Empirical" medicine eschews such "laws" as idealizations and abstractions. Empirical doctors work from long individualized traditions of observing sequences of pathology and cure and recording the responses of different organisms to discrete remedies. Where a rationalist may find only one symptom, a single effect, an empiricist usually sees a codon that has a variety of meanings depending on its placement and stage in a larger epiphenomenal sequence. The "empirical" laws of cure are thus a deciphering of the layered and submerged syntax of living substance. Every remedy has a "meaning" and consequences that radiate through the rest of nature and the duration of the organism's life. Since cure is natural, the doctor's role is to recognize and foster an intrinsic

All systems have aspects of the seven levels of cure, so placement is a function of which aspect predominates. The lower the number, the more active the person treated has to be—the more he or she has to cure himself or herself. The higher numbers are, by degree, relatively quicker and more mechanical. A pathology in the seventh category is dealt with in a matter of months or even seconds. The first level requires years (though spontaneous cures of faith are possible). As one moves up the scale the treatments allow more passivity by the patient, the healer substitutes cultural mechanisms for the internal force.

The chart should be viewed flexibly, as an intuitive guide not a taxonomy. Although the first and seventh levels are extremes, those in between differ by minute degrees depending on how they are practiced. Most medicines are multilayered and combinatorial, and include elements of self-reflection, activity, diet, and healing by the senses. Massage can be done subtly at the level of chanting. Acupuncture can soften to dō-in. Even coarse factory drugs have some curative herbal properties in them, for they are based on herbs historically and pharmaceutically.

The pure vitalist medicines are left off the chart because they could be considered at any level depending on interpretation. They are herbs if one chooses the metaphor with pills and infusions, and they are prayers if one thinks of them by analogy with the "currents" of faith-healing. Drugs, radiation, and surgery are not outside the spectrum but at the opposite pole from meditation. "People get the medicine they deserve," said Paul Pitchford, now an Idaho-based acupuncturist and Chinese herbalist, when he arranged the original series on which this one is based.[20]

MECHANICAL MEDICINE

Healers at the seventh level work on a physical/mechanical plane. The image of them as money-hungry hacks is simply a New Age cartoon. Most of them want to heal, and most of them use excellent judgement on the plane on which they work. Almost any of

---

process. The "rational" laws of cure extrapolate a localized and temporally simplified sequence of cause and effect; there is only a rudimentary knowledge of the far-reaching and holistic effects of any remedy, thus the everpresent danger of iatrogenic disease.

them are capable of saving lives and relieving extraordinarily painful
and debilitating ailments. It would be useless for them to try acupuncture or praying over patients; they would be no better than a
shaman at surgery. In fact, it is dangerous when healers at this
level are attracted by the holistic fad. Unless they transform their
whole experiential base, they simply turn other methods into metaphors of mechanical medicine.

For most people in the West today, medicine at the seventh
level is perfectly acceptable; even its failings are acceptable. People
require immediate change at any cost, and that is what they get.
They are "advertisers" laying out hundreds of thousands of dollars
for the seconds of a prime-time ad on TV, which happens to be
their lives; so they expect gross change within a conventional frame
of time. Time is money, but most true healing does not occur in
the usual denominations of space-time.

Those who prefer the seventh level are the same people who
reach nervously for a cigarette, a cup of coffee, or the symptomatic
relief of their jobs or social lives. Heart surgery is another hit for
the home-improvement, standard-of-living junkie in all of us. We
go on amassing artifacts of externalization. And yet we live, some
of us for a long time.

Carton-a-day smokers, victims of organ diseases and successive
operations, and workers in carcinogenic factories may well outlive
some faith-healers and yogis who die of stomach cancer or leukemia
at relatively young ages. Genetic and karmic factors are imponder-
able, and pure longevity is not the major criterion for depth of life
experience. Because a particular monk who fasted and meditated
regularly then died at forty does not mean that we should not
practice yoga or manage our diets according to therapeutic principles. We do not know all the factors in his case or ours. Because
a *t'ai chi* master died suddenly in middle age does not mean that
t'ai chi is not curative. A brilliant homoeopath may develop a serious physical disease that has emotional roots not touched by the
remedies, but his cures of other people may regularly reach that
depth. Whatever keeps people alive and well does so for unique
and individual reasons, and for different reasons in different people.
If George Burns, after smoking all those cigars, survives to sing at
eighty: "I wish I were eighteen again, going where I've never been,"
and to play the role of God in a movie with comic grace, then

something keeps him alive, perhaps the original vaudeville elixir. Something else keeps Bob Hope and Ronald Reagan alive in this same parable.

MEDITATION, PRAYER, SELF-REFLECTION: ACUPUNCTURE

If matter and energy are linked by mind, and matter and mind through energy, then "thoughts" should be able to penetrate the organs and even the cells. No one questions "psychosomatic disease," or that feelings affect health. However, the proposition of direct will reversing malignancy, either in one's self or another, is outside the pale of conventional medical science.

If mind can shape matter aboriginally and on some level outside of space and time, then the world becomes an unexplored place. Yet such hypothetical powers are apparently not under our control: psychokinesis is predominantly unconscious. So if we are to seek the directed medicines of mind into matter, we must look for them in unconscious faces of conscious activity.

Meditation

Meditation is a conscious method for entering unconscious matter and transforming it through concentration. For the practitioner his thoughts are not just images but a kinesthesia of breath, organs, and mind. Distances appear as they actually are according to inner reality, so external obscurities can be located and clarified according to internal phenomenology. It is not the mind of thoughts that is cultivated but the thoughtless mind that penetrates the whole body. An image held in duration at its own beginning transcends itself until what is held is the quality of mind and being. Conscious breath can then be directed to organs in needs of healing. One Ceylonese master writes: "This method of allowing the simple facts of observation to speak and make their impact on the mind will be more wholesome and efficacious than a method of introspection that enters into inner arguments of self-justifications and self-accusations, or into an elaborate search for 'hidden motives.' "[21] To work on an illness, meditation must cut deeper than the illness and must avoid being trapped in the intrinsic arguments of that illness at any level of body/mind. The pain of disease is necessarily one of the foci of mindfulness, and it should not be anesthetized. It is the most direct connection to not only the ailing organ but the ailing principle of mind/body holism.

Most diseases for most people fall beyond the realm where meditation of which they are capable can heal. Yet the commitment to meditation, even in the first halting try to listen to a thought, is a step onto a path that leads ultimately to the point where mind and disease meet—if we have "world enough and time."

Prayer

Prayer is a different sort of medicine from meditation, though the two come together in mantras in all the languages of the world. Whereas meditation arises from knowing and being, prayer arises from faith and ritual. When Jesus says, "Your faith has healed you," he means not an obedient act of thought but a spontaneous meditation that changes one's nature to the universe. For prayer to heal, one must have faith in the gods inside oneself and in the forces of the cosmos to which they correspond. Submission may be an instantaneous act, but the capacity to submit takes much of a lifetime.

Prayer often works in a community context, as with Navaho sandpainting rituals and Christian faith-healings. A group of people create a common mind in which individuals among them can be touched. The "mind" includes supernatural beings and mythological events, so it penetrates deeply into the cultural identity of the group where much disease originates. The following prayer, part of the Navaho Beautyway Ceremony, retains its power even in translation:

Prayer to Big Snake Man at Dropped-out Mountain

Young man this day I gave you my tobacco, at Dropped-out Mountain, Young Man Big Snake Man, Head Man!

Today I have given you my tobacco, today you must make my feet and legs well, my body, my mind, my sound, the evil power you have put it into me, you must take it out of me, away, far away from me!

Today you must make me well. All the things that have harmed me will leave me.

I will walk with a cool body after they have left me.
Inside of me today will be well, all fever will have come out of
me, and go away from me, and leave my head cool!
I will hear today, I will see today, I will be in my right mind
today!
Today I will walk out, today everything evil will leave me, I will
be as I was before, I will have a cool breeze over my body,
I will walk with a light body.
I will be happy forever, nothing will hinder me!
I walk in front of me beautiful, I walk behind me beautiful,
under me beautiful, on top of me beautiful, around me
beautiful, my words will be beautiful!
I will be everlasting one, everything is beautiful![22]

Self-Reflection

Self-reflection is the continuous act of noting and internalizing
events—not narcissistically but as a token of one's objective presence
in the world. Every interaction—a purchase at a market, a stray
image of a building on a side street—is reexperienced silently for its
unstated assumptions, its physiological background, its passage into
body/mind: dreams, making love, dealing with children; even washing the dishes becomes a careful exercise.

Self-reflection changes one's frame of knowing and being and thus
changes the matrix within which health and disease occur. This
process will differ from person to person, and some will no doubt
substitute clever habitual thinking for true self-reflection. Gurdjieff
claimed that, despite the strong desires of individuals, it was impossible to cultivate a true will without a specific shock or tension to
break with the abstract polarity imposed on life. Only such a jolt
could separate a "third force" and release us from our dualism and
existential mirage.[23]

The hope of all therapies of image, prayer, and reflection is that
the healer or sick person can break into the original dialogue of
psyche and soma. In the cases of immune system diseases such as
lupus and multiple sclerosis, and nervous ailments such as strokes
and epilepsies, there is a clue that the biological language has gone
awry; perhaps an unconscious replica of embryological code, a primitive and shamanic speaking in tongues can restore the psychochem-
istry of the failed connection.

Acupuncture

Acupuncture shifts the meridians rather than reaching to the organs through mind. Since it involves an outside operator, a "surgeon" of the meridians, we have placed acupuncture on the heavy side of the spectrum. However, while surgery moves the organs themselves and sometimes even removes them, acupuncture alters only the meridians and the flow of energy through them; and, since the meridians encompass the whole mind/body, it remains on the level of holism. There is no "bad" energy; energy is simply in the wrong place: perhaps the mind has stolen from the heart and lungs through the nervous system; the stomach has bloated itself from the intestines; the kidney is overactive, the triple heater lethargic.

It could be argued reasonably that acupuncture belongs at a subtler level than heavy bodywork because the needles are so fine— fine enough to be cousin to the homoeopathic potencies and other energy medicines. They may be subtle, but they are deep. Heavy bodywork, even rolfing, is less surgical than acupuncture, for the body/mind more gradually incorporates the levels of realignment proposed by the treatment.

In acupuncture the needles go directly into the body's mind. They feel like bee-stings, but their actual locations are redistributed by the field they create. It is not so much the pain of the needles that is uncomfortable but the overall sense of being out of alignment, of being torn between two selves. The old self withdraws, and a new self that burns like the poisons goes deeper than the perceived physical body. The pain of even the smallest motion is intense. Even thought hurts, for the same thoughts can no longer come in the old way.

It is, Paul Pitchford says, like irrigation.[24] One makes a new grid for the river. After the treatment the river will gradually return toward its familiar bed, but it will have been slightly redirected. Over time, through recurrent acupuncture treatments, herbs, t'ai chi, or other remedies, the river may form a new channel. Whatever this river is made of—nerves, blood, *chi*, mind, or some unknown fluidity of the primeval body—it carries the organs with it, for they are elementally subsequent. At every portion of experience a distortion of current is felt because the entire field of the meridians is being realigned. Each needle changes the field, the person's sense of who he is.

ACTIVITY: BODYWORK

Activity is the somatic counterpart of self-reflection, or in the unity of the mind/body, it is the quality of reflection moving through the organism. This includes regular activity such as walking, standing, breathing, talking, tensing, relaxing, eating—"life style," as it is contemporarily defined. Where does our energy for being in the world come from? How do we experience it as we use it? How deep do our functions go? Do we act from roots? Or do we act from the surface, feeding ourselves symptomatically, moving anxiously, and adrenalizing our emotions?

The relation between life style and disease has been reemphasized in a recent fad of studies linking certain types of behavior to heart disease and cancer. A new awareness of movement, aerobics, and exercise has generated a range of cultural events from mass public jogging to movie star fitness parlors and "jazzercise" classes. These are the innovations of lucid self-reflections, but our actual pathology is more than just a lack of action; it is a distortion, and when a new activity is added without deep internalization, the imbalance is simply shifted.

Dō-in

There is a more formal series of activities akin to medicine itself. These exist in every culture and subculture, but a few have become newly prominent in holistic medicine. Dō-in is an ancient form of Oriental self-massage and daily exercise. A practitioner regularly familiarizes himself with his body/mind, breaking through the collective abstraction by interacting with the surfaces, bones, and organs, draining waste, removing callouses and surface deposits, breathing, praying, making sound. The whole body is included: the spiral of the ear; every joint of every finger and toe and the space between them; every orifice, freckle, and wart. This activity establishes a harmony and cleanses mind and body. The connections of all the organs and meridians at the ears, the eyes, on the feet, and at numerous other points are used for diagnosis, stimulation, and sedation [25]

Some of the separate exercises are like mantras; others are primal calisthenics and chiropractic. In one set of movements, eyes look into the infinite distance while the person kneels with hands clasped at the level of the heart. Sounds are heard, but not any particular sound. The hands are clapped clearly and sharply. The body is twisted around. The teeth are beaten together. In a related sequence, the tongue is used to collect and taste saliva from the upper region of the palate. In another, each finger is rotated at the point where it connects to the hand. The fists are drummed on the back with the spine held straight: to relieve not only sciatic nerve pains but throat congestion and hemorrhoids.[26] We should remember that the point of each exercise is not to strengthen any particular muscle or capacity but to redistribute vital energy and balance elements. Dō-in is physical movement directed toward spiritual movement—to clear the mind and to move fear and anger while wastes are drained from the body.

T'ai Chi Ch'uan

T'ai chi ch'uan is a specific set of exercises in a regular sequence for addressing simultaneously the internal gravity of the body and the external field of the Earth. Skeletal organs and meridians mediate between the zones, so the form itself is directed toward removing their tension. Some mistake t'ai chi as just the position and force of the body vis a vis a real or imagined opponent; they miss how the form includes the internal organs in their viscosity and contiguity, how the skeleton and muscles crowd the organs or give them space. The external power of the form comes from raising the internal vital force from the abdominal region with self-generated heat through the zone of conception, the nervous and circulatory systems, simultaneously into the meridians of the body. This current is blocked by imbalanced posture and unclear thoughts, the distortion translated to the organs. Precise and exacting, the exercises work on this distortion, effecting a gradual alignment through a repetition day after day and year after year. As the movements are internalized, the meridians are irrigated, and over time the circulation of the medicinal chi allows the spine to straighten and the organs to soften. It may take ten years of practice to achieve just the slightest change of a fraction of a degree in the angle of the spine and the fluidity of the organs, but this change, so minute from an external perspective, reflects an enormous shift for organs contained in the small spaces of the body cavity.[27]

This precision makes *t'ai chi* very different from jogging. The movements cannot be done mechanically; the external form is learned only to create an internal set of movements that have far greater leverage and angular momentum. Even paralyzed people have been known to learn a form of *t'ai chi* from observation and to replicate it inside their bodies without visible external motion. Ultimately the most advanced masters move internally without doing the outward form. When used martially, the most internal *t'ai chi* seems ghostlike, psychokinetic.

The movements apparently originated from an external meditation on the movements of living animals and other entities. The association of medicinal forms with things martial is neither accidental nor unfortunate. How one deals with an external opponent —a daily aspect of the world for primitive man—is translated into a very different kind of centering activity through internalization. Language itself may be an internalization of interjections shouted during battle and other crises. Suddenly actions which are semiconsciously and habitually ejected from the mind/body are rediscovered in internal echoes. Martial activities are basic because they teach survival against a deadly enemy, be it animal, human warrior, or spirit. Disease is a far more subtle and grievous opponent who must be dislodged the same way. At the meeting point of internal and external, there is only the self, seeing both ways that the enemy is one's own imbalance and tension.

Not all martial activities are healing. Football hardly leaves the meridians of the players in better condition than before they began the "exercise." Most warfare puts its disciples up against opponents far more lethal than they have developed the power to handle— today far more lethal than they could develop the corresponding move in a thousand lifetimes. *T'ai chi, aikido, pa kua, capoeira,* and related forms teach martial acts only as applications of basic principles of nature. Fighting is not encouraged; these are systems for the internal warrior rebalancing the organism and the external warrior rebalancing the society.

Chanting

Chanting, which is an aspect of *dō-in* and of many native war dances, uses the organs just as other activities do. The deepest chants involve not only the breath and the throat muscles but heart, intestines, and the leg muscles at the root of their mandrake cry. Through the unity of the body the chant changes the anatomy, partly through the breath, partly through the integration of the meridians, and partly in the long-term relationship between the voice and the frame of meaning in the society. Mind/body disease can be the disease of language, of myths; disciplined chanting can reach these areas and make changes. The mind does not always understand the chant. Margaret MacKenzie reports that shamans in the Cook Islands lapse into ancient languages only they and the sick person understand, and then only during the actual moment of chanting.[28]

It may be idealistic to think that we can drive out the wolf of lupus by chanting, but it *is* possible to meet diseases on their own battlefields in an active mode. A prose song (abridged below) was generated by a lupus victim working in curative eurythmy with the internal L which represented her own name Laura and the name of her disease (as well as light and life). She was on a journey from the pathological L to the healing L: "To summon inside—The brave shining warrior, glittering hero of the skies with flaming sword, astride a horse so white, you *know* you are ready, to meet and overpower the dreadful. I've got my firm together now, my word drawn up, to hold and to swing into warning. Big 'L's' begin lifting, for lightness and levity, raising the sediments Up in the body. L is for *lucia*, I said with my slipper, for all of the liquid that rises forever and falls into falls to further the flowing to keep us in motion. . . . The globe itself hovers there before you. Yes, you can touch it, give it a little 'L.' "[29]

Bodywork

Bodywork is "activity" generated by a healer—the heavier and deeper the response to the healer's touch or instructions, the closer it comes to the sixth level; the lighter and more self-originated, the closer to the second level. Many forms of bodywork have both active and passive poles, so they fluctuate. The deep physical pressure of rolfing and *shiatsu* is proto-surgical; the stimulation of the organs by touch is "*dō-in*."

Polarity is generally categorized under "bodywork," but it is a

New Age recombination of a number of traditional methods, including Ayurvedic diet and *tridosha* theory, acupuncture points, American Indian herbalism and shamanism, alchemical medicine, *shiatsu*, Reichian bodywork, and chiropractic. The founder, Dr. Randolph Stone, has travelled around the world in an attempt to make a modern "planet medicine." Polarity, like *t'ai chi*, diagnoses blocks on a mind/body level, and attempts to restore organ balance. With its Ayurvedic roots, it works from the uniqueness of each person's tension and integrates diet with massage. Eating is an aspect of regular daily activity, like breathing and moving, and food carries out internal massage. In external polarity massage, the body is treated as an expression of the five elements and an electromagnetic field with positive and negative poles (however we understand these).[30] Within such a magnetic *tridosha* field, massage and organ treatment are polar, and primal intelligence of the cells directs mind through the meridians. No other form of massage so literally treats the body as a magnet, though, interestingly, Eduardo the Peruvian speaks of the bioelectromagnetic power (*poder bioelectromagnético*) which gives potentiality to his staffs of power in the healing *mesa* (*potencialidad a la vara*). The staffs then vibrate precisely according to the account, the reason for the sickness (*la cuenta, a la razón de la enfermedad*).[31] At the elemental level, the bioelectromagnetic field, the work of massage and herbs, and the chanting become the transit of meridians and light, and bodywork becomes spiritual healing—the degree depending on the nature of the patient and the qualities cultivated in the healer.

DIET AND HERBS: HEALING BY THE SENSES

Diet

Few things are as basic to health as diet, whether one considers food on a physical plane as supplying the actual material of life or on an elemental level as potentiating the forces necessary to balance the energy in the body. The primary vectors and substances that make us up also express themselves in the environment and the foods we eat. We are sustained or made over again from matter by the relationship between food and constitution.

Much of the medicinal practice of diet takes place on the simplest physical level. According to some systems, meat and other strong foods should be avoided as sources of poisons. Wastes shunted off to the cells must eventually return as disease. Just because they are hidden and because the body invariably compensates does not mean that the organism is functioning well. Grains, fruits, and vegetables are chosen for their direct effect on the organs, simultaneously as nutrition and medicine. Eating and digesting are internal yoga. If we feed the body meaty protein and processed foods we pretend to do for it in advance what it must do for itself, and so we rob it of its vitality. Stimulants are regarded as disease agents because they liberate certain forces at the expense of others. Diet must be seasonally attuned, balanced elementally, and grounded in an intuitive realization of the effects of food. Most Oriental healing systems study food closely, as a matter of overall philosophy as well as etiology of disease. The roles of the allergist and nutritionist are absurd in the ancient sense: we are supposed to be able to *feel* which foods harm us.[32]

"Eating" occurs on the psychological and spiritual levels too. Our state of mind affects how food enters our system; eating must approach prayer to happen consciously and assimilate fully. Chewing is important, first to mix the food with saliva and change it chemically, and second for the internal experience of developing a relationship with that food. It is important too to realize and experience the suffering and death of animals that goes into meats, not only as sympathy for fellow sentient beings, but as a decision not to numb ourselves to the reality of our situation. If we numb ourselves to the nature of our food, we cut ourselves off from our own nature; our foods become heavy and deadening, producing wastes on all planes. It is not just a matter of gulping down unknown and unnamed substances in hunger—the classic American posture of well-being, even in gourmet circles. On a mass cultural level Americans end up choosing Colonel Sanders and the chefs at MacDonald's as their teachers, along with Coors beer barons and the corporate heads of canned food conglomerates—instead of the Ayurvedic chefs and the raw vegetables and mineral water of the Earth.

The mistake of the West is always to think of mechanical aspects only. Eating and digesting are processes, modes of integration; as we get older we must move away from what Da Free John calls the "celebrants" of our twenties, the meat and alcohol and coffee, to the fine elemental strands on which life is strung, the etheric being.

Fasting is another level of yoga. Da Free John writes: "The stress of fasting favors healthy or growing cells. Defective cells do not function well under the stress; they die shortly and are eliminated. Thus, the body literally 'eats' its own wastes and diseased or dying cells, and it fully eliminates whatever it cannot consume."[33]

There are many other foods. The air is a food. Rain is a rich tea even when absorbed subtly from the atmosphere without drinking. Heat and cold pass through the pores into the body too. Everything in the environment is taken in and assimilated in our organisms—sounds, images, tastes: impressions (as Gurdjieff called them collectively). How we take substances, coarse and fine, into the mind and lungs and stomach determines who we are and what we are becoming. We do not have the leisure to be passive in relationship to all of these "foods" and "herbs," for without our conscious aid they would overwhelm us.

Herbs

Herbs can be defined as "medicinal foods." They are foods which serve primarily as catalysts for the natural functions of the organs, so they are prescribed to reactivate lethargic processes or slow down overactive ones. Some are given according to homoeopathic principles (fever-causing herbs for fever), and others are prescribed by the law of opposites. All foods are herbs, and all herbs are foods. Homoeopathic remedies are "herbs," not foods, which are meant to affect the body and mind only on a vital level; unlike foods they provide no substance for the organs and tissues to digest. Foods (herbs included) start with substance which has potential energy in it but which becomes energy only through its relationship to the organs. Herbs incarnate replicas of the elements to be given as medicines. They have more energy and less substance. In another sense, they are simply the substances of the world "proven" one by one and region by region over millennia for their profound internal leverage and mild side-effects. They are the cream of empirical medicine.

As internal doctors, herbs begin the treatment, but the patient must complete the cure by gradually responding. Drugs, contrarily, are antibiotic or anesthetizing "herbs" that are meant to "replace" the organs in carrying out a process in relation to a particular pathology. Their after-effects are intrinsic to their nature: the body/mind can respond to them only as outsiders, initially as brilliant physicians from out of town, but secondarily as thieves who have left the organs with only relative powers to carry out their own functions. Herbs transfer power, so they are rarely iatrogenically pathological. They are unconscious yogis and ancient rural doctors with signatures in the living world.

Flowers are among the most visible physicians: blossoms of clover, dandelion, saffron, yarrow to purify the blood. Herbal berries include rose hips, quisqualis, may apple for tumors; seeds are poppy, wild carrot, pumpkin, oat straw. Fennugreek, flax, and fennel make a strong intestinal mixture with comfrey root for absorbing liquids and eliminating wastes. The leaves of horsetails, raspberry, and parsley are common herbal ingredients; the leaves of mugwort are burned into the meridian points in moxibustion. Apple bark is used to lower blood pressure, cherry bark as an astringent, bayberry bark for ailments of the gall bladder.[34]

Garlic is a famous cure-all and oxygen-bearer, but no root is a more honored physician than ginseng. Apparently wild ginseng is such a deep rejuvenating medicine that it was stalked to extinction, and all we have left are the semidomesticated varieties. Stephen Fulder describes ginseng as a true stimulant, a medicine that restores energy and harmony and gives long life and true yang rather than draining these like pills and coffee. He quotes from a Russian writer's description of finding one of the last wild roots in 1934:

"I sat with the Chinese and we were all staring, when to my great amazement I noticed that the root had a human form: here was a separation between the feet, there were hands, and there, a neck, and on it the head and even a little plait. The fibres of the hands and feet were like long fingers.

"I was . . . overwhelmed by these seven people wrapped in contemplation of the root of life . . . I could hardly bear their faith. The lives . . . of millions of people seemed to me to be in relation to the enduring faith like the waves are to the sea. The waves began rushing towards me, the living, as to a beach, begging me to grasp the power of the root. Not with my flesh, because that will soon go, but with the wisdom of the stars and the constellations and maybe something beyond that."[35]

Can one doubt the intimation of the planet shaman in this root?

Other herbs include olive oil; wheat germ oil; walnut husk tincture; bamboo sap as an expectorant; honey; crystal; bear gall; fungi of all varieties; kelp, kombu, and other sea vegetables for diseases of the nervous system; haliotis and oyster shells; pearls for headache and insomnia; animal excrement; rhinocerous horn and toad secretion to cool and detoxify the blood; the scorpion as a nerve tonic; and the fossilized bones of dinosaurs as tranquilizers and antispasmodics. In China a variety of substances is used to cure different fevers: the whole earthworm, the exuviae of the cicada, the rhizome of the cnidium, and the tortoise shell. The Chinese also use human hair calcined and powdered as an astringent and dried human placenta for impotence, infertility, and ailments that do not improve with other treaments.[36]

Cinnibar, sulphur, fluorite, and other minerals are used medicinally. Ayurvedic physicians form very pure and fine wires of metals like gold, silver, copper, and tin, and after dousing them in plant juices, make them into a powder which is then mixed with other herbs. Supposedly metal can be given in this fashion without aggravation. Iron enters the blood faster than in an allopath's intravenous injections and without gastric side-effects.[37]

Salt is a great herbal shaman, but true salt with its many trace minerals cannot be sold in this country as a food. First it must be purified so that it is toxic; then it makes the front pages of national magazines as an assassin. Such is our strange alchemy.[38]

There are strong herbs just as there are powerful chanters, but they do not work indiscriminately. Diagnosis is as crucial to herb science as preparation and assimilation. When enthusiasts hear that an herb is cleansing they often rush to the "word" with the same obsessiveness and unconsciousness with which they have accumulated disease. Too weak to respond to treatment, they simply become weaker. Hallucinogens and tonics do not always bring clarity and power, even to those with much internal energy. There is no solution to our dilemma, no sure way to be home free. To have great power is to approach the diseases of great power. All around us, the worlds of medicine (herbs included) stand in total balance with reality and phenomena, and there is only that balance to return to through their aid.

Healing by the Senses

Each of the medicines we have discussed to this point have aspects of healing by the senses. Internalized imagery, either in the colored fields of healing ceremonies or the interior focus of meditation, uses the sense of sight. Chanting uses the path of the ear and sound vibrations into the body/mind. Taste is an element of healing by diet and herbs. Various types of aromatherapy have been used in both Western and non-Western ceremonies. Touch is present in virtually every cure, but often so ubiquitously it is part of the background (even though we may be totally unconscious of it and incapable of being conscious of it). It marks the continuous point of contact between any herb and the body—on cellular, molecular, and atomic levels. Touch also occurs on an organic level in massage, bodywork, and chiropractic—lightly when used to heighten one's response to a particular area; deeply painful when used for cleansing, deep breathing, and crying.

Beyond the basic five senses, there are other more complex sensual ranges. Wilhelm Reich considered sexual pleasure, genitalized and spread through the body, the one universal medicine. Massage and chiropractic work beyond the simple sense of touch on an overall kinesthesia of breath, body balance, symmetry, and polarity. Memory is another collective sense: even an amnesiac has a connected feeling of speech and action. Through our memory we are surrounded in a blanket of senses, a cognitive field that joins all the other senses together in a coherent reality. Healing must take place in the memory as well as in the present knowing. Psychoanalysis could be considered specifically a medicine of the memory, for it changes people by changing their histories.

From the collectivity of internal and external senses mind/body is capable of knowing itself and being its own physician much of the time. The doctor stands outside this body, outside its universe, but the sick person experiences the disease directly and changes it with each internal gesture—the deeper the gesture the deeper the change. More than ninety-nine per cent of all medicine is such self-healing.

Paranormal and unconscious "senses" such as telepathy, intuition of distant events, instincts, and archetypes, may also be medicinal; but, in our failure to locate and define them we both fear and hope that they exist at all. Finally, though, we must assume that the conscious memory-field is only a small part of our being; we are also things we are not conscious of. Whether such realms actually exist and are part of our sensual knowledge is an epistemological question, but most healing systems assume a reservoir of deep knowledge and autonomic power. We are not the conscious organism; we are a being immersed in a world of unknown phenomena experiencing directly only the outer layer of existence. Different systems perceive the underlying layers according to their own modes of knowledge and beliefs.

Western science conceives of a primordial sequence of instincts inherited biologically from our ancestors much the way birds inherit capacities of navigation and spiders the ability to find food immediately after birth. Many Western systems also postulate a collective unconscious of presymbolic matrices. The Jungian doctor attempts to put the sick person in touch with archetypal imagery, which becomes medicine in the same way it manifests originary growth and form in nature. Other systems claim memories of specific ranges of phenomena; for instance, scientology may or may not believe in an available cosmic memory going back billions of years to events in other galaxies, but it uses the pretense of such a memory curatively. Non-Western systems routinely accept past lives, not only as the causative substratum of this life but as a level contactable through meditation; to regain this memory is to heal this entire life by putting it in its actual frame: diseases then truly become guides between incarnations. In native systems, awareness of the collective lineage of ancestors and mythological beings is cultivated through an interchange with these beings in rituals and vision-quests. Healing then becomes a mediation between conscious forces of being and unconscious forces of nature—personal, collective, and cosmic. The mythological level is intentionally aroused through a particular ceremony or hallucinogen; it is one mode of entering unconscious frames without having to become conscious. "The shaman, himself, is important, primordial," says Eduardo Calderon, "and without substitution in the field of curing. He uses the San Pedro which affects special points of a person, and gives him a 'sixth sense' in accord with the topic with which he is dealing. Taking San Pedro makes him leap into a special dimension."[39]

We can see this in Hopi healing ceremonies, African myth-enactments, and Australian Aborigine Emu Dances—initially through bright feathers, pigmentation on the dancers, chanting to open the interior field of sound, incense, herbs, rhythmic dancing, and secondarily through the collective invocation of mythological "memory."

"The mesa," says Eduardo, "is nothing more than a control panel by which one is able to calibrate the infinity of accesses into each person."[40]

The complexity of this mode can overwhelm us, so we should remember the simple initial case: the senses are orifices into the body; they are active channels to contact the part of us which is sentient, the part of us that is human. In healing through the senses, we are contacting the epiderm not only of consciousness and memory but of the elemental process becoming refined and individualized, and, through these vectors, the polar field of the body.

The second thing to remember about the senses is that they are points of focus and surprise in healing. Gurdjieffians separate the "third force"; the faith-healer awakens the lameness, the deafness; the healing shaman presents the visible form of the disease; the emetic "vomits"; Eduardo shoots a sudden spray of holy water from his mouth in the moonlight; the psychotherapist invokes the moment of trauma—these are bolts of energy, allopathic or homoeopathic shocks. Surgery and drugs offer such "shocks" too, but (as in the telltale case of shock treatment) they work to deaden the senses, away from pain; they remove the symptom without kinesthesia and elemental awareness. In a material age, the doctor who does not arouse the senses is a hero.

The third point is that healing by the senses is quite active. The process begun by the shock or by a particular image or aroma must be digested and integrated. The more intensely surprise is able to penetrate the stasis and get into the viscera, the deeper its impact and the more healing processes are activated.

Dreams are a form of spontaneous healing through the senses. Physiologists now tell us in their own words the old esoteric truth: nightly dreaming maintains psychosomatic equilibrium and prevents serious mind/body ailments. Whether the images of sleep inspire the auto-medicines or the medicines autonomically require dreams that the mind must provide, images and chemistry are linked in synchronous process.

Of course all the senses work curatively at all times. Such is the medicinal phenomenology of life. The gestalt of our being is vital, and if we do not resist being lived by it, it will carry us through most crises—that is, we will carry ourselves through these crises; we will die with the scars of many fatal diseases we cured that we did not even know we had.

But the dreamwork, like the senses, can also be made active, whether through focusing on the dream images after the dream or by actually trying to wake within the dream (as yogis and shamans do). In either case, we assume that the events that happen within the dreaming are not the arbitrary by-product of hormonal balancing, a movie show to distract us while the real business is going on biochemically. They are instead the symbolic and archetypal counterpart to the underlying curative elixir of sleep; they correspond in the holism to a deeper rejuvenation and transformation than a simple study of chemistry can reveal.

The dreamer—or more specifically, the ancestor and shaman within the dream—can be taught by a dream therapist. Such beings do not respond to direct commands like: "Pay attention now to this problem!" or "Heal this!" Resistance is stronger than the suggestion of change—the dilemma of the superficial hypnotherapist. The Freudian laws of the unconscious are the dream's laws of gravity, so the suggestion must be given through a distortion or reversal that mirrors the system of reversal and distortion in the dreamwork. If transformation is to occur, it must correspond to the transformation already occurring on another level in the dream, even if the desired healing is syntactically stuck in that transformation in such a way that it repeats the pathology and alters it only in surface features. We will consider some examples:

A man is working with a dream teacher, but for many months his advice has no impact on the dreams. Then suddenly the teacher appears in a dream as a guide through its events. His message is necessarily one of which neither teacher nor dreamer is consciously aware. The teacher-guide is conducting a dream class on swimming in a strange heavy medium from which one propels oneself into the air; it is an ordinary swimming pool at an old Y. Students from all over the country have come here for this lesson. The dreamer is standing by the ocean trying to find something very complex happening in the waves. The guide appears and makes a banal comment; the dreamer tells him he will no longer do. The guide stands there looking silently at the sea. His presence leads the dreamer to the complexity in the waves. He is replaced in successive dreams by a master of martial arts, a naive female social worker, and an authoritarian baseball manager. The true identity lies within the multiple phenomena, and change can happen only by being experienced, and can be experienced only gradually through a rebus—can be experienced, in a sense, only as some other thing.

Another mode is through integrating repulsive or toxic objects in dreams. The dream guide teaches that all elements of the dream express aspects of the dreamer—the lost children in him or her, the undeveloped creatures, the hostile shadow-beasts, the magnificent fields and blue skies, and even the remote planetary systems of his uncompleted self. Attention to this material forces the dream to deepen, for although dreaming must allow some of the unconscious to become conscious, it can never allow unconsciousness itself to become conscious. A repulsive man—bald, ugly, and covered with a sickly oil—is chasing children from his house with a shotgun. Before the dream is over, the dreamer must embrace him and hold him close. In another dream during an illness for which the dreamer seeks herbal aid, a possible holistic doctor has been replaced by a huckster at a fair handing out antibiotic tablets in plastic wrappings with the dreamer's name on them. The dreamer seeks his guide for advice; the teacher suggests taking the tablets because the dreamer can remedy any side effects later with vitamins. So he does. A dramatic change occurs in waking life. In dream language these tablets are herbal remedies, homoeopathic potencies, exactly by not being them; they are the thing one would not consider in waking, which makes them the actual medicine within dreaming. An act of reconciliation is carried out on an unconscious level with substances of the very pharmacy one is trying to avoid conceived of as symbolic poisons. But dreams heal by representing the medicine as exactly what it is not so they can then transform it through the distortion into elixir.

The vitamins may never appear as actual pills, but later, in another dream, a flood of icy water comes over a previously dry and sterile yard, and it is filled with exotic flowers and has moved closer to the sea so that bright-colored fish are now mating in it. Trees drop purple and pink paper maché blossoms into the water. Whether these are the symbolic Bach waters or the dreamer's own auto-medicine, they now carry out an actual healing through the dreaming process. A few dreams later the dreamer finds himself in an egg, which he recognizes as an egg because huge fields of yolk are separating around him; he has the sense of his entire self shifting in relation to unconscious elements. A few nights later he uses the swimming technique taught months ago at a seedy pool in a dream Y to swim toward the stars. Now it is the cosmic field shifting; a curative relationship is evolving between the embryology of individuation and the entire archetypal and unconscious field of the self behind the dreamer. This may be as close as he comes to experiencing the elements and meridians sensually.

The dreamer now decides that he no longer needs a guide; he is tired of working on a symbolic level and would prefer heavy body-work. Pushing the dreamwork aside, he engages in herbs, massage, and acupuncture. Suddenly the dreams flower. He is led almost by the hand through a demonstration of the whole "disease." The symptoms are so graphic and didactic that no guide is necessary. The ailing organs are the rooms and streets of the dreams. The decision to drain and heal on a physical level has relieved the pressure of literal symbolism, freeing the dream to complete its own process of transformation. The dream reflects the bodywork, as the bodywork reinvokes the dream.[41]

This is how the multiple healing systems work together. As one progresses through layers of confusion, unclarity, and disease, one requires and accepts different levels of work at different times, different types of therapists and different therapies. Long-term processes like meditation, *t'ai chi*, and diet are maintained throughout but change their relationships to the specific remedies. A homoeopathic dose blends with dream analysis so that the remedy is partially expressed through a series of archetypal images in sleep. The *t'ai chi* student goes to a rolfer to open a block of which he had no awareness before the second year of *t'ai chi* and which is preventing further progress in the form. As an adjunct to a particular acupuncture treatment, a client is given a prescription of cleansing and sedating herbs. A woman who has changed enormously through two years of Reichian bodywork suddenly feels overwhelmed by the confrontative aspect of herself and herself in the world; life has lost some of its richness even in becoming richer. A breathing exercise leads her to meditation; she switches modes and a whole new apperception, far gentler and exploring a different interior, arises.

There is a unity within, and the different medicines and therapies express their variant harmonies of it. In the dream the herb may be personified as a magician, the magician becomes a chiropractor, the chiropractor moves a rock that represents the sick organ, but the rock turns into the archetype for a homoeopathic remedy, and all this is still a shadow play for a deeper process of mind, matter, and energy. The woman in a sexual dream fantasy is not a woman at all; she is a medicine. But she is so alluring, the dreamer's desire for her is so strong she transcends her nature and suggests a new symbolic frame. She may be seen again among the bee-stings during an acupuncture treatment. She is also the unintegrated female element of the dreamer, intuited as he thumps lightly on his ear during dō-in, setting up a vibration in the jawbone: a presence behind vision.

The arts and the sciences have failed us: do not be fooled any longer. Once experimental art, philosophy, and radical politics were our cutting edge, the paths to new worlds. But they became arrogant and inflexible; they did not change our lives, and they denied that anything could change our lives. They laughed at the first of the new healers for their unexamined syntax and pompous mythology. "Lots of loose talk about *chakras*," said the artist from New York. "This stuff will go down in Boise. But not for me."⁴² And yet even he changed before the decade was out. It no longer matters that the new healer is naive about politics; he will make politics over. It no longer matters that his art is naive; clever artists have made their own prisons. Before long he will not even call himself a healer.

We are back to the synthesis. We see anew that medicine is real not because it alone heals or because it can finger the agent or the cure, but because it alone contains the metaphor for change. Despite their failings the new medicines fill us with joy and hope and give us something to do during the long hours. When the clouds descend to ground zero and we cannot find a surface or a direction, they provide the skin with which to inhabit and shape the fog. All other materials and events fall back into the relativism of the world and the mystery of not knowing who we are and how we got here.

Planetary Healing

This book already carries such a layering of enigmas and their negations that there is no gainful way to extend its territory. Even my ongoing experience is foreshadowed dormantly in prior text. I have also had the surprise of finding myself working therapeutically with readers who then tell me they have developed parts of their practice out of earlier editions.

Insofar as the 1982 Epilogue and 1987 Foreword (and other internal revisions) provide expanded frames for viewing the original 1976-1978 work, the only viable addition now is in continuing to excavate contemporary modes of diagnosis and healing. After all, despite the fact that there are no easy or definitive answers to the mystery of disease, we confront a globalizing civilization (our own) that suffers profoundly from its failure to take rational, long-term action in the face of epidemic suffering. If this crisis draws me into a naively literal diatribe I hope it will more bemuse than anger the Sphinx.

RESOURCES

I can speak confidently only of the schools and centers with which I have direct experience, most of them in Northern California. In truth, there are relatively few nondenominational training centers that deal with mind, body, and spirit together. Lomi School (at various sites in Marin and Sonoma Counties) and Heartwood Institute in Garberville (Humboldt County) are my own favorites. Lomi's strength lies in the integration of psychotherapy, martial arts, spiritual practice, and body-work: one can deepen and expand his or her own breath/existence while learning to teach other people how to move and dissipate mental and physical blocks. Lomi Work combines neo-Reichian therapies, gestalt, Feldenkrais exercises, various traditions of massage, acupressure, mantra, neuromuscular adjustment, and even some unexpected forms like straight sports and singing. Its techniques are surprising and unconventional.

Heartwood Institute for the Healing Arts is located in the wilderness of Humboldt County and is an accredited facility for a wide-ranging curriculum in alternative medicine. Resident and visiting staff cover bodywork and massage including structural balancing, polarity, and lymphatic massage, shiatsu, and the application of *chi* and meditation to massage. Heartwood also trains the full range of Oriental healing arts along with various forms of hypnotherapy and radical psychotherapy, and it seasonally incorporates Native American practices (herbs, psychotropics, sweat lodges, story-telling, musical instruments, chanting, and general ceremony). It has an extensive dietary and kitchen training program: Paul Pitchford (whose work is described in this book) has been teaching "Food as Consciousness" there since 1987.

American College of Traditional Chinese Medicine in San Francisco is less psychotherapeutic in orientation than the afore-mentioned but has a tough medical-school level program in many holistic disciplines, integrating Oriental techniques with Western physiology, biochemistry, and laboratory work.

There are naturopathic colleges (with homoeopathic programs) in Portland, Seattle, and other North American cities, spawning a growing network of new qualified homoeopaths, many of them with M.D.s. It appears that for the decade of the '90s (and, one hopes, beyond) we will have access again to homoeopathic treatment on a national basis. It will be nothing like the florescence of the Civil War years, but then we are no longer in the mechanical and sectarian model of that era.

Reborn homoeopathy is more sophisticated and refined than its forebear (as well as more integrated into other holistic disciplines). Now that practitioners generally accept (even if they do not fully understand) that microdoses do not and cannot work according to a standard allopathic paradigm, they are free to move outside Hahnemannian strictures and begin to explore actual efficacies and inefficacies. The Hahnemann Clinic in Berkeley, California, and Holistic Family Medicine in Spokane, Washington, are two facilities I would recommend from experience.

CONTEXT AND TIMING

Cures are not always dispensed in linear time and space. There is a mistaken tendency to expect healers of all schools—conventionally allopathic, herbal, psychic—to diagnose a condition and offer its remedy in the form of a pill, regimen, physical adjustment, prayer, or some more esoteric currency; the petitioner assumes that he or she "gets" it then.

This is often the case. Yet on another level medicines may contact such deep-seated conditions that some of their effects will not be felt for years, or even decades (this is axiomatically true for autogenic "medicines" like dreams, life experiences, and sudden insights). Thus, any medicine is simultaneously short-term and long-term, exoteric and esoteric, activating and internalizing. While a dose of comfrey instantly energizes an intestinal condition a concurrent use of barley grass or microflora may begin flushing the liver of deeper-seated toxins. The person may experience some degree of immediate relief from the comfrey (more ease digesting, less frequent constipation), but also a painful intensification of other symptoms (chronic pain, emotional distress, uncomfortable changes in taste and appetite, burning tears) that betray longer-term cleansing. This hypothetical example pinpoints a more subtle generality:

The information in this book—or in any book of medicinal theory or self- help—exists disguised on a number of synchronic levels in relation to any reader, including the author. Perhaps a person seeks both homoeopathic and psychotherapeutic treatments at one stage of life and recognizes a mellowing/empowering along with a gradual relief of her explicit somatic symptoms. (A homoeopathic remedy often *requires* concurrent psychological work; otherwise the condition it was treating may lapse into unconsciousness, reenergize, and return, either in its previous guise or as some other ailment. A successful microdose—or herb, or pill—does not eliminate the requirement of changing awareness and discipline; it merely makes the commitment to them more accessible.) Years later the same person may perceive that, having previously removed red meat from her diet (with some pride), now merely replacing biweekly chicken with a dish combining brown rice, miso, seaweed, and carrots deepens a change begun on *seemingly* more internal vital and psychological planes. The shift of attention and metabolism brought about through diet reexamination after psychological work is newly capable of rousing something *pre–psychic* in the organism; yet dietary attention alone (originally) would not have initiated a character change and might not have even had the same healthful physical effect.

One cannot do everything, so it is hard to know where to begin. All around us are various orthodoxies proclaiming: eat macrobiotic food . . . take out mercury fillings . . . primal therapy (by trademark) to clear early trauma (or rebirthing or orthodox Reichian work—equally by trademark) . . . only a homoeopath can handle serious inherited miasms . . . breathe in the belly . . . get your spine realigned . . . most oils are rancid, or have the wrong cholesterol (for some people) . . . filter fluoridated water to guard your immune system . . . replace milk with whey to avoid heart disease . . . plus, keep checking with your physician to catch pathologies early. It becomes crazy-making because healing cannot be *instead* of living. An ocean of creature experience and biological process, by definition unexamined and beyond remediation, underlies any medicinal directive. Thus, attention and refinement are far more critical than any modes of meticulous selection or advocacy. If one tracks his own process, ideally he is drawn from psychotherapy to diet to meditation, or, in other instances, the reverse way (that is, as a condition changes, so must one's level of attention, and that is the only guide to direction of cure). Some paths even usefully include radiation and allopathic drugs. There is no "healing authority" that declares which treatments are health-bearing and which ones are iatrogenic or otherwise pathological. The outcome rests in the mystery of individual process. Listening is the key to both life and healing—staying with the path a particular event (or act of attempted cure) initiates and following its effects to the next stage of diagnosis or insight.

Recently a friend with a lung/chest condition sought explanation and relief from a succession of allopaths, eliciting diagnoses ranging from exotic respiratory parasites to lupus (biomedically trained physicians are just as prone to mistake their own specialties for the facts of a disease). Then, with her pain so searing and her mood so oppressive she was at the point of suicide, she went to a homoeopath, got diagnosed according to different parameters (as having the disorder currently euphemized as Chronic Fatigue Syndrome), was given potentiated microdoses, and experienced marked improvement, especially in her suffocating pain and despair. However, only a form of Korean finger acupuncture relieved her next deeper level of symptoms. Later, a different doctor offered a series of dō-in exercises and diet changes (eliminating all sugars and meats). This not only ameliorated symptoms; it redefined the very life she was living. Her next stage might be to seek a form of Jungian therapy to disclose the layer of self that accepted the disease on an archetypal level.

By this point in the patient's quest the original pathology has been reconceived as a harbinger of growth, a deathlike blow dislodging an even more profound systemic morbidity. Admittedly, I have posed an optimistic succession, but then this is a fictionalization of an actual case, plus in general in this book I am trying to propose what is possible when things *work*, not to recount the all-too-well-known ravages of incurable pathology. This progression—or even anything resembling it—may also have no dynamism for another person diagnosed with the so-called "same" Chronic Fatigue Syndrome but living a different constitution, individuation process, or etiology.

In another example, a naturopath may hand her client a note-page full of remedies—herbs, dietary changes, modes of exercise, a homoeopathic constitutional, a biweekly bathing ritual, and points on the body on which to do self-acupressure. The sincere patient may well attempt all of these things but forget about regularly pressing two Intestine points at the creases of his elbows. Ten years later another healer from a different tradition may emphasize *only* those points—and suddenly the person remembers, and the result is a more sustained degree of cure. That does not mean healing was not taking place all along: awakening to an already-ongoing process meets another octave within the process.

It is also possible a different person might never explicitly recall those two points but then unknowingly (and efficaciously) incorporate them in a sequence of *chi-kung* exercises, perhaps as part of a sound, a "kaaa!" or "ssss" intoned within a cycle of "animal-form" motions, breath-awareness, and light massage of the heart meridian. Again, this is why attention itself is more important than attention to any one orthodoxy. As in many of the internal martial arts, if one moves with spirit and fills the holes as they appear, then the big questions are answered without having to be asked. A physician merely isolates and objectifies a natural *"chi-kung"* when the body/mind has lost its way.

Students of *t'ai chi ch'uan* often remark how their form changes over the years even though they were ostensibly always doing the form. One practitioner told me he was startled only after some five hundred classes to realize, "That's what the teacher means by 'move from the center.' He doesn't mean, 'Get an image of the center and sort of shift that way.' He means—there really is a center to the body."

Likewise, the master instructs the student to "sink." But how? Peter Ralston, a proficient martial artist, recalled that for many years he tried to lower his body in every imaginable mechanical and mental way, using different exercises and images, and then suddenly one day he let go of an unexamined image on which he was relying without realizing it: then his entire being sank as though on its own.

On the level of disease and cure the body-mind probably goes through a similar process of training and reeducation unconsciously. For instance, Ralston continued his tale with another story: "You know you're there when a car whips around the corner and there's no time to think. Instead of jumping up, which is perhaps first instinct, you go right to the ground and stride past. It's faster than thought. You don't think, 'Oh, car! I better do what my teacher says and sink!' You find yourself having sunk because you know it at the deepest level."

I imagine every serious medicine gives us the same opportunity. As we have discussed, even homoeopathic and herbal remedies, which are received passively, ultimately require fairly profound internal adjustments.

The actual healer is always the self—the same hologram of independent cells orchestrated as tissues and organs that formed embryogenically from the seeds of the zygote and continues to unfurl in mystery. Transit across a lifetime is itself a passage into the inner, unrevealed chambers of a sanctum — and this process is unique and inscrutable in each person. It cannot be generalized or socialized according to the formulas of demography or even genetics. The unconscious, unarticulated shadow animal never visits the physician, or at least never declares itself when the social persona brings it there. The most intransigent diseases lurk in this shadow, but also the most intransigent cures. They exist on the primordial level of a crocodile or wild mouse, which do not even address their existences ontologically, let alone their ailments and dying.

I suspect that a large number of people develop illnesses, even potentially fatal ones, then heal them endogenously without ever knowing they had such a disease or were involved in a mode of self-treatment. The choices they make in their daily activities, seemingly based on other issues, turn out to be, synchronistically, the correct medical decisions too. The unbroken flow of mind and body through blood, breath, metabolism, human contact, imagination, and dream is always far more potent than an exogenous treatment or substance, for it contains the larval sea worm, its gut and heartbeat—the existential link to the desire to live at all.

As I have noted in a number of places in this book, the successful healer presents an "other" in the form of either a concrete medicine or his (or her) own presence that enables the "sick" person to "perceive" his own health. And this "perception" may be conscious or unconscious, biochemical or psychospiritual, highly cathected and painful or silent and brief as a breeze over a field of clover. The same mystery that lies in the twaining of healer and patient marks autonomous self-healing. We all live out our own individual stories which, by the living, we turn into families, diseases, cures, works of art, technologies, and whole cultures.

SUBTLE MEDICINE

Perhaps one reason the simple essences of oil that the French use in their medical aromatherapy are effective is that scents such as lavender, orange, and rose arouse the primal olfactory lobes of the brain, replicas of tissue that once experienced the anonymous earth healer directly, molecularly. The true language of smell can never be resurrected in primate philosophy because it is prior to a complex three-dimensional manipulation of the environment. Yet the sublime flavors and elixirs sought by alchemists and herbalists may have always resided innately in the concentrated aromas drawn from substances. Even without a formal system of smell diagnosis we walk along city streets (in sun or in rain) and are altered profoundly in mood and depth by elusive aromas— why not in metabolism and health too? Gardens, jungles, ponds, shifts in wind, visits to the beach, even stale office buildings carry both raw pathogens and medicines. This subtle play of scent won't necessarily cure an existing disease, but it continuously retunes the fluctuating matrix from which either vitality or degeneration later emerge.

When aromatherapist John Steele was asked to address a conference of corporate perfumers in early 1990, he knew it was a radical departure for them even to invite him. He shared the podium with marketing experts and executives from Fabergé, Calvin Klein, and Revlon, but whereas the speeches they delivered concerned only the promotion of scents as business, he proposed a notion of layers of consciousness activated by smell. "Most of them hadn't the slightest idea of what I was talking about," he told me, "but a few were really excited—like this was something they always suspected but had no idea how to talk about."

"What did they think aromas were if not consciousness?" I asked him.

"The usual things—sexual attractiveness, power, commerciality, the manufacture of desire. They are totally cynical in that sense. They presume that it's all a seduction and that the goal is to market scents in such clever disguises that people will be attracted to them but also basically fooled because they are really—well, nothing—you know, wisps of flavored air, immaterial gas." He pressed his fingers in a poof! "It was as though perfumes couldn't be real, so they better keep repackaging them to keep everyone fooled."

"But those things are consciousness based. Do they think desire is only artificial and manipulable?"

"I, like you, forget that anyone still thinks that way," he laughed, "but of course, they do. Notions like 'the earth is alive' or 'the reptilian brain is what responds to scents' would strike them as the most outrageous sort of California nonsense."

Herbs are more "material" than aromas, but are still quite subtle for this culture. Commercial pharmaceuticals are both gross and abstract—gross in their chemistry but abstract in their relation to the body-mind's actual dynamics of survival. These highly synthesized medicines are more semantic than substantial; they originate in and then generate clichés and presumptions that unconsciously alter so-called objective biochemical research and prescribing. One often ingests someone else's fantasy, a cumulative guess as to what a standard condition and its range of potentiation are.

The simplicity of most herbs makes them concrete as well as precise. If one eats iris or black cohosh or quercitrin tree bark, they are supplying their organs with raw building blocks that contributed to the genesis of these plants, albeit in elaborately mingled and synchronized fashion. Of course, the organs of the body will not make plants out of them, but they will use them in ways that would be impossible if the molecules did not originate herbally.

Refined pharmacy changes the characteristics of its "herbs" into more immediately activating substances that are less subtle and probably less creative, hence more toxic (for their lack of adaptability). The classic medicinal smell of the hospital is really the fragrance of the industrial laboratory.

We often miss that what is subtle is also basic, like the olfactory sensors in the reptilian brain. Herbs contain fundamental "messages," presemantic signatures from the heart of nature. We can even taste aspects of these. A blend for calming the liver based on peony root has a unique orange-clay flavor; dandelion root is earthy too but sweeter. The spotted colors and tangled horns of foxglove suggest heart arhythmia. The sparkle of phosphorus evokes the fragile hypersensitivity of its remedy. Reality is so basic it is a wonder we lose it in background abstractions.

Recently Paul Pitchford directed me to a traditional pharmacy in Oakland Chinatown. From the moment I stepped into the shop I was charmed and astonished to see how raw and unadorned its substances were: parts of animals hanging from the ceiling and walls—horns, antlers, fur, cuttlebones; micaceous earth; grasshoppers and cicadas; bear galls; dried earthworms and smaller worms; huge chunks of fungus, rind, and bark; roots of all sizes and topologies; whole fish; and other unidentifiable items that looked disconcertingly like the exports of cannibals. (One might wish we had access downtown to Australian Aborigine and African pharmacies too.)

When I asked for my prescription of abalone shell the clerk couldn't find it, and I had to wait for her to get the proprietor to consult his chart to the many drawers that lined the wall behind the counter. This was carried out uncertainly and in painstaking English with the help of other customers. Any fear I had that the language barrier might lead to my getting the wrong "herb" was quickly dispelled when he opened a seemingly random drawer and pulled out a handful of distinctive whole shells glistening iridescently. He slid them into a sack, weighed them quickly on a delicate balance he held in the air, then said, "Fifty cents."

I wasn't ready for such a literal response, so I tried to explain that I needed to make a tea. He agreeably unwrapped them and dumped them in a metal mortar; then he beat and crushed them with a pestle until they were chips and powder. Every tenth stroke he hit against the side of the mortar, setting it ringing. This demonstration of the transposition of raw shells into "medicine" was quite powerful. The abstraction was certainly demolished, so that when I poured hot water over the remains I knew what I was drinking. I even imagined the mineral shimmer asking interesting questions of my cells as they encountered it—questions they may not have heard for many years.

A medicine can be basic in the way "sinking" is for the practice of *t'ai chi ch'uan*. One tries to get down under, to beneath the rapt but insensible qualities of their own tendencies to move and consume. When the right hand forming a needle has been placed and taken from sea-bottom, then one's arms are spread like a fan from the roots, and one *is* briefly an herb: intrinsic energy patterns change. But it is difficult to keep this in mind, in heart—or to remember, as the old musical avowed (though not necessarily about abalone shells), "The moon belongs . . . to everyone."*

In our suicidal civilization there is some question of how many of us want to transform the poison and go on living. Most people it seems would rather manufacture more and more poison so that they can die more quickly and anonymously, with the least pain. But cure is always change; it always involves suffering: separation before new unity. It is far easier to live and die on the surface and accept that existence comes

---

*"The Best Things in Life Are Free" from Good News.

from the oblivion of universal cell life and deteriorates into the oblivion of catabolic dissociation. No doubt part of the attraction of modern science is that it disdains a universe of karma (with all its necessary growth and struggle) and replaces it with a sterile panoply of atoms and molecules. At least those atoms and molecules are under interdict to obey *our* mechanical laws. So the bad news of medical science is always that we are obliterated in the end, but the good news is that at least we get to have "the big sleep," the ultimate disease.

Conventional medicine works on the same level as mechanical physics: it prefers to alter (temporarily) the substratum of molecules and cells while ignoring the mystery of life itself. But that is not to say conventional medicine doesn't also awaken the dragon. After all, the universe operates not by name tags and ideologies; it sets its own esoteric levels among realms of consciousness and unconsciousness, and we discover the realities of conditions often where we least expect. No one can usefully rate doctors for purity and holism just as no one can rate them according to the applicability of their scientific training and the technologies to which they have access. Existence is primal and pagan, and Coleridge's "negative capability" is probably still a more accurate gauge of our potential for growth and change (and cure) than even the most healthy regimen of Whole Earth Medicine. The Osage Rite of Vigil (with its vapor baths, Sun Turtles, sacred moccasins, war clubs, and House of Mystery)—or the Navaho Beautyway Ceremony (with its Mountain Gods, Magic Tobacco, Big Snake with No End, and Monster-Slayers)—remain the micro-encoded infrastructures for a true BIG "planet medicine" yet to be born.

Or, as the same song promises more succinctly, "And love can come . . . to anyone. . . . "

Recently I had an opportunity to participate in a Native American ceremony conducted by a Western woman who had trained with a Cheyenne medicine man. Well into the rite she took up a small hoop-shaped drum and began beating it in rhythmic sequences punctuated by pauses. We had already burned cedar and chanted, shook a rattle, and diagnosed by a hawk feather. The drum was so engulfing and powerful that the seriality of its beat and texture of its thumps resonated at different levels of my mind and body. The intellectual in me wondered why I never included a drum in *Planet Medicine* (afterwards, I looked in the index and realized in fact I had). "I could see your mind being chased by my drum," the medicine lady told me. "So slippery you are, so tricky; you have so many ways and places to hide, so many ways to pretend to

the drum you are there when you are not."
'Right,' I thought. 'All through *Planet Medicine* as well, I run.'
"Your mind does you no good at this point. You must turn, embrace
it, and carry it to your heart."
So now, the unruly drum.

ECOLOGICAL CRISIS

To a degree that had not been so explicit at the time of my original
writing, planetary disease threatens the continuation of our species and
all others on our world. We cannot exist indefinitely in an escalating car-
bon-dioxide climate with a frayed ozone layer and an increasingly devi-
talized biosphere—even assuming the legendary acupuncture and
homoeopathy of masters this book at least proposes. After all, faith healers and shamans cannot turn Mars or Venus into habitable planets on the
physical-incarnate sphere. Even leaving aside matters of intra- and inter-
species slaughter (in the names of science and nation), even conceding
nuclear winter and radioactive waste as politically addressable issues,
there remains an undaunted, ongoing erosion of farmland, jungle, and
atmosphere, a poisoning of the layers of life, and an extinction of species
(and with them, their unique ecospheres, genes, and spirits). One com-
mentator has observed that the planet itself now has AIDS, its immune
system weakened to a degree even Gaia cannot reconstitute it without
hard yoga from its inhabitants.

If this is the case, as sooner or later it will be, then the big medicinal
task of the coming decades is to understand that issues of individual health
and planetary health are inextricably linked in increasingly shorter and
simpler cycles. It is probably not too late for people to heal themselves
and then begin healing the environment (and vice versa for those of more
activist bent), but both are necessary. Just like the body, the world
responds to realities not ideologies, to molecules of carbon and oxygen
and photons radiating from the sun. The ecological crisis has no agenda;
in fact, it is no more a crisis than chlorophyll or fog are. Thus, it cannot
ultimately be located in a political arena of discourse and diagnosis.

A civilization of drugged junk-food addicts working at psychospir-
itually vacuous jobs will not respond to the crisis in time—no matter
how many newspapers they read, contributions they make to Green-
peace, and aluminum cans they recycle. When the patient has AIDS you
don't simply berate the manufacturers of fluorocarbons. You speak to
the hollow at the heart of the modern world.

FOOD

Pharmaceuticals, psychotherapies, vital substances, and modes of touch
can all engender impressive cures, but eventually one must make an
attempt to consume whole foods and unpolluted water and minerals; to
stop eating meat, fatty and rancid oils, sugar and artificial sweeteners, and
pesticided food. Unquestionably some people override this one, just burn
right through the modern cyberworld on a steed of metabolized energy,
many of them keeping the economy going at the expense of their bodies.
But most people are going to get weaker from the modern civilized diet
and stronger even just from the conscious attempt to treat food as a matter
of practice rather than a neutral body and emotion fuel. That is, unexamined stuffing of material into one's system is a kind of phenomenological
poisoning that may even intensify the molecular effects of the food itself.

Fasts (even short ones) can be surprisingly strong medicines. The effect
on the body is obvious: the organs have more time to assimilate and cleanse;
digestion goes deeper into the static layers of tissue, reaching older congestion. The effect on the mind is subtler and probably more profound. A constant readiness to eat (to take in food as pleasure)—an "I consume" mentality
ranging from snacks and coffee breaks to gourmet meals—suffuses existence
with dolor and inertia. We become the victims of our hungers, thus never sati-
ate them. It is not just a matter any longer of avoiding gluttony; our collective
malady is one of addictively flooding taste cells and tissue with dense
superficial medicines in order to relieve an existential disease of the soul.
It is a pathology most difficult and unpleasant to face. Those in the West certainly mean to protect their consumption empire from the face of Kali which
stares into it from every Third World portal (not to mention the eternal
famine of unconscious mind and its representation in the night).

A person might consider walking past those bagel and donut shops he usually frequents. Instead of stopping to consume, he simply breathes the aromas
and imagines what it is he craves. Microdose replaces compulsive overdose.
Suddenly his senses become alert to the many different textures and layers
of existence. Hunger turns out to be subtler than a desire for food. It is
satisfied by scent, by image, eventually even by fast. Yogis who famously
breathe the air for chi and "drink" from sun with their skin not only prophesy
a planet with a healthier ecosphere, they likely taste the intrinsic qualities
(sour, bitter, salty, sweet), the elemental yin and yang that Western civilization gets only symptomatically from its roast ribs and chocolate fudge cake.

One must assume that Buddha and Jesus were not merely spouting pieties
on this issue. Buddha in fact skips over all the subtler and more psychological

issues of modern existential Buddhism and says simply, "Don't eat meat." We don't have to take that admonition literally or assume that all discussion of the matter stops there, but there is a possible interpretation of his teaching in which diet is prior to philosophy, even in matters of enlightenment.

One of the most striking symptoms of our civilization is that it is almost impossible (especially in the capitalist countries of the First World and those that imitate them) to find ordinary food. Try driving down the streets of any city or town in North America and look at what the super-markets and restaurants advertise and offer as normal—synthesized by-products with overdoses of preservatives, hormones, and artificial flavors to create the illusion of prosperity and satisfaction. It is consumption addiction, not eating. Or perhaps it is one more face of the petroleum rush that locates us in our shallow and desolate materialism—a materialism that does not even deign to examine the internalization of the images it floods us with, let alone the substances we ingest through those images.

Our political and elite establishment would prefer to face petty crises of economics and military adventurism than to change the real patterns of our existence. The reality that is served with the morning newspaper and chatters twenty-four hours a day on radio and television runs a meaningless gamut from left-wing to right-wing, from greed to humanitarianism, from nihilism to ecstasy, but it is all a single mirage in place of real activity, of chi-flow and mind-breath. In terms of overall impressions and mind-sets, the Hollywood/Madison Avenue complex is as deadly as the Military/Indus-trial one. We are fed images that destroy our sense of well-being, our mental health, our uniquenesses, and our ability to act from the heart.

Fasting is a form of silence, and silence is the beginning of feeling. From feeling, the tissues and organs know one another and their intrinsic unity. Feeling is what accumulates in our nervous systems to fire as homeostatic as well as cognized intelligence. To cut off sensation is to give disease its first foothold, is the beginning of not wanting to live.

I violate the neutrality of my text to make this one suggestion: if you are sick, change your diet—of impressions as well as of food and drink. At least practice a consciousness of consumption. Challenge unexam-ined, undifferentiated omnivorousness.

DRUGS AND VACCINATIONS

Antibiotics kill germs, but they do so at the expense of the immune system and the overall vitality of body/mind. While nature breeds healthy organisms, antibiotics (and pesticides) breed more and more virulent germs (and "pests"). Our mindless attack upon the imagined world of germs and parasites has left us weaker than our supposed enemies, for we not they are the ultimate victims of relentless mutations. There is a growing belief that the host of newer immunity-related diseases are at least partially the side-effects of antibiotic residues in people's systems. Such toxic medicines may sometimes be necessary (even as guns may be necessary in the face of a direct adversary), but they are never a strengthener of overall health and should not be sought as curealls.

Vaccinations (especially the routine childhood DPT shots) may be even more hazardous than antibiotics. Although no links to serious ailments have been proven, a number of researchers believe that treated disease products have far deeper somatic and psychological consequences than simply to immunize against specific diseases. They may transpose aspects of pathology into overall systemic activity and thereby set in motion more intractable and exotic neurological disorders. One would be advised to consult the references available on this topic and carefully weigh the pros and cons before taking any "shot."

Sedatives, anti-depressants, anti-anxiety drugs, psychotropics, and the like are stopgap measures that numb one's being to pain, hence to the real crisis. They are police measures in a security- and property-conscious state.

The other "drugs"—crack, heroin, ice, etc.—are hardly the toys of a kick-happy society. They are last-resort medicines for people who cannot handle the input of a materialized, external-value, bottom-line-only lifestyle in which family and community are already nostalgias. Environmentally we may have some margin left, but psychically and in our inner life we have reached *Blade Runner* and *Mona Lisa Overdrive*. Drugs are medicines of despair not fun. "Just say, 'No!'" is the most ironical of jokes when everyone who takes these medicines addictively has already said a far deeper "No!" than Nancy Reagan or George Bush could fathom. Crack and heroin are the coffee and tobacco of a less leisurely and gracious time.

PSYCHOTHERAPY

I don't accept the "pre-psychotherapeutic" trashing of therapy. If one has little sense of an internal life or of the cause-and-effect relationships of their emotions, then they can change themselves in remarkably healthful ways by therapy with someone who is artful beyond the diagnostic manual. However, there is a "post-psychotherapeutic" criticism well worth expounding, particularly in a book likely to be read by people favoring depth analysis.

Once one has a sense of an inner life and an intuition of personal symbols, yet still feels depressed, anxious, or otherwise hampered, only more radical and energy-oriented therapies will catalyze a change. Contemporary psychotherapy too often provides a person with a story, a new fiction to replace the so-called wounded one he or she is carrying around. That fiction can be based upon the Freudian notion of an "original trauma," or it can be highly visioned, as many of the Jungian versions are, with gods and goddess functions, Amazons and heroes, ancient myths and socially constructed images of masculinity and femininity. The goal of even such benignly expansive therapy is always adaptation to a therapeutic story. And by whose authority is one tale truer than another? (Even the stories of Christ and other great teachers have been scandalously abused by various denominations of preachers as well as by Church hierarchies themselves for centuries, i.e., have been used to steal people's own mysterious lives and replace them with blind allegiance to a literalized account that can be managed and exploited by authorities.)

The person seeking therapy is reduced finally to choosing among models of co-dependency, primal violation, archetypal quest, and the like. But what about the actual and immediate life he or she is also leading? Does it just become a shadow of therapeutic reality? Can such immediacy be lived without first shattering therapeutic authority and its act of clan initiation? It would seem that our soul-doctors have blundered into just the confusion of psychological and spiritual authority our Constitution sought to guard against by separating Church and State.

Tithing to a therapist for personal growth and vision is perhaps only superficially removed from tithing to a priesthood for the same. And who is to say that the psychiatric profession is not the priesthood reendowed? Oftentimes traditional divinatory methods (like Navaho myth-chanting and sand-painting) or oracular therapies (like the *I Ching*) can have a more profound and creative impact by supplying totally novel images in circumstances where an imposition of Jungian archetypes or Westernized shamanisms would represent only a continued assault of authoritarian consciousness. And this is because the unconscious answer is always liberating, always a process-oriented response to the mysteries of psyche.

The casting of astrological charts, for instance, has the possibility of revealing cycles which are beyond consciousness and unconsciousness both (and are routinely ascribed to stars and planets for lack of any other metaphor). "Uranus and Venus in opposition" or "three planets in the twelfth house" are potentially radicalizing challenges, not programmatic myths. (Jung himself would likely be appalled by the present worship of the archetypes—its fantasies of goddess-dom and male warrior-shamans. He was at least clear that real danger and wisdom lay in the soul itself as opposed to the exotic images generated through the course of individuation.)

But I emphasize—this is not a hardhat anti-therapy position; it is an anti-authoritarian position. I would recommend polarity therapies, various forms of bodywork and neo-Reichian methods, and, in some instances, gestalt and other interactional therapies—in other words, therapies that energize one to make a new life rather than tell a new version of an old story. In the end life itself is what the gods of Egypt (or any nome) measure on the scales; they make no dispensation for sanity or insanity, no extraneous distinction between myth and reality.

VITALISTIC MEDICINES

This one is, as they say, still conceptually up for grabs. Homoeopathy, acupuncture, chiropractic, curing by sound and vision, faith healing, and their allies have certainly not been proven even mildly effectual by the mainstream scientific credentialing process. In fact, there have been innumerable assertions by skeptics that certain of these processes are now conclusively debunked. Proof or disproof in this genre changes nothing. We do not live long enough and are not objective enough to see the universe blink.

I believe we are energy bodies. That is, I believe we are more than tissue formed by cell growth and differentiation, or that that tissue is imbued with a subtle prana current. But in our time this must be a matter of faith not quantification. If you believe in the existence of the energy body and have enough courage to set your star by it, then the above medicines are ultimately your true pharmacy (and even surgery). They are forerunners of an era (at least we can hope) in which men and women will aspire to be more than well-kept machines.

But do not expect vitalism to replace technological medicine in this generation. Do not even expect it to engage professional allopathy in a substantial dialogue. Concede the spoils to the AMA. Use vitalistic medicine only to treat actual disease. Cede the reign of quantity and proof to the neo-sophists and computer hacks.

A system like homoeopathy cannot work as substance. It is in fact a medicine of the *shadow* of technology. Its validity—its capacity to heal—must come at least in part from its denial of the overendowed material and substance flooding the modern world, i.e., its defiance of biochemical priority. I would imagine that even a medicine of "nothing"—which is what the AMA considers homoeopathy—has tremendous potential power in an age choked with overproduction and vapid data. Homoeopathy tells us that the whole bureaucracy is "nothing" also, the life it endows "nothing" as well. It (and the other energy medicines) carry the full power of the uncompensated-for spirit inside us. They are allopathy's true enantiodromia.

There is unquestionably a certain amount of quackery and fraud posing as vitalist medicine—and this makes it far too easy for the medical establishment to remain smug in their model of the body-mind. But much of science is simply cleverly disguised and sophisticatedly funded quackery— academic semantics without an object. Yes, a chiropractor may well miss diabetes—and even worse—attempt instead to treat his own mythological version of the disease. But a urologist might likewise miss the basis of a thirst introducing too much liquid in noting mere excess urination. Errors of diagnosis and cure finally transcend professional boundaries.

As I pointed out earlier, the scientific model of our existence is almost religious in its dread of an unbounded universe of psyche and energy. For the weary scientist so far along in his professional life, death of spirit is the only way out. So the two camps of a potential "planet medicine" remain substantially isolated. Vitalistic medicine operates without currency, and allopathy has become pure deficit spending. Some future generation will have to render the verdict (see below).

But, remember, there are no guarantees in the world of spirit. There are at least limited guarantees in the search-and-destroy world, and in the end one must make the bargain they can live with.

The Health Establishment

The experiment on the populace in the name of health care is becoming so uncontrollably expensive that we may not be able to afford it much longer. Even as the establishment is getting more and more skillful at targeting loci of disease, new diseases are springing up epidemically and the overall quality of life and spirit is deteriorating. One can certainly find a decent physician in the health establishment, but the old-fashioned combination of clarity and compassion are now the exception rather than the rule. Ultimately our civilization must redefine health care, along with its redefinitions of education, employment, and politics.

Although it borders on incendiary to compare the medical system to the practices of the Nazis (even metaphorically), I feel that one of the most distinctive marks of our century is an unfortunate living out of the discovery that bodies can be made into objects and used for purposes other than lives. People are converted to statistics hundreds of times over, as if this were the natural consequence of existence in civilization. Genocide is mere social policy. A planeload of innocent people can be exploded to make a statement about a whole other thing (admittedly, the passengers are in some way implicated or they wouldn't be there, but then everything is implicated in everything else, and that proves nothing).

From birth in the hospital to death in the morgue our bodies are potential victims of a science that ostensibly seeks to give them longevity while gaining knowledge about itself. Dozens of diagnostic exams provide each individual with "significant" information about his or her own being: the biological computer has replaced the Oracle at Delphi, and it speaks a stochastic language exiled from a universe of vital energy or gods.

There is literally "no way out," and the recent movie of that title provides a series of images for the dilemma: not only are we trapped like the hero (Kevin Costner) by a computer that will reconstruct us from a single cell (and likewise destroy us through the secrets of our genetic material), but we are tracked even after our death like the heroine (Sean Young) by the actual molecules extracted from our digestive system. In an age of gene-mapping and splicing we are mesmerized in the illusion that we are by-products of our own existence. Any way you look at it, the goal is to make us into products and to replace our freedoms with service to the most conventional images of the state machine—all under the guise of health care (or other "well-fare"). We may intuit the degree to which we are sexually manipulated by the media (as well as by the perfumers and food-and-drink merchants), but we probably do not realize that this is just a minor chord in the overall biological manipulation. Our body-minds are spies who *cannot* come in from the cold.

The so-called AIDS epidemic is another instance of this intrusion. Unquestionably a serious immune-oriented illness has spread globally, but the explanation that its symptoms are the result of the Human Immunodeficiency Virus is quite possibly as much a myth as anything of which a materialist might accuse an astrologer. The only advantage that HIV causation confers is the creation of a research empire based on this virus and overseen by the ostensible discoverer (even this "fake" discovery has been challenged as theft by the French government protecting the interests of its own scientists). But if the accused virus is only a late scavenger of a diseased immune system, then the whole wild goose chase becomes one more symptom of our preference of images and ideologies over realities. Even negative concepts (like an explicit AIDS virus) are more easily (and hysterically) marketed than the complicated realities they disguise.

People are led to fear becoming sick almost to the degree they fear being arrested. Either way freedom is coopted by the establishment; the body is turned over to the authorities for their disposition, and the treatment may well make the person far sicker (or terminally depressed). What is most askew with the health establishment is that it is operating more and more invasively on the physical by-products of our existence and less and less on the mystery and spirit of life itself.

The fierceness of the Tibetan Siamukha figurines, devouring infants and skulls and bearing flayed humans on their backs, is precisely the gentleness available when we adopt their demeanor in confronting the real enemies (who generally come with smiling visages these days). We face so many genial assassins that compassion requires a fierce internalization, a wrathful embodiment from the spectrum of energy, devouring obscurity to the dharma and serving as a manifestation of enlightened mind. We have no other way of confronting the false priests and physicians, the real devourers of souls. Perhaps the current fad of horror movies reflects our initial healing response to a civilization that has embalmed its bodies in junk-food and fashions and merchandized alienation from them at every level.

Mainstream psychoanalysis has fallen into the same morass that gene-mapping and fictive viruses portend on the somatic side of the scale. It would be quite a surprise if a society willing to lose millions of acres of farmland a year and dumping radioactive materials into its offshore waters were willing to engage in long, careful episodes of insight therapy with members of the populace. I see no place for the dialogue between therapist and patient, even in its most stereotyped and watered-down Oedipal version, in a society satisfied by TV sitcoms, Trump palaces, media presidencies, and multi-million- dollar sports contracts. In 1969 we could go to the Moon with esprit; little more than a decade later we barely cared enough to put viable O-rings on a space shuttle or, failing that, to hold the launch at least till the icicles melted. So why would an analyst sit for hours and years with his patient trying to track down the unknowable origins of trauma (except, as mentioned earlier, to found a profitable church)?

Most psychoanalysts now barely care enough to do that. Why bother with creative fictions when one can simply prescribe an anti-anxiety or anti-depression drug? When symptoms suggesting incipient schizophrenia or panic reactions are noted in children now, a regimen of medication is routinely adopted to "manage" the disease. If everything in the life can be reduced to the biochemistry of one's genome, then searching for insight and writing philosophy are big wastes of time.

Children growing up in an era of chemical dependency, genocide, recreational murder, nations armed with nuclear weapons, ozone-layer destruction, and portending drought *should* suffer anxiety. Does it really serve the planet—or even our species—to drug and addict them to expensive, psychoreductive substances? And what happens if the guinea pigs ever try to break free of their medications? What will they confront then in the form of personality breakup and panic? And how hard will it be for them to distinguish between the original conflicts in their souls and the dark moods they associate addictively with the alleviation of the drugs?

If we routinely take to prescribing medication for fear and the shadow world, we will have no Faulkner, or Kierkegaard, or Doris Lessing, or R. D. Laing, but long before that we will have no world at all.

ACTION

There is little doubt that such things as aerobics, jogging, and general exercise are healthier than general "couch potato" sloth. However, even in strengthening our bodies and beginning to move our sluggish parts, we have a tendency to give our allegiance to the most explicit, showiest options and to miss the level at which we are being duped by overacting (or duping ourselves). Just jogging or moving to music in an exercise class or using weights in a health club, while certain to tonify the outer neuromusculature, may later stiffen or subtly injure organs, or, more insidiously, engender a sense of duty and mindlessness through which the vast middle ground of existence is lost. In such a state only strong gestures and feelings seem to count, only exaggerations of our lives—conditioning to a peak and surviving marathons become the goals worth achieving. Ordinariness and dailiness are devalued. And, despite the grueling crosstown jogs and grunts on the Nautilus, one axiomatically is never hard on oneself in the way that they most require it. Resistance to change is always stronger than willed intentions. There are places where even the most spirited and well-trained marathon runner hides out from deepening awareness, from even the looseness and freedom of her own body.

We cannot always act strategically to make ourselves healthier. Sometimes we must learn *not* to act—to mourn, to relinquish, to fail and experience long sorrows. Such middle ground ultimately is the body of health.

Although it is presumptuous to judge anything on face value, it is generally true that various forms of internal martial arts (mostly based on *t' ai chi ch' uan, hsin-i ch' uan,* and *aikido*) provide more integrated alternatives to such typical exercise. Internal martial arts integrate *chi- kung* breathing modes, subtle response to gravity, the roots extending into the earth under one's feet, and fundamental principles of motion and energy— integrate these phenomena into acts of confrontation and blending with real opponents. The experience of a center *is* the center, a punch comes from compression into the ground, and yielding is only in response to feeling. The martial-arts practitioner must stay in the middle ground because he or she must respond to and blend with an actual opponent rather than a regimen, fiction, or even the agenda one might project on an opponent (whether overfearful or overconfident). Speed alone and force alone are famously ineffective where grounding, attention, timing, and filling holes as they occur are the effective tools. Suddenly it is no longer a case of speculatively trying out forms of exercise but of working functionally toward a shadow realm in which one is blocked and unknowingly rigidified.

Internal martial arts, in a sense, reenact the therapeutic situation— the classical psychoanalytic one as well as the more conventional doctor-patient exchange. But in the martial situation the participants are equalized — healer and patient, both sources of transference, both exchangers of activating energy.

The importance of actuality (as concretized by combat and blending) cannot be underestimated in a hype-oriented society. There is no symbolic trauma finally—the so-called trauma is reenergized again and again as the simultaneous block and the attack of the opponent, and one must blend each time originally, and, despite exhaustion and distraction, summon up resources to deal with this living partner. In that circumstance the sources of impediment are discovered autonomously. In fact one discovers not only the obvious physical blocks but limitations he or she did not know existed, discovers them simply by breaking through (via a rollback, throw, or retreat) into open territory beyond.

It is possible that this can be done through pure exercise—and no doubt is—but *t' ai chi ch' uan* and *aikido* place it in a hierarchical system of self-discovery and initiation, and they also clearly distinguish between ideas and opinions of effectiveness on the one hand and actions on the other—a distinction which would appear to be obvious but isn't. Better to get instructions from a master of *chi* than an Olympic athlete or New Age trainer. By engaging with a master in a tradition going back generations one at least is not naively or arrogantly trying to reinvent all of practice.

Psychotherapy classically tries to locate trauma in affective event and then expiate it through understanding. *T'ai chi ch'uan*, on the other hand, provides a set of affectless moves—aggressions and their neutralizations, punches and their feints, uproots and their dodges, and a map for locating where one's soul bottoms out in the tricks of one's body. All these skills function from a growing capacity for subtle feeling, which they also heighten by providing personal images, sometimes quite profound ones, that come from layers of memory and are not part of the traditional system of training.

In the flow of form and the impersonal moves of an opponent, primal events are reenacted and transformed, especially if the practitioner respects these levels of feeling, sensations coming from the energy of his opponent, clues of his own tension, and the constant of gravity itself. Thus traumas may be reexperienced, cathected, and healed (even as Freud or Reich would have had it). Whereas in therapy this is mediated by words and symbols, in martial play it is evoked through movement and energetic interaction.

In a culture where words and symbols make up the trap, discussion of them (and through them) is not always the way out of the trap. The so-called "soft" martial arts are silent, but they are also truly martial, for people must fight their way not only through the imagined danger of the streets but out of a swamp of therapeutic images and reassurances. Where the soul bottoms out, the shadow is no longer an *idea* of a nightmare, a memory of damage done; it is the actual inability to strike or defend. And yet it is a block that one can engage creatively and energetically.

Still the ritual must be real. To do amateur psychotherapy and call it Indian magic is no better. Many of the current male and female initiation rights (notably the empowered males drumming and dancing to confront their weak fathers, and their counterparts, the newly shamanized females) are simply ideas and opinions masquerading as acts. This playing at being shamans shows how we overendow image and product, how we are incorrigible spiritual materialists— and it is finally embarrassing in light of where real danger and real disease are coming from currently in this world.

NATIVE MEDICINE

There are some vision quests it is still possible to take. Ayahuasca has gotten new attention not only as a healing agent but a tool in shamanic diagnosis of disease. Aboriginally used in the Upper Amazon, the Orinoco Plains, and the Pacific coast of Colombia and Ecuador it has now spread through urban areas of Brazil, Colombia, and Peru to the cities of North America. It was a feat for an ancient trans-Amazonian culture to invent this brew at all, since, in order to be active, it requires two distinct agents, the stem of a jungle vine which is cooked together with the leaves of one or another plant (depending on the region).

Ayahuasca is an antiparasitic, antimalarial herbal mix, but most crucially its ingestion reveals other medicines in the form of plant, animal, and celestial spirits, and it is used by shamans for insight into methods of curing. In fact, one anthropologist (Luis Eduardo Luna) reports that ayahuasca has given shamans the ability to hear the whole Amazon crying out along with the spirits of individual plants and animals. If this is so, then we might listen not only to the voices of responsible scientists warning us about the destruction of the rainforest but the jungle itself, which may contain an epigrammatic wisdom available through initiation.

Luna's main informant, the shaman Pablo Amaringo, pointed to the center of a photograph of a galaxy I was showing him recently and spoke a cosmology I would render from his own rough English as: "There is where I have gone. It looks like this on the outside; but inside, in the mind, it is a series of waves undulating eternally from the bark on the outside of the cosmos, bark like a tree. Those waves are dynamic and have terrible dark places in them, voids so great I thought I was going to die." He went on to explain that these waves pass through plants and the etheric levels of animals even as they simultaneously enter the unconscious aspects of our minds and fill them with a knowledge that must be decoded through experience and translated through traditional knowledge. In a universe of pure intelligence, surely stars and vines and even molecules of water speak too.

During a recent speech to a homoeopathic conference, Edward Whitmont remarked, "All of the illness and growth potentials of man, the microcosm, are also to be found in the macrocosmic information of body of our mother, the Earth. We are like aspects, microcosmic replications of a vast cosmic form process.

"Perhaps it is not too far-fetched then to consider whether our attitudes, and illnesses, may not also be forms of communion with the Earth planet, particularly as we resort to the help of external medicinal substance fields. Perhaps, in some way which we still do not understand, some form of consciousness development occurs and is of use to the planetary process rather than only to ourselves. I leave it to you to ponder what this may mean in terms of the ways in which our chemical and drug technology current pollutes and poisons the Earth as well as our own organisms."

Shamans apparently linger elsewhere, in the Australian deserts and the remaining wilderness of Africa and Asia, but collectively at the moment we have as much chance of hearing them as of hearing a conversation on Neptune. We are trenchantly tuned to other channels, and we are in trouble. But as Ted Enslin warned, now many years ago, "Of course it's impossible. Therefore, do it!"

Notes

CHAPTER I

I am grateful to Dr. H. Robert Bagwell of the Mental Health Division of the Oregon Department of Human Resources in Salem for reading and criticizing the material in this chapter from the standpoint of professional medicine.

1. This insight comes in part from my work with Stanley Keleman and the ideas he has presented in professional colloquia in Berkeley, Calif., during 1978.

2. See note 1.

3. My source for this is the tape of Charles Olson's reading/talk before the University of California (Berkeley) Poetry Conference, in Wheeler Hall, July 23, 1965.

4. See note 1.

5. The American recognition of China, since the writing of this text, further clarifies the example. An actual relationship between the two nations proceeds, quite apart from and, in a sense, in defiance of the ultraradical and ultrareactionary images different people impose.

6. See note 1.

7. Edward Schieffelin, research associate in medical anthropology, University of California, Berkeley; personal communication.

8. Michel Foucault, *The Birth of the Clinic*, trans. from the French by A. M. Sheridan Smith, Pantheon, New York, 1973 (originally published in France in 1963), p. 3.

9. I have written on this issue at much greater length elsewhere. Note particularly Richard Grossinger, *Martian Homecoming at the All-American Revival Church* (North Atlantic Books, 1974), p. 82; *The Slag of Creation* (North Atlantic Books, 1975), p. 237; *The Unfinished Business of Doctor Hermes* (North Atlantic Books, 1976), pp. 54, 79, and 85; and *Ecology and Consciousness*, ed. Richard Grossinger (North Atlantic Books, 1978). (Both North Atlantic Books

and the journal *Io* are edited and published by the author of this book. The locations of publication have been Amherst, Mass., 1964–66; Ann Arbor, Mich., 1966–69; Mount Desert, Me., 1969–70; Cape Elizabeth, Me., 1970–72; Plainfield, Vt., 1972–77; Oakland, Calif., 1977; and currently, 1978 et seq., Richmond, Calif. Places of publication of North Atlantic Books will be omitted from the notes in this book to avoid confusion.)

10. Gregory Bateson, "Restructuring the Ecology of a Great City," *Io/#14, Earth Geography Booklet No. 3, Imago Mundi,* 1972, p. 141.

11. It might make sense to spell out here the idea that there are two different types of disease: those that occur from external forces, injuries, poisons, germs, malnutrition, etc.; and those that arise from the organism being in battle with its own mind/body. The first category is generally considered accidental (though not without argument), and it is the prime concern of humanitarian technology. It is when that technology attempts to cure a disorder of the second type *as if it were* a disease of the first category that it is overmatched and disruptive—for the forces which caused the disease will continue to erupt as long as they are untended and unresolved. It is not always possible to distinguish functionally between the two categories, and they overlap in any organism—but the idea of this distinction should clarify both our criticism and praise of modern professional medicine.

12. See references in note 9.

13. A story told me by Peter Ruddick in Plainfield, Vt.

14. Kathleen Goodwin, "Alternative Medicine: A Note of Caution," *City Miner* (Berkeley, Calif.), Vol. 3, No. 3, 1978.

CHAPTER II

1. Most of this material about early human society is rewritten from notes taken at graduate school lectures delivered by Dr. Roy A. Rappaport in ecological anthropology at the University of Michigan in Ann Arbor.

2. I am developing anew here, in terms of my own topic, many of the arguments of Claude Lévi-Strauss on the structural study of myth and totemism particularly as advanced in his books *The Raw and the Cooked* and *From Honey to Ashes.*

3. S. A. Barrett, *Pomo Bear Doctors,* University of California Publications in American Archaeology and Ethnology, Vol. 12, No. 11, July 11, 1917, University of California Press, Berkeley.

CHAPTER III

1. A. E. Waite, trans., *The Hermetic and Alchemical Writings of Paracelsus,* James Elliot, London, 1894.

2. D. Jenness, "The Carrier Indians of the Bulkley River," Bulletin No. 133, Bureau of American Ethnology, Washington, D.C., 1943; quoted in Claude Lévi-Strauss, *The Savage Mind,* University of Chicago Press, Chicago, 1966.

3. Waite, op. cit.

4. The information behind this "story" comes from Frank G. Speck, *A Study of the Delaware Indian Big House Ceremony,* Vol. II, Publications of the Pennsylvania Historical Commission, Harrisburg, Pa., 1931.

5. Kekulé's dream famous in psychoanalytic annals; James Watson referred to this in his book *The Double Helix,* Atheneum, New York, 1968.

6. Michael J. Harner, *The Jívaro*, Doubleday/Natural History Press, Garden City, N.Y., 1972, pp. 138–39.

7. The information behind this and the succeeding stories comes from William Wildschut, *Crow Indian Medicine Bundles*, ed. John C. Ewers, Museum of the American Indian, Heye Foundation, New York, 1975.

8. Ibid., pp. 9–10.

9. For the ethnoastronomy, see Alexander Marshack, *The Roots of Civilization*, McGraw-Hill, New York, 1972.

10. Lévi-Strauss, op. cit.

11. R. B. Fox, "The Pinatubo Negritos: Their Useful Plants and Material Culture," *The Philippine Journal of Science*, Vol. 81, Nos. 3–4, 1953; quoted in Lévi-Strauss, op. cit., pp. 4–5.

12. This material comes in part from discussion with Dr. Donald Lathrap of the Department of Anthropology, University of Illinois, Urbana.

13. This issue is taken up in great depth in my essay "Origin of the Human World," *Io/#23, An Olson-Melville Sourcebook*, Vol. II: *The Mediterranean*, North Atlantic Books, 1976, pp. 5–91.

14. Brian Inglis, *A History of Medicine*, World Publishing Co., Cleveland, 1965, p. 6.

15. Victor W. Turner, *Lunda Medicine and the Treatment of Disease*, Occasional Papers of the Rhodes-Livingstone Museum, No. 15, Livingstone, Northern Rhodesia [Zambia], 1964, pp. 61–62.

16. See Grossinger, *The Unfinished Business of Doctor Hermes*, pp. 102–3.

17. Marshall Sahlins, *Stone Age Economics*, Aldine-Atherton, Chicago, 1972, p. 2.

18. Ibid., p. 37.

19. Ibid., p. 4.

20. Loc. cit.

21. Ibid., p. 36.

22. Ibid., p. 4.

23. The discussion on this and the following pages deals with the writings of Carlos Castaneda, primarily *The Teachings of Don Juan: A Yaqui Way of Knowledge*, University of California Press, Berkeley, 1969; *A Separate Reality*, Simon and Schuster, New York, 1971; *Journey to Ixtlan*, Simon and Schuster, New York, 1972; and *Tales of Power*, Simon and Schuster, New York, 1974.

24. Castaneda, *Journey to Ixtlan*, p. 107.

25. Edward Dorn and Gordon Brotherstone, trans., "The Aztec Priest's Reply," *New World Journal*, Vol. 1, Nos. 2/3, 1977; p. 52.

26. Speck, op. cit., p. 65.

27. Owen Barfield, *Unancestral Voice*, Wesleyan University Press, Middletown, Conn., 1965.

28. Theodore Enslin, "Journal Note," quoted in Grossinger, ed., *Alchemy: Pre-Egyptian Legacy, Millennial Promise*, North Atlantic Books, 1979.

CHAPTER IV

1. Claude Lévi-Strauss, *From Honey to Ashes*, trans. from the French by John and Doreen Weightman, Harper & Row, New York, 1973, pp. 57–58.

2. Discussion with Donald Lathrap; see note 12, Chap. III, above.

3. See Richard Grossinger, "Origin of the Human World," especially pp. 34–48.

4. See Grossinger, ed., *Alchemy: Pre-Egyptian Legacy, Millennial Promise,* Chap. 7, n. 11.

5. Ven. Rinpoche Jampal Kunzang Rechung, *Tibetan Medicine,* University of California Press, Berkeley, 1973, pp. 82–84.

6. *Huang Ti Nei Ching Su Wên,* trans. Ilza Veith as *The Yellow Emperor's Classic of Internal Medicine,* University of California Press, Berkeley, 1966, Introduction, pp. 2–3.

7. Ibid., general text.

8. For a fuller discussion of this episode from a conversation with a participant, see Grossinger, *The Unfinished Business of Doctor Hermes,* pp. 144–45.

CHAPTER V

1. Edward Dorn, *Recollections of Gran Apachería,* Turtle Island, Berkeley, Calif., 1974.

CHAPTER VI

1. Erwin H. Ackerknecht, "Problems of Primitive Medicine," *Bulletin of the History of Medicine,* XI (1942), Johns Hopkins Institute of the History of Medicine, Baltimore, Md.; quoted in William A. Lessa and Evon Z. Vogt, eds., *Reader in Comparative Religion,* Harper & Row, New York, 1958, p. 399.

2. Benjamin Rush, *Medical Inquiries and Observations,* Vol. I, Pritchard and Hall, Philadelphia, 1789, p. 29; quoted in Harris Livermore Coulter, *Divided Legacy,* Vol. III, Wehawken Book Company, Washington, D.C., 1973, p. 40.

3. Coulter, op. cit.

4. George Way Harley, *Native African Medicine,* Harvard University Press, Cambridge, Mass., 1941, p. 85.

5. E. S. Craighill Handy, Mary Kawena Pukui, and Katherine Livermore, *Outline of Hawaiian Physical Therapeutics,* Bernice P. Bishop Museum, Bulletin 126, Honolulu, 1934, pp. 17–19.

6. Miguel Covarrubias, *Island of Bali,* Alfred A. Knopf, New York, 1937, pp. 352–53.

7. Morton C. Kahn, *Djuka: The Bush Negroes of Dutch Guiana,* Viking Press, New York, 1931, pp. 154–55.

8. Paul Pitchford, at a seminar on Chinese medicine, Berkeley, Calif., August 1976. Notes of my own conversations with Pitchford appear in Grossinger, "The Tablets of the Sphynx," *The Unfinished Business of Doctor Hermes,* pp. 126–45.

9. Harley, op. cit., p. 38.

10. Simon Ortiz, "That's the Place the Indians Talk About," in Grossinger, ed., *Ecology and Consciousness,* pp. 108–11.

11. William Wildschut, *Crow Indian Medicine Bundles,* p. 7.

12. Gladys Tantaquidgeon, *Folk Medicine of the Delaware and Related Algonkian Indians,* Pennsylvania Historical and Museum Commission, Harrisburg, 1972, pp. 22–23.

13. Handy, Pukui, and Livermore, op. cit., p. 14.

14. Ibid.

15. Shway Yoe, *The Burman*, Macmillan, London, 1910, p. 421.
16. Gladys A. Reichard, *Navaho Religion*, Bollingen Foundation, Pantheon, New York, 1950, p. xxxvi.
17. Yoe, op. cit., p. 421.
18. Handy, Pukui, and Livermore, op. cit., p. 13.
19. Ibid.
20. Michael Gelfand, *Medicine and Custom in Africa*, Livingstone, Edinburgh, 1964.
21. John R. Swanton, *Religious Beliefs and Medical Practices of the Creek Indians*, 42nd Annual Report to the Bureau of American Ethnology, Smithsonian Institution, 1924–25.
22. Covarrubias, op. cit., p. 353.
23. Gerald Cannon Hickey, *Village in Vietnam*, Yale University Press, New Haven, 1964, p. 81.
24. *Huang Ti Nei Ching Su Wên*.
25. Swanton, op. cit.
26. Dorothy M. Spencer, *Disease, Religion and Society in the Fiji Islands*, Augustin, New York, 1941.
27. Gelfand, op. cit., pp. 56–57.
28. A. P. Elkin, *Aboriginal Men of High Degree*, Australasian Publishing Company, Sydney, 1944, pp. 29–30.
29. Ven. Rinpoche Jampal Kunzang Rechung, *Tibetan Medicine*, p. 89.
30. Elkin, op. cit., pp. 15–16.
31. Ibid., p. 50.
32. Walter B. Cannon, " 'Voodoo' Death," *American Anthropologist*, XLIV, 1942; republished in Lessa and Vogt, eds., op. cit., pp. 321–27.
33. Ibid., p. 326.
34. Ibid., p. 327.
35. Claude Lévi-Strauss, "The Sorcerer and His Magic," in *Structural Anthropology*, trans. from the French by Claire Jacobson and Brooke Grundfest Schoepf, Doubleday/Anchor, Garden City, N.Y., 1967.
36. Franz Boas, *The Religion of the Kwakiutl Indians*, Part II: *Translations*, Columbia University Press, New York, 1930, pp. 17–18.
37. Ibid., p. 19.
38. Ibid.
39. Lévi-Strauss, op. cit.
40. Ackerknecht, op. cit., p. 400.
41. Harley, op. cit., p. 156.
42. Ibid., p. 157.

CHAPTER VII

1. A. R. Radcliffe-Brown, *The Andaman Islanders*, Free Press, Glencoe, Ill., 1948.
2. Michael J. Harner, *The Jívaro*, pp. 161–63.
3. Gerald Cannon Hickey, *Village in Vietnam*, p. 76.
4. Miguel Covarrubias, *Island of Bali*, pp. 324–25.
5. Dorothy M. Spencer, *Disease, Religion and Society in the Fiji Islands*.
6. Knud Rasmussen, *Intellectual Culture of the Iglulik Eskimos: Report of*

the *Fifth Thule Expedition to Arctic North America*, Gyldendalske Boghandel, Nordisk Forlag, Copenhagen, 1929, p. 56.

7. George Way Harley, *Native African Medicine*, p. 14.

8. Ibid.

9. Ibid., pp. 17–18.

10. Ibid., p. 137.

11. Spencer, op. cit.

12. This thesis about Melville is developed at great length in Richard Grossinger, "Melville's Whale: A Brief Guide to the Text," *Io/#22, An Olson-Melville Sourcebook*, Vol. I: *The New Found Land*, North Atlantic Books, 1976, pp. 97–152.

13. Herman Melville, *Moby Dick*.

14. The full passage from Melville's journals is quoted in the Grossinger essay cited in note 12, pp. 104–5.

15. Carlos Castaneda, *Journey to Ixtlan*, p. 114.

16. Ibid., pp. 114–15.

17. Alfred F. Whiting, *Ethnobotany of the Hopi*, Northern Arizona Society of Science and Art, Museum of Northern Arizona, Bulletin 15, Flagstaff, 1939.

18. A. P. Elkin, *Aboriginal Men of High Degree*, p. 113.

19. Harley, op. cit.

20. Ibid., p. 202.

21. Gladys Reichard, *Navaho Religion*, p. 5.

22. Ibid., p. xxxiv.

23. Ibid., p. 116.

24. Rasmussen, op. cit., p. 69.

25. Reichard, op. cit., p. xxxvii.

26. Ibid., p. 707.

27. Ibid., pp. 652–53.

28. Réné de Berval, *Kingdom of Laos*, France-Asie, Saigon, 1956, p. 423.

29. Israel Regardie, *The Eye in the Triangle*, Llewellyn Publications, St. Paul, Minn., 1970, p. 220.

30. Aleister Crowley, *The Confessions of Aleister Crowley*, ed. John Symonds and Kenneth Grant, Hill and Wang, New York, 1969.

31. Louis Mars, *The Crisis of Possession in Voodoo*, trans. from the French by Kathleen Collins, Reed, Cannon & Johnson, Berkeley, Calif., 1977.

32. Gladys Tantaquidgeon, *Folk Medicine of the Delaware* . . .

33. Spencer, op. cit.

34. Shway Yoe, *The Burman*, pp. 425–26.

35. Reichard, op. cit., pp. 99–100.

36. E. S. Craighill Handy, Mary Kawena Pukui, and Katherine Livermore, *Outline of Hawaiian Physical Therapeutics*.

37. De Berval, op. cit., p. 302.

38. Omar Khayyam Moore, "Divination—A New Perspective," *American Anthropologist*, LIX, 1957, pp. 69–74; republished in William A. Lessa and Evon Z. Vogt, eds., *Reader in Comparative Religion*, pp. 377–81.

39. Roy A. Rappaport, "Sanctity and Adaptation," *Io/#7, Oecology Issue*, 1970; republished in R. Grossinger, ed. *Ecology and Consciousness*, pp. 114–15.

40. Coles, William, "Adam in Eden, or The Paradise of Plants," republished in Io/#5, *Doctrine of Signatures*, 1968, pp. 39–45.
41. William Wildschut, *Crow Indian Medicine Bundles*, pp. 105–6.

CHAPTER VIII

1. Werner Heisenberg, "The Relationship Between Biology, Physics and Chemistry," in *Physics and Beyond*, trans. from the German by Arnold J. Pomerans, Harper & Row, New York, 1971, p. 113.
2. I. S. Shklovskii and Carl Sagan, *Intelligent Life in the Universe*, Delta Books, New York, 1967, p. 227.
3. Ibid., pp. 243–44.
4. Heisenberg, op. cit., p. 114.
5. Loc. cit.
6. Shklovskii and Sagan, op. cit., p. 184.
7. Paracelsus, quoted in Harris Coulter, *Divided Legacy*, Vol. I, p. 478.
8. A. E. Waite, *The . . . Writings of Paracelsus*, Vol. II, p. 59.
9. Ibid., pp. 22–23.
10. Ibid., p. 24.
11. I have omitted detailed discussion of alchemy from this book because of a concurrent book I have written entitled *Alchemy: Pre-Egyptian Prophecy, Millennial Promise*, North Atlantic Books, 1979.
12. For a fuller description of this theory, see my primary source: Frances Yates, *The Rosicrucian Enlightenment*, Routledge & Kegan Paul, London, 1972.
13. For a fuller description of the New Alchemists, see my book on alchemy cited above in note 11; also "The Rosicrucian Pony Back at the Barn" in Grossinger, *Martian Homecoming at the All-American Revival Church*, pp. 87–95, and *The Slag of Creation*, pp. 197–202.
14. Robert Kelly, in a letter to the author (January 24, 1979), provided some of the insights in this paragraph.
15. Jule Eisenbud, in an interview conducted by Richard Grossinger, January 8, 1972, originally published in Io/#14, *Earth Geography Booklet No. 3*, reprinted in Grossinger, ed., *Ecology and Consciousness*, p. 168. (For another brief interview by the author with Eisenbud [1975], see Grossinger, *The Unfinished Business of Doctor Hermes*, pp. 14–15.)
16. Ibid., pp. 168–69.
17. Ibid., p. 169.

CHAPTER IX

1. Philip Wheelwright, ed., *The Presocratics*, Odyssey Press, Indianapolis, 1966, p. 72.
2. Ibid., p. 268.
3. The information on this and the following pages comes from Ven. Rechung Rinpoche Jampal Kunzang, *Tibetan Medicine*.
4. The information on this and the following pages comes from *Huang Ti Nei Ching Su Wên*.
5. Ibid., p. 15.
6. Ibid., p. 108.

7. Ibid., pp. 108, 117.
8. Rechung, op. cit., p. 32.
9. The Academy of Traditional Chinese Medicine, *An Outline of Chinese Acupuncture*, Foreign Languages Press, Peking, 1975, pp. 69–70.
10. The information on this and the following pages comes from Baba Hari Das and Dharma Sara Satsang, "Ayurveda: The Yoga of Health" in *The Holistic Health Handbook*, Berkeley Holistic Health Center, And/Or Press, Berkeley, Calif., 1978, pp. 53–61.

CHAPTER X

For the concepts of Empiricism and Rationalism and much of the factual information in this chapter, I have relied on an excellent and not usually acknowledged book, the first volume in Harris Livermore Coulter's three-volume history of medicine entitled *Divided Legacy* (published by Wehawken Book Company, 4221 45th Street, N.W., Washington, D.C. 20016). Volume I covers the period from Hippocrates to Paracelsus.

1. See note 3, Chap. I, above.
2. Aulus Cornelius Celsus, *De Medicina*, quoted in Coulter, op. cit., p. 274.
3. If the Hippocratic writings stand in relation to medicine as the *Odyssey* and *Iliad* do to literature, then certainly James Tyler Kent's *Lectures on Homoeopathic Philosophy*, published originally in 1900, is the *Moby Dick* of homoeopathy —the great American medical book; see note 1, Chap. XII, below.
4. Philip Wheelwright, ed., *The Presocratics*, p. 272.
5. Hippocrates, *Medical Works*, quoted in Coulter, op. cit., p. 62.
6. Paracelsus, quoted in Coulter, op. cit., p. 358.
7. Ibid., p. 359.
8. Jan Baptista van Helmont, *Oriatrike, or Physick Refined*, London, 1662; quoted in Coulter, op. cit., Vol. II, p. 15.
9. For further discussion of Paracelsus and the preparation of alchemical medicine, see Grossinger, *Alchemy: Pre-Egyptian Legacy, Millennial Promise*.
10. Paracelsus, quoted in Coulter, op. cit., p. 354.
11. Van Helmont, quoted in Coulter, op. cit., p. 33.
12. Théophile de Bordeu, *Oeuvres*, Caille and Ravier, Paris, 1818; quoted in Coulter, op. cit., pp. 241–42.

CHAPTER XI

1. My sources for this chapter are recapitulated in Chapters XII–XIV, on homoeopathy. However, much of my own insight comes from ten years of research, fieldwork, discussions, and interviews. I am grateful to the following people for the verbal teaching and practical experience in homoeopathy they took the time to give me: Theodore Enslin, Dana Ullman, Edward Whitmont, Randall Neustaedter, Stephen Cummings, Michael Medvin, Wolfgang Kailing, Don Gerrard, and Prakash Mehta.

In particular, Randall Neustaedter and Stephen Cummings made it possible for me to sit in on cases and consultation at the Hering Family Clinic in Berkeley during the fall of 1978.

I have also relied on the three-volume history of medicine, *Divided Legacy*, by Harris Livermore Coulter, cited at the beginning of the notes to Chapter X.

CHAPTER XII

1. James Tyler Kent, *Lectures on Homoeopathic Philosophy* (1900), republished by North Atlantic Books, 1979, p. 39.
2. Samuel Hahnemann, *The Organon of Medicine*; quoted in Coulter, *Divided Legacy*, Vol. II, pp. 385–86.
3. Ibid., p. 12.
4. George Vithoulkas, *The Science of Homeopathy: A Modern Textbook*, Vol. I, Athens, Creccc, A.S.O.H.M., 1978, pp. 134–35.
5. Hahnemann, *The Lesser Writings*; quoted in Coulter, op. cit., p. 375.
6. See primarily M. L. Tyler, *Homoeopathic Drug Pictures*, Health Science Press, Holsworthy Devon, England, 1942. This is one of the best attempts to write up the homoeopathic symptom clusters as character studies of patients and disease-remedy types.
7. Claude Lévi-Strauss, *Totemism*, trans. from the French by Rodney Needham, Beacon Press, Boston, 1963.
8. Alfred North Whitehead, *Process and Reality*, Macmillan, Toronto, 1929.
9. Hahnemann, *The Organon of Medicine*; quoted in Coulter, op. cit., p. 380.
10. Vithoulkas, "The Science of Classical Homoeopathy," lecture series delivered at the California Academy of Sciences, April–May 1978.
11. Hahnemann, *The Organon of Medicine*; quoted in Kent, op. cit.
12. Ibid.
13. Hahnemann, *The Lesser Writings*; quoted in Coulter, op. cit., Vol. III, p. 19.
14. Theodore Enslin, speaking at a seminar at Goddard College, Plainfield, Vermont, May 1977.
15. Kent, op. cit., pp. 253–65.
16. Hahnemann, *The Lesser Writings*; quoted in Coulter, op. cit., Vol. II, p. 389.
17. For a recent discussion of the bowel nosodes, see Stephen Cummings, "History and Development of the Bowel Nosodes," *Journal of Homeopathic Practice*, Vol. 1, No. 2, 1978.
18. Kent, op. cit., p. 96.
19. See note 14, above.
20. Wyrth P. Baker, Allen C. Neiswander, and W. W. Young, *Introduction to Homeotherapeutics*, American Institute of Homoeopathy, Washington, D.C., 1974.
21. Edward Whitmont, "Toward a Basic Law of Psychic and Somatic Interrelationship," *The Homeopathic Recorder*, February 1949, p. 206.
22. Carl Jung, *Psychology and Alchemy*, trans. from the German by R. F. C. Hull, Routledge & Kegan Paul, London, 1953, p. 132.
23. Whitmont, "The Analysis of a Dynamic Totality: *Sepia*," *The Homeopathic Recorder*, reprint, 1948–1955, p. 232.
24. Ibid., p. 233.

25. Whitmont, "Natrum Muriaticum," *The Homeopathic Recorder*, 1948, p. 119.

26. Whitmont, "Phosphor," *The Homeopathic Recorder*, April 1949, p. 265.

27. Rudolf Hauschka, *The Nature of Substance*, trans. from the German by Mary T. Richards and Marjorie Spock, Stuart and Watkins, London, 1968, pp. 136–37.

28. Whitmont, "Lycopodium: A Psychosomatic Study," *The Homeopathic Recorder*, 1948, pp. 264–65.

29. Whitmont, "Psycho-physiological Reflections on Lachesis," *British Homeopathic Recorder*.

30. Whitmont, "Non-causality as a Unifying Principle of Psychosomatics— Sulphur," *The Homeopathic Recorder*, 1953, p. 32.

CHAPTER XIII

I have reconstructed Samuel Hahnemann's biography primarily from Richard Haehl, *Samuel Hahnemann, His Life and Work*, Vol. I, Homeopathic Publishing Co., London, 1922. General information from the text will not be cited but specific quotations will.

1. Haehl, op. cit., p. 10.
2. Ibid., p. 11.
3. Ibid., p. 36.
4. Ibid., p. 35.
5. Ibid., p. 58.
6. Ibid., p. 63.
7. Ibid., p. 64.
8. Ibid., p. 322.
9. Ibid., p. 126.
10. Harris Livermore Coulter, *Divided Legacy*, Vol. III, p. 170.
11. Ibid., p. 171.
12. Quoted in Haehl, op. cit., p. 100.
13. Samuel Hahnemann, *The Chronic Diseases, Their Peculiar Nature, and Their Homeopathic Cure*, Boericke & Tafel, Philadelphia, 1904, p. 12.
14. Ibid.
15. Ibid., p. 38.
16. Haehl, op. cit., p. 179.
17. Ibid.
18. Ibid., p. 222.

CHAPTER XIV

Much of the information in this chapter comes from the third volume of Harris Livermore Coulter, *Divided Legacy* (see notes for Chapter X, above).

1. Coulter, op. cit., pp. 62–63.
2. Ibid., p. 180.
3. Ibid., p. 106.
4. Ibid., p. 168.
5. Ibid.

6. Ibid., p. 169.
7. Richard Haehl, *Samuel Hahnemann: His Life and Work*, p. 187.
8. Coulter, op. cit., pp. 264–65.
9. Ibid., pp. 269–70.
10. Ibid., p. 403.
11. Ibid., p. 411.
12. Ibid., p. 414.
13. Ibid., p. 438.
14. Ibid., p. 441.
15. Ibid., pp. 447–48.

CHAPTER XV

1. Jacques Derrida, *Of Grammatology*, trans. from the French by Gayatri Chakravorty Spivak, Johns Hopkins University Press, Baltimore, 1976; see also Derrida's "Freud and the Scene of Writing," trans. from the French by Jeffery Mehlman, *Yale French Studies*, Yale University Press, New Haven, n.d., p. 116.
2. Sigmund Freud, *An Outline of Psychoanalysis*, trans. from the German by James Strachey, Norton, New York, 1949, p. 11.
3. Ibid., p. 9.
4. Ibid., p. 13.
5. Claude Lévi-Strauss, *Totemism*, pp. 1–2.
6. Freud, *The Interpretation of Dreams*, trans. from the German by James Strachey, Basic Books, New York, 1955.
7. Ibid., p. xxxii.
8. Ibid., p. 88.
9. Ibid.
10. Ibid.
11. Ibid., p. 92.
12. Ibid., p. 211.
13. Ibid., p. 366.
14. Ibid., p. 267.
15. Ibid., p. 215.
16. Ibid., pp. 389, 391, 392.
17. Ibid., p. 548.
18. Ibid., p. 264.
19. This is recalled by the author from a film shown during a psychology course at Amherst College taught by Robert Birney.
20. In the 1971 Yugoslav film *WR: Mysteries of the Organism*, directed by Dušan Makavejev, Robert Ollendorf, a Reichian physician, stands on the deck of an ocean liner, with Manhattan in the background, and says: "If any sane man or woman would be produced by a doctor suddenly, what would be the consequences? Well, this is very simple; he, very likely, would commit suicide!"
21. I have written two essays on this subject in "Body-Count from the Indo-European Front" and "The Bicentennial Malpractice Suit," in *The Unfinished Business of Doctor Hermes*, pp. 74–97.
22. Sandor Ferenczi, *Thalassa: A Theory of Genitality*, trans. from the German by Henry Alden Bunker, Norton, New York, 1968, pp. 99–101.

Chapter XVI

1. Wilhelm Reich, *The Function of the Orgasm*, translated from the German by Vincent R. Carfagno, Farrar, Straus and Giroux, New York, 1973, p. 62.
2. Ibid., p. 85.
3. Ibid., p. 210.
4. Mary Higgins and Chester M. Raphael, editors, *Reich Speaks of Freud*, Farrar, Straus and Giroux, New York, 1967 (interview occurred in 1952), p. 90.
5. Reich, op. cit., p. 85.
6. Ibid., p. 145.
7. Wilhelm Reich, *Character Analysis* (Third Edition), translated from the German by Vincent R. Carfagno, Farrar, Straus and Giroux, New York, 1972, p. 340.
8. Reich, *Function*, p. 6.
9. Ibid., p. 102.
10. Ibid., pp. 105-6.
11. Higgins and Raphael, op. cit.
12. Ibid., p. 31.
13. Reich, *Character Analysis*, p. 325.
14. Reich, *Function*, p. 120.
15. Reich, *Character Analysis*, p. 244.
16. Reich, *Function*, p. 173.
17. Reich, *Character Analysis*, p. 319.
18. Reich, *Function*, pp. 77-78.
19. Higgins and Raphael, op. cit., p. 85.
20. Ibid, p. 47.
21. Ibid., p. 70.
22. Reich, *Character Analysis*, p. 381.
23. Ibid., p. 396.
24. Higgins and Raphael, op. cit., p. 123.
25. Reich, *Character Analysis*, p. 353.
26. Higgins and Raphael, op. cit., p. 127 (footnote).
27. Reich, *Function*, pp. 383-85.
28. Ibid., p. 187.
29. Wilhelm Reich, *Cosmic Superimposition*, translated from the German by Therese Pol, Farrar, Straus and Giroux, New York, 1973, pp. 220-21.
30. Reich, *Cosmic Superimposition*, pp. 167-70.
31. Lois Wyvell, "Orgone and You," *Living Tree Journal*, 1986, pp. 7-8.
32. James DeMeo, Richard Blasband, Robert Morris, "Breaking the 1986 Drought in the Eastern United States," *The Journal of Orgonomy*, Vol. 21, No. 21, pp. 14-41; Robert Harman, "Current Research with SAPA Bions," ibid., pp. 42-52; Courtney Baker, Robert Dew, Michael Ganz, Louisa Lance, "Wound Healing in Mice (Part I)," *Annual of the Institute of Orgonomic Science*, September, 1984, Vol. 1, No. 1, pp. 12-32; Jutta Espanca, "The Effect of Orgone on Plant Life (Part 7), " *Offshoots of Orgonomy*, Spring, 1986, No. 12, pp. 45-50; Jesse Schwartz, "Some Experiments with Seed Sprouts and Energetic Fields," *Living Tree Journal*, 1986, pp. 34-9.
33. Peter Reich, *A Book of Dreams*, Harper & Row, New York, 1973, pp. 23-27.

34. Myron Sharaf, *Fury on Earth: A Biography of Wilhelm Reich*, St. Martins Press, New York, 1983, p. 454.

CHAPTER XVII

1. Georg Groddeck, *The Book of the It*, trans. from the German by V.M.E. Collins, Funk & Wagnalls, New York, 1950.
2. "Sex Between Therapist and Patient," transcript of a meeting of the APA, June 21, 1976, *Psychiatry*, Vol. 5, No. 12.
3. Benjamin Lo, verbal comments during a *t'ai chi* class in San Francisco, 1978.
4. A. P. Elkin, *Aboriginal Men of High Degree*, p. 125.
5. Miguel Covarrubias, *Island of Bali*, p. 334.
6. Stanley Keleman at a professional colloquim, October 29, 1977.
7. Lee Sannella, *Kundalini—Psychosis or Transcendence?* Dakin, San Francisco, 1976.
8. Ibid.
9. Ibid.
10. J. G. Bennett, *Gurdjieff: Making a New World*, Harper & Row, New York, 1973, p. 191.
11. R. Katz, "Education for Transcendence: Lessons from the !Kung Zhu Twasi," *Journal of Transpersonal Psychology*, Nov. 2, 1973; quoted in Sannella, op. cit., p. 14.
12. See note 6, above.

CHAPTER XVIII

1. Franz Boas, *The Religion of the Kwakiutl Indians*.
2. Brian Inglis, *The Case for Unorthodox Medicine*, Putnam, New York, 1965, pp. 109–12.
3. Paris Flammonde, *The Mystic Healers*, Stein & Day, New York, 1974, p. 71.
4. Ibid., p. 153.
5. Ibid., pp. 153–54.
6. Ibid., pp. 143–44.
7. Ibid., pp. 165–66.
8. John G. Fuller, *Arigo: Surgeon of the Rusty Knife*, Crowell, New York, 1974; reprinted by Pocket Book, 1975, p. 20.
9. Ibid., p. 234. See also Grossinger, *The Unfinished Business of Doctor Hermes*, pp. 13–20 ("Waiting for the Martian Express"), for a fuller discussion of this incident.
10. Jacques Derrida, *On Grammatology*.
11. Evon Karonoff, personal communication, Berkeley, 1978.
12. Felix Mann, *Acupuncture: The Ancient Chinese Art of Healing and How It Works Scientifically*, Random House, New York, 1973, pp. 166–71.
13. *Huang Ti Nei Ching Su Wên*, p. 163.
14. Ibid., pp. 147–48.
15. A Veronica Reif, "Eurhythmy and Curative Eurhythmy," Berkeley Anthroposophical Society, 1978.
16. Benjamin Lo, comments during a *t'ai chi* class, San Francisco, 1978.

17. Paul Pitchford, see note 8, Chap. VI, above.
18. Peter Tompkins and Christopher Bird, *The Secret Life of Plants*, Harper & Row, New York, 1973, pp. 46–49.
19. Robert K. G. Temple, *The Sirius Mystery*, St. Martin's Press, New York, 1976.
20. Robert Anton Wilson, *Cosmic Trigger*, And/Or Press, Berkeley, Calif., 1977.

CHAPTER XIX

1. Faith Mitchell, *Hoodoo Medicine: Sea Island Herbal Remedies*, Reed, Cannon & Johnson, Berkeley, Calif., 1978.
2. Jane Roberts, *The Seth Material*, Prentice-Hall, Englewood Cliffs, N.J., 1970.
3. James Hillman, *The Myth of Analysis*, Northwestern University Press, Evanston, Ill., 1972, pp. 39–40.
4. Chögyam Trungpa, *Cutting Through Spiritual Materialism*, Shambhala, Berkeley, Calif., 1973.
5. Ibid.
6. Ibid., pp. 235–36.
7. Wilhelm Reich, *The Function of the Orgasm*, op. cit., pp. 358–59.

CHAPTER XX

1. Carl Jung, *Psychology and Alchemy*, pp. 95–98.
2. A story told to me by Ian Grand in 1978.
3. See note 2, above.
4. G. I. Gurdjieff, *Views from the Real World: Early Talks*, Dutton, New York, 1975, p. 273.
5. Ibid., p. 274.
6. Theodore Enslin, at a seminar at Goddard College, Plainfield, Vt., 1977.
7. Stan Brakhage, personal communication, 1964.
8. Robert Kelly, personal communication, 1965.
9. William Carlos Williams, "Asphodel, That Greeny Flower," from *Pictures from Brueghel and Other Poems*, New Directions, New York, 1962.

EPILOGUE

1. Jule Eisenbud, *Paranormal Foreknowledge: Problems and Perplexities*, Human Sciences Press, New York, 1982.
2. Ibid., p. 231.
3. Ibid., p. 229 (material in parentheses from previous paragraph).
4. For instance, Bruce Holbrook, *The Stone Monkey: An Alternative Chinese-Scientific Reality*, Morrow, New York, 1981.
5. See pp. 242–43.
6. See p. 354.

7. Eduardo Calderon, Richard Cowan, Douglas Sharon, and F. Kaye Sharon, *Eduardo el Curandero: The Words of a Peruvian Healer*, North Atlantic Books, Richmond, California, 1982, p. 38.

8. Harris L. Coulter, *Homoeopathic Science and Modern Medicine: The Physics of Healing with Microdoses*, North Atlantic Books, Richmond, California, 1981.

9. Calderon et al., op. cit., p. 41.

10. Richard Grossinger, "Cross-Cultural and Historical Models of Energy in Healing," paper delivered at a conference entitled *Conceptualizing Energy Medicine: An Emerging Model of Healing*, University Extension and School of Public Health, University of California, Berkeley, March 28, 1981.

11. Philip M. Chancellor, *Handbook of the Bach Flower Remedies*, C. W. Daniel Co., London, England, 1971.

12. From a conversation with Eric Love, Lela Center, Eureka, California, March 1982.

13. Dr. Chandrashekhar G. Thakkur, *Ayurveda: The Indian Art & Science of Medicine*, ASI Publishers, New York, 1974, pp. 16–17.

14. Gerrit Lansing, "Fundamentals of Indian Medical Theory," from *Notes on Structure and Sign in Ayurveda*, unpublished manuscript.

15. Thakkur, op. cit., pp. 23, 31–32.

16. Ibid., p. 34.

17. Ibid., p. 39.

18. Lansing, op. cit.

19. Thakkur, op. cit., p. 94.

20. From a lecture at Pacific College of Naturopathic Medicine, San Rafael, California, January 1982.

21. Nyanaponika Thera, *The Heart of Buddhist Meditation*, Samuel Weiser, Inc., New York, 1969, p. 71.

23. Father Berard Haile, recorder and translator; in Leland C. Wyman, ed., *Beautyway: A Navaho Ceremonial*, published for the Bollingen Foundation by Pantheon Books, New York, 1957, pp. 141–42.

23. J. G. Bennett, *Gurdjieff: Making a New World*, Harper/Colophon, New York, 1973, p. 202.

24. See note 20.

25. Michio Kushi, *The Book of Dō-IN: Exercise for Physical and Spiritual Development*, Japan Publications, 1979.

26. Jacques de Langre, *Dō-in 2: The Ancient Art of Rejuvenation Through Self-Massage*, Happiness Press, Magalia, California, 1978.

27. Class teachings of Martin Inn, Inner Research Institute, San Francisco, California, March 1982; see also Benjamin Lo, Martin Inn, Robert Amacker, and Susan Foe, *The Essence of T'ai Chi Ch'uan: The Literary Tradition*, North Atlantic Books, Richmond, California, 1979.

28. From a lecture at Pacific College of Naturopathic Medicine, San Rafael, California, March 1982.

29. Laura Chester, "In a Motion," unpublished manuscript.

30. Gregory Vlamis, "Interview with Pierre Pannetier," *Well-Being Magazine*, Issue #28, 1978.

31. Calderon et al., op. cit., pp. 45–46.

32. Kushi, op. cit.; Bubba Free John (Da Free John), *The Eating Gorilla Comes in Peace: The Transcendental Principle of Life Applied to Diet and the Regenerative Discipline of True Health*, The Dawn Horse Press, Middletown, California, 1979.

33. Bubba Free John, op. cit., p. 178.

34. Michael Tierra, *The Way of Herbs*, self-published, Ben Lomond, California, 1977.

35. Stephen Fulder, *The Root of Being: Ginseng and the Pharmacology of Harmony*, Hutchinson Publishing Group, London, 1980, p. 86.

36. Dr. Hong-Yen Hsu: *How to Treat Yourself with Chinese Herbs*, Oriental Healing Arts Institute, Los Angeles, 1980.

37. Thakkur, op. cit., p. 109.

38. Jacques de Langre, lecture at a healing ceremony, Santa Creek, Idaho, June 1981.

39. Calderon et al., op. cit., p. 42.

40. Ibid., p. 45.

41. Some of this dream information comes from my conversations with Charles Poncé during 1981 and 1982.

42. This is an actual quote from a participant at a healing workshop Paul Pitchford gave in Boise, Idaho in 1980.

Bibliography

References in the "Epilogue" are not included here. See "Notes."

The Academy of Traditional Chinese Medicine. *An Outline of Chinese Acupuncture*, Foreign Languages Press, Peking, 1975.

Ackerknecht, Erwin H. "Problems of Primitive Medicine," *Bulletin of the History of Medicine*, XI (1942).

Baker, Wyrth P., Allen C. Neiswander, and W. W. Young, *Introduction to Homeotherapeutics*, American Institute of Homoeopathy, Washington, D.C., 1974.

Barfield, Owen. *Unancestral Voice*, Wesleyan University Press, Middleton, Conn., 1965.

Barrett, S. A. *Pomo Bear Doctors*, University of California Publications in American Archaeology and Ethnology, Vol. 12, No. 11, July 11, 1917, University of California Press, Berkeley.

Bateson, Gregory. "Restructuring the Ecology of a Great City," *Io/#14, Earth Geography Booklet No. 3, Imago Mundi*, Cape Elizabeth, Me., 1972.

Berkeley Holistic Health Center. *The Holistic Health Handbook*, And/Or Press, Berkeley, Calif., 1978.

Boas, Franz. *The Religion of the Kwakiutl Indians*, Part II: *Translations*, Columbia University Press, New York, 1930.

Bordeu, Théophile. *Oeuvres*, Caille and Ravier, Paris, 1818.

Cannon, Walter B. "'Voodoo' Death," *American Anthropologist*, XLIV, 1942.

Castaneda, Carlos. *Journey to Ixtlan*, Simon and Schuster, New York, 1972.

———. *A Separate Reality*, Simon and Schuster, New York, 1971.

———. *Tales of Power*, Simon and Schuster, New York, 1974.

———. *The Teachings of Don Juan: A Yaqui Way of Knowledge*, University of California Press, Berkeley, 1969.

Celsus, Aulus Cornelius. *De Medicina*, trans. W. G. Spencer, Loeb Classical Library, Harvard University Press, Cambridge, Mass.

Coles, William. "Adam in Eden, or The Paradise of Plants," republished in *Io/#5, Doctrine of Signatures*, Ann Arbor, Mich., 1968.

Corbin, Henry. *Creative Imagination in the Sūfism of Ibn 'Arabi*, trans. from the French by Ralph Manheim, Bollingen Foundation, Princeton University Press, Princeton, 1969.

Coulter, Harris Livermore. *Divided Legacy*, Vol. I: *The Patterns Emerge: Hippocrates to Paracelsus*; Vol. II: *Progress and Regress*: *J. B. van Helmont to Claude Bernard*; Vol. III: *Science and Ethics in American Medicine, 1800–1914*, Wehawken Book Company, Washington, D.C., 1973–77.

Covarrubias, Miguel. *Island of Bali*, Alfred A. Knopf, New York, 1938.

Crowley, Aleister. *The Confessions of Aleister Crowley*, ed. John Symonds and Kenneth Grant, Hill and Wang, New York, 1969.

Das, Baba Hari, and Dharma Sara Satang. "Ayurveda: The Yoga of Health," reprinted in *The Holistic Health Handbook*, Berkeley Holistic Health Center, And/Or Press, Berkeley, Calif., 1978.

De Berval, Réné. *Kingdom of Laos*, France-Asie, Saigon, 1956.

Derrida, Jacques. "Freud and the Scene of Writing," trans. from the French by Jeffery Mehlman, *Yale French Studies*, Yale University Press, New Haven, n.d.

———. *Of Grammatology*, trans. from the French by Gayatri Chakravorty Spivak, Johns Hopkins University Press, Baltimore, Md., 1976.

Dorn, Edward. *Recollections of Gran Apachería*, Turtle Island, Berkeley, Calif., 1974.

———, and Gordon Brotherstone, trans. "The Aztec Priest's Reply," *New World Journal*, Vol. 1, Nos. 2/3, 1977.

Eisenbud, Jule. "Interview conducted by Richard Grossinger, 8 January 1972," originally published in *Io/#14, Earth Geography Booklet #3, Imago Mundi*, republished in Richard Grossinger, ed., *Ecology and Consciousness*, 1979.

Elkin, A. P. *Aboriginal Men of High Degree*, Australasian Publishing, Sydney, 1944.

Enslin, Theodore. "Journal Note," in Richard Grossinger, ed., *Alchemy: Pre-Egyptian Legacy, Millennial Promise*.

Ferenczi, Sandor. *Thalassa: A Theory of Genitality*, trans. from the German by Henry Alden Bunker, Norton, New York, 1968.

Flammonde, Paris. *The Mystic Healers*, Stein & Day, New York, 1974.

Foucault, Michel. *The Birth of the Clinic*, trans. from the French by A. M. Sheridan Smith, Pantheon, New York, 1973.

Fox, R. B. "The Pinatubo Negritos: Their Useful Plants and Material Culture," *The Philippine Journal of Science*, Vol. 81, Nos. 3–4, 1953.

Freud, Sigmund. *An Outline of Psychoanalysis*, trans. from the German by James Strachey, Norton, New York, 1949.

———. *The Interpretation of Dreams*, trans. from the German by James Strachey, Basic Books, New York, 1955.

Fuller, John G. *Arigo: Surgeon of the Rusty Knife*, Crowell, New York, 1974; Pocket Book, 1975.

Gelfand, Michael. *Medicine and Custom in Africa*, Livingstone, Edinburgh, 1964.

Goodwin, Kathleen. "Alternative Medicine: A Note of Caution," *City Miner* (Berkeley, Calif.), Vol. 3, No. 3, 1978.

Groddeck, Georg. *The Book of the It*, trans. from the German by V. M. E. Collins, Funk & Wagnalls, New York, 1950.

Grossinger, Richard. *Martian Homecoming at the All-American Revival Church*, North Atlantic Books, Plainfield, Vt., 1974.

———. *The Slag of Creation*, North Atlantic Books, Plainfield, Vt., 1975.

————. *The Unfinished Business of Doctor Hermes,* North Atlantic Books, Plainfield, Vt., 1975.

————, ed. *Alchemy: Pre-Egyptian Prophecy, Millennial Promise,* North Atlantic Books, Richmond, Calif., 1979.

————. *Ecology and Consciousness,* North Atlantic Books, Richmond, Calif., 1978.

————. *An Olson-Melville Sourcebook,* Vol. I: *North America.* Vol. II: *The Mediterranean,* North Atlantic Books, Plainfield, Vt., 1976.

————. *Io,* 1964–79, Amherst, Mass.; Ann Arbor, Mich.; Mount Desert, Me.; Cape Elizabeth, Me.; Plainfield, Vt.; Oakland, Calif.; and Richmond, Calif.

Gurdjieff, G. I. *Views from the Real World: Early Talks,* Dutton, New York, 1975.

Haehl, Richard. *Samuel Hahnemann: His Life and Work,* Vol. I, Homoeopathic Publishing Co., London, 1922.

Hahnemann, Samuel. *The Chronic Diseases, Their Peculiar Nature and Their Homoeopathic Cure,* trans. from the 2d enlarged German edition of 1835 by Louis H. Tafel, Boericke & Tafel, Philadelphia, 1904.

————. *The Lesser Writings of Samuel Hahnemann,* coll. and trans. R. E. Dudgeon, Radde, New York, 1952.

————. *The Organon of Medicine,* 6th ed., trans. William Boericke, M.D., Roysingh, Calcutta, 1962.

Handy, E. S. Craighill, Mary Kawena Pukui, and Katherine Livermore. *Outline of Hawaiian Physical Therapeutics,* Bernice P. Bishop Museum, Bulletin 126, Honolulu, 1934.

Harley, George Way. *Native African Medicine,* Harvard University Press, Cambridge, Mass., 1941.

Harner, Michael J. *The Jívaro,* Doubleday/Natural History Press, Garden City, N.Y., 1972.

Hauschka, Rudolf. *The Nature of Substance,* trans. from the German by Mary T. Richards and Marjorie Spock, Stuart and Watkins, London, 1966.

Heisenberg, Werner. "The Relationship Between Biology, Physics and Chemistry," in *Physics and Beyond,* trans. from the German by Arnold J. Pomerans, Harper & Row, New York, 1971.

Hickey, Gerald Cannon. *Village in Vietnam,* Yale University Press, New Haven, 1964.

Higgins, Mary, and Chester M. Raphael, eds. *Reich Speaks of Freud,* Farrar, Straus and Giroux, New York, 1967.

Hillman, James. *The Myth of Analysis,* Northwestern University Press, Evanston, Ill., 1972.

Hippocrates. *Medical Works,* trans. by W. H. S. Jones, Loeb Classical Library, Harvard University Press, Cambridge, Mass.

Huang Ti Nei Ching Su Wên. Trans. from the Chinese by Ilza Veith as *The Yellow Emperor's Classic of Internal Medicine,* University of California Press, Berkeley, 1966.

Inglis, Brian. *The Case for Unorthodox Medicine*, Putnam, New York, 1965.

———. *A History of Medicine*, World Publishing Company, Cleveland, 1965.

Jenness, D. "The Carrier Indians of the Bulkley River," Bulletin No. 133, Bureau of American Ethnology, Washington, D.C., 1943.

Jung, Carl. *Psychology and Alchemy*, trans. from the German by R. F. C. Hull, Routledge & Kegan Paul, London, 1953.

Kahn, Morton C. *Djuka: The Bush Negroes of Dutch Guiana*, Viking Press, New York, 1931.

Katz, R. "Education for Transcendence: Lessons from the !Kung Zhu Twasi," *Journal of Transpersonal Psychology*, Nov. 2, 1973.

Keleman, Stanley. *Living Your Dying*, Random House, New York, 1974.

———. "Professional Colloquium," in Richard Grossinger, ed., *Ecology and Consciousness*, 1978.

Kent, James Tyler. *Lectures on Homoeopathic Philosophy* (1900), North Atlantic Books, Richmond, Calif., 1979.

Lessa, William A., and Evon Z. Vogt. *Reader in Comparative Religion*, Harper & Row, New York, 1958.

Lévi-Strauss, Claude. *From Honey to Ashes*, trans. from the French by John and Doreen Weightman, Harper & Row, New York, 1973.

———. *The Raw and the Cooked*, trans. from the French by John and Doreen Weightman, Harper & Row, New York, 1969.

———. *The Savage Mind*, University of Chicago Press, Chicago, 1966.

———. "The Sorcerer and His Magic," in *Structural Anthropology*, trans. from the French by Claire Jacobson and Brooke Grundfest Schoepf, Doubleday/Anchor, Garden City, N.Y., 1967.

———. *Totemism*, trans. from the French by Rodney Needham, Beacon Press, Boston, 1963.

Lo, Pang Jeng, Martin Inn, Susan Foe, and Robert Amacker. *The Essence of T'ai Chi Ch'uan*, North Atlantic Books, Richmond, Calif., 1979.

Makavejev, Dušan. *WR: Mysteries of the Organism*, Avon, New York, 1972.

Mann, Felix. *Acupuncture: The Ancient Chinese Art of Healing and How It Works Scientifically*, Random House, New York, 1973.

Mann, W. Edward. *Orgone, Reich and Eros: Wilhelm Reich's Theory of Life Energy*, Simon and Schuster, New York, 1973.

Mars, Louis. *The Crisis of Possession in Voodoo*, trans. from the French by Kathleen Collins, Reed, Cannon & Johnson Co., Berkeley, Calif., 1977.

Marshack, Alexander. *The Roots of Civilization*, McGraw-Hill, New York, 1972.

Meek, George W. *Healers and the Healing Process*, Theosophical Publishing House, Wheaton, Ill., 1977.

Melville, Herman. *Moby Dick*, 1851.

Mitchell, Faith. *Hoodoo Medicine: Sea Island Herbal Remedies*, Reed, Cannon & Johnson, Berkeley, Calif., 1978.

Moore, Omar Khayyam. "Divination—A New Perspective," *American Anthropologist*, LIX, 1957.

Olson, Charles. *Muthologos*, Vol. I, Four Seasons Foundation, Bolinas, Calif., 1978.

Oyle, Irving. *The New American Medicine Show*, Unity Press, Santa Cruz, Calif., 1979.

Paracelsus. *The Hermetic and Alchemical Writings of Paracelsus the Great*, trans. by A. E. Waite, James Elliott, London, 1894.

Psychiatry. Vol. 5, No. 12, transcript of the June 21, 1976, meeting of the American Psychiatric Association entitled "Sex Between Therapist and Patient."

Radcliffe-Brown, A. R. *The Andaman Islanders*, Free Press, Glencoe, Ill., 1948.

Rappaport, Roy A. "Sanctity and Adaptation," *Io/#7, Oecology Issue*, 1970; in Richard Grossinger, ed., *Ecology and Consciousness*, 1978.

Rasmussen, Knud. *Intellectual Culture of the Iglulik Eskimos: Report of the Fifth Thule Expedition to Arctic North America*, Gyldendalske Boghandel, Nordisk Forlag, Copenhagen, 1929.

Rechung, Ven. Rinpoche Jampal Kunzang. *Tibetan Medicine*, University of California Press, Berkeley, 1973.

Regardie, Israel. *The Eye in the Triangle*, Llewellyn Publications, St. Paul, Minn., 1970.

Reich, Peter. *A Book of Dreams*, Harper & Row, New York, 1973.

Reich, Wilhelm. *Character Analysis*, 3d ed., trans. from the German by Vincent R. Carfagno, Farrar, Straus and Giroux, New York, 1972.

———. *Ether, God & Devil–Cosmic Superimposition*, trans. from the German by Therese Pol, Farrar, Straus and Giroux, New York, 1973.

———. *The Function of the Orgasm*, trans. from the German by Vincent R. Carfagno, Farrar, Straus and Giroux, New York, 1973.

Reichard, Gladys A. *Navaho Religion*, Bollingen Foundation, Pantheon Books, New York, 1950.

Reif, A. Veronica. "Eurhythmy and Curative Eurhythmy," essay accompanying lecture at the Berkeley Anthroposophical Society, 1978.

Roberts, Jane. *The Seth Material*, Prentice-Hall, Englewood Cliffs, N.J., 1970.

Rush, Benjamin. *Medical Inquiries and Observations*, Pritchard and Hall, Philadelphia, 1789.

Sahlins, Marshall. *Stone Age Economics*, Aldine-Atherton, Chicago, 1972.

Sannella, Lee. *Kundalini—Psychosis or Transcendence?* Dakin, San Francisco, 1976.

Shklovskii, I. S., and Carl Sagan. *Intelligent Life in the Universe*, trans. from the Russian by Paula Fern, Delta Books, New York, 1967.

Speck, Frank G. *A Study of the Delaware Indian Big House Ceremony*, Vol. II, Publications of the Pennsylvania Historical Commission, Harrisburg, Pa., 1931.

Spencer, Dorothy M. *Disease, Religion and Society in the Fiji Islands*, Augustin, New York, 1941.

Swanton, John R. *Religious Beliefs and Medical Practices of the Creek Indians*, 42nd Annual Report to the Bureau of American Ethnology, 1924–25, Smithsonian Institution, Washington, D.C., 1928.

Tantaquidgeon, Gladys. *Folk Medicine of the Delaware and Related Algonkian Indians*, Pennsylvania Historical and Museum Commission, Harrisburg, Pa., 1972.

Temple, Robert K. G. *The Sirius Mystery*, St. Martin's Press, New York, 1976.

Tompkins, Peter, and Christopher Bird. *The Secret Life of Plants*, Harper & Row, New York, 1973.

Trungpa, Chögyam. *Cutting Through Spiritual Materialism*, Shambala Publications, Berkeley, Calif., 1973.

Turner, Victor W.: *Lunda Medicine and the Treatment of Disease*, Occasional Papers of the Rhodes-Livingstone Museum, No. 15, Livingstone, Northern Rhodesia [Zambia], 1964.

Tyler, M. L. *Homoeopathic Drug Pictures*, Health Science Press, Holsworthy, Devon, England, 1942.

Van Helmont, Jan Baptista. *Oriatrike, or Physick Refined*, London, 1662.

Veith, Ilza. *See Huang Ti Nei Ching Su Wên*, above.

Vithoulkas, George. *The Science of Homeopathy: A Modern Textbook*, Vol. I, A.S.O.H.M., Athens, Greece, 1978.

Waite, A. E., *See Paracelsus*, above.

Westlake, Aubrey T. *The Pattern of Health*, Shambala Publications, Berkeley, Calif., 1973.

Wheelwright, Philip, ed. *The Presocratics*, Odyssey Press, Indianapolis, 1966.

Whitehead, Alfred North. *Process and Reality*, Macmillan, Toronto, 1929.

Whiting, Alfred F. *Ethnobotany of the Hopi*, Northern Arizona Society of Science and Art, Museum of Northern Arizona, Bulletin 15, Flagstaff, 1939.

Whitmont, Edward. *Psyche and Substance: Essays on Homoeopathy in the Light of Jungian Psychology*, North Atlantic Books, Richmond, Calif., 1979.

Wildschut, William. *Crow Indian Medicine Bundles*, ed. John C. Ewers, Museum of the American Indian, Heye Foundation, New York, 1975.

Wilson, Robert Anton. *Cosmic Trigger*, And/Or Press, Berkeley, Calif., 1977.

Yates, Frances. *The Rosicrucian Enlightenment*, Routledge & Kegan Paul, London, 1972.

Yoe, Shway. *The Burman*, Macmillan, London, 1910.

Index

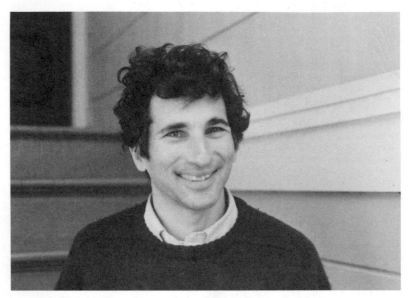

Photograph of author by George Leonard

Richard Grossinger was born in New York City in 1944 and raised there. He attended Amherst College and the University of Michigan from which he received a Ph.D. in anthropology for a study of fishing in Maine. Afterwards he taught for seven years at the University of Maine at Portland-Gorham and Goddard College in Plainfield, Vermont. He is the author of a number of books, including *The Long Body of the Dream, The Slag of Creation, The Unfinished Business of Doctor Hermes, The Night Sky, Embryogenesis,* and *Waiting for the Martian Express.* Since 1977 he has lived in Berkeley, California, with his wife, Lindy Hough, who is a writer and teacher, and his son Robin and daughter Miranda.